THE YOGA MECHANIC

How to Tune Up or Jump Start Your Yoga Practice

KAT HENDRIX
PhD, ERYT500

Photographs by Lea Austen

Second Edition September, 2022
First Edition published under the title, Yoga Tune-Up, March 2022, ISBN 978-0-9834487-7-8

Book design by Andie Reid

Photography by Lea Austen

ISBN 978-0-9834487-9-2

www.kathendrix.com
www.yoga-mechanic.com

For everyone who can't put their foot behind their head.

CONTENTS

INTRODUCTION

I wrote this book for all the people who think yoga isn't for them, and for everyone who's become discouraged, bored, or injured practicing yoga. Many people don't think they can do yoga, and I completely understand why. Its public image is intimidating—just look at the thousands of photos online showing young, super-fit people (mostly women, and mostly white) pulling off difficult poses in skin-tight workout clothes. Yikes.

The fact is, most people take up yoga to just stretch, and to get in a little better shape—not to learn how to put their foot behind their head. Along with all those photos, there's a dizzying online galaxy of yoga websites, tweets, and blogs, touting everything from gut-cleansing diets to new translations of ancient texts. No wonder people who have never done yoga are nervous about starting. I get it. Planet Yoga looks weird.

I'm here to tell you that none of that stuff is necessary to have a safe, effective yoga practice that improves your physical and mental health. In other words, you don't have to become a "yogi" to benefit from doing some yoga. You don't have to chant mantras, say OM, become vegetarian, or touch your toes in order to reap positive health returns from a regular practice. One day, you might want to find out more about the other, more philosophical aspects of yoga. One day you might even consider yourself a yogi. But it's always best to start with the basics.

This book is intended to be a touchstone for the foundation of your yoga practice. In these pages we'll explore how to find the right class and teacher for you, and how to do the poses in a way that strengthens and stretches your body and your mind. With that knowledge, you can take your yoga practice in any direction you want. It's yours to grow and enjoy.

I've taught yoga for sixteen years, but first and foremost I'm a medical science writer. So this book explains yoga from an anatomical perspective. We'll look at how doing yoga poses improves your health, how to avoid injury, and what to do if you are injured. My aim is to help you build a practice that best suits your own body, goals, and lifestyle.

This book also celebrates the wonderful people I've met through yoga. The people in the photographs are real students who take my classes. They're of all ages, shapes, and sizes, and they come from all walks of life as teachers, retailers, pilots, assembly-line workers, home makers, lawyers, artists, and cabinet-makers. The youngest of them is 26, and the oldest is 86. Each started doing yoga for a different reason, but they all found that it helped them get through life's physical and mental ups and downs. I hope you recognize yourself in them, and use this book as a guide to tune up or start up your own yoga practice.

—Kat

HOW TO USE THIS BOOK

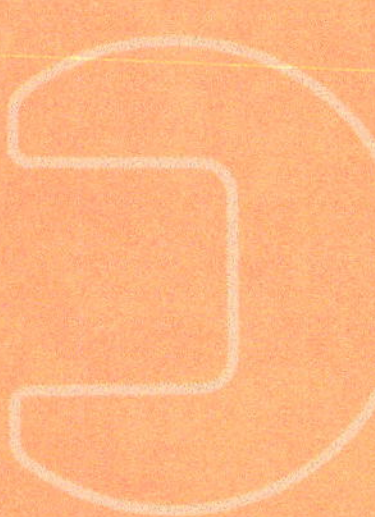

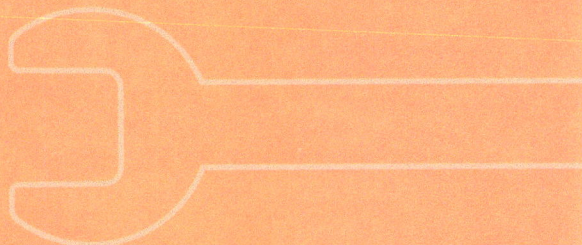

This book is meant to help you jumpstart and tune up your yoga practice. Think of it like a repair and maintenance manual for your car. It covers basic anatomical information so you understand how your body is put together, how it moves, and how its parts work with each other. But, just like a car manual doesn't teach you how to drive, this book doesn't give you step-by-step instructions for doing poses you've never seen or tried to do before. In my opinion, it's always best to first learn new poses in person, from an experienced instructor, rather than from a book, video, or internet site. An instructor can watch how you're approaching that pose and give you real-time feedback and advice, so you avoid bad habits and injuries.

Use this book as a companion guide to help make your yoga practice as good as it can be for your overall health and well-being. After you read all the way through, you'll be able to jump to certain sections as needed to review a variation or get tips on doing a specific pose. If you're an instructor, I hope you find these pages to be a helpful source for ideas to help your students make progress.

We'll start by laying out the basics and dispelling some common misconceptions. Then we'll take a close look at how breathing works in yoga, so you understand how important it is to your practice. From there, subsequent chapters will examine a selection of poses, working from the ground up—your feet to your shoulders—explaining how each stretches or strengthens particular parts of your body, and describing ways to make them more effective. And then we'll finish with some general advice for teachers and students.

Ready? Let's get started!

CHAPTER 1

KEY CONCEPTS FOR A SAFE, EFFECTIVE PRACTICE

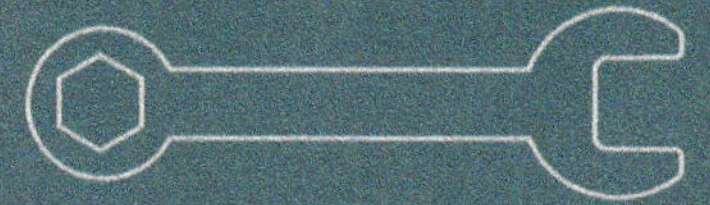

When most people hear the word "yoga," they think of the physical poses and movements (called *asanas*). If you're practicing yoga already, that's where you probably started.

Yoga asanas (there are hundreds of them) were developed over several centuries, by lots of different people who were interested in how movement, strength, and flexibility in the physical body can promote a clear, steady, mental state. Even today, the way that we understand and teach yoga poses continues to evolve, which is why I like to think of yoga as a living, physical art form. But if you don't understand the true purpose of the asanas, you'll cheat yourself out of the full benefits of a yoga practice. And you might even be setting yourself up for frustration and injury. So before we discuss specific poses, we're going to spend this chapter understanding the purpose behind the poses, and how they can help you. Then we'll talk about using that knowledge to find the yoga class that fits you best, and get you started on tuning up your practice for the best possible results.

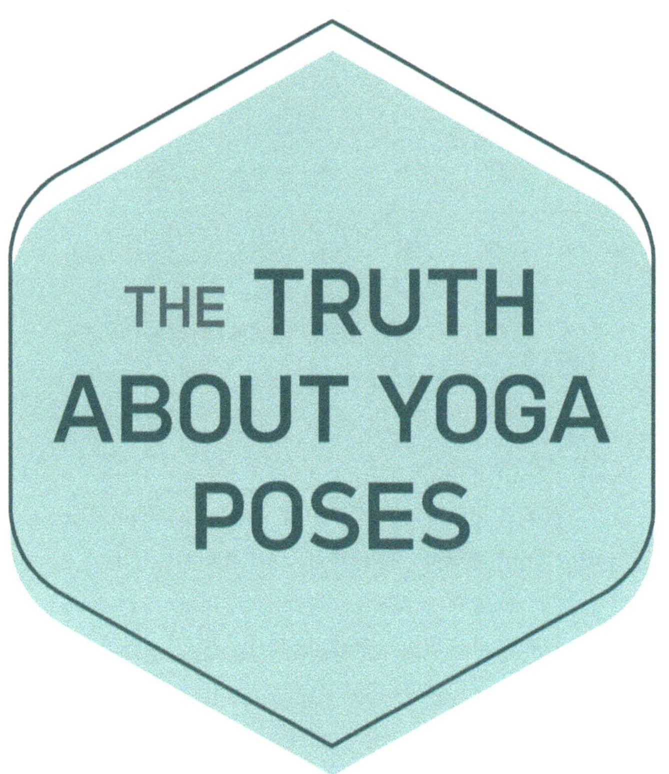

THE TRUTH ABOUT YOGA POSES

Because most people start with the physical poses, a lot of folks think that mastering these positions is the whole point of doing yoga. And it's true that establishing an intelligent physical practice lets you experience for yourself how much better you can feel with even a little yoga in your life. But if you focus only on the physical poses, you miss the bigger picture. The asanas are not just gymnastics. They are tools, designed to turn down the volume on all those thoughts banging around inside your head. In fact, the yoga poses were originally developed to help philosophers and sages sit still and meditate for long periods of time.

And that is the true end game in yoga. It's much more useful to be able to quiet your mind and stay calm in a crisis, or think things through before you say or do something you might regret, than to put your foot behind your head.

People who misunderstand this deeper purpose often end up getting injured, because their enthusiasm to accomplish these physical feats makes them impatient. The truth is, practicing the physical poses of yoga without controlling your breathing and focusing your mind is a dangerous habit. Occasionally, a student comes to me after class and says, "Such and such pose hurt me." My reply is always, "I'm sorry that the way you did the pose hurt you. Let's take a look and see what's going on." Most of the time, this happens because they were speeding; rushing to do a position before they have enough strength, flexibility, and focus to succeed.

Patience and humility are the lessons that yoga poses teach us, over and over again, no matter how many years we've been practicing, and no matter how strong and flexible we become. That's why anyone who practices yoga, from a first-lesson beginner to a ten-year teacher, needs to keep these principles in mind: Be patient. Pay attention. Know the limits of your strength and flexibility and stop there. Breathe.

Intense or Advanced?

Yoga poses have different degrees of difficulty. But I prefer using the word "intense" to describe more difficult poses, rather than "advanced." Progress in your yoga practice does not depend on moving from doing "beginner poses" to doing "advanced poses." That's a false hierarchy. The point is not to master the most so-called advanced variation of each pose. The point is to learn to do *every* pose—the simple ones and the difficult ones—with the same level of clarity, focus, and calm.

Approach intense poses slowly and methodically, because taking on the most difficult poses when you're not physically or mentally prepared leads to injury. Remember, every body, and every day, is different. When my mind is particularly distracted or my body is achy, I don't do the most intense version of every pose. There's always tomorrow for that. Be alert to yourself, and be patient. Don't speed. Just like driving a car, adjust your practice to the conditions.

MECHANIC'S NOTE: PLAN YOUR TRIP

Approach intense poses like you're preparing for a long journey, and you'll reap great rewards, no matter how long it takes or where your journey ends:

Plan your route. Read about the pose, and ask people who can do it well how they learned to do it.

Gather your supplies. Practice less intense variations to build the physical strength and flexibility you'll need for an intense pose.

Pack efficiently. Sharpen your mental ability to stay focused and calm all the way through class, by setting your eyes on a single focal point (called a *drishti*) in each pose, and evening out your inhales and exhales.

Start with a single step. Practice one stage (called a *krama*) of the pose at a time, until it feels quite calm and easeful.

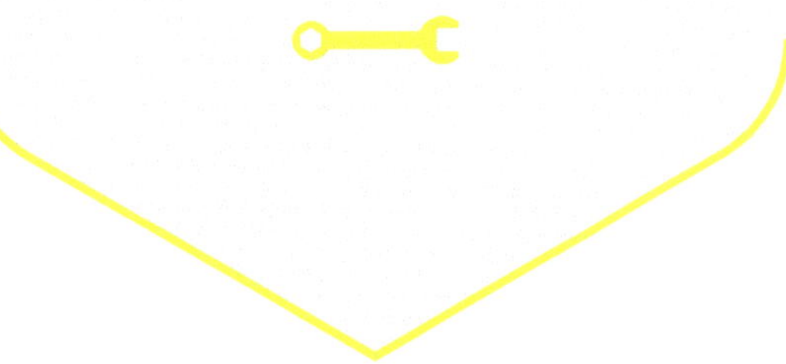

Accomplishing poses that require a lot of strength and flexibility does not necessarily mean that you have an "advanced" practice. Progress is measured by how well you keep your mind focused and your breath steady.

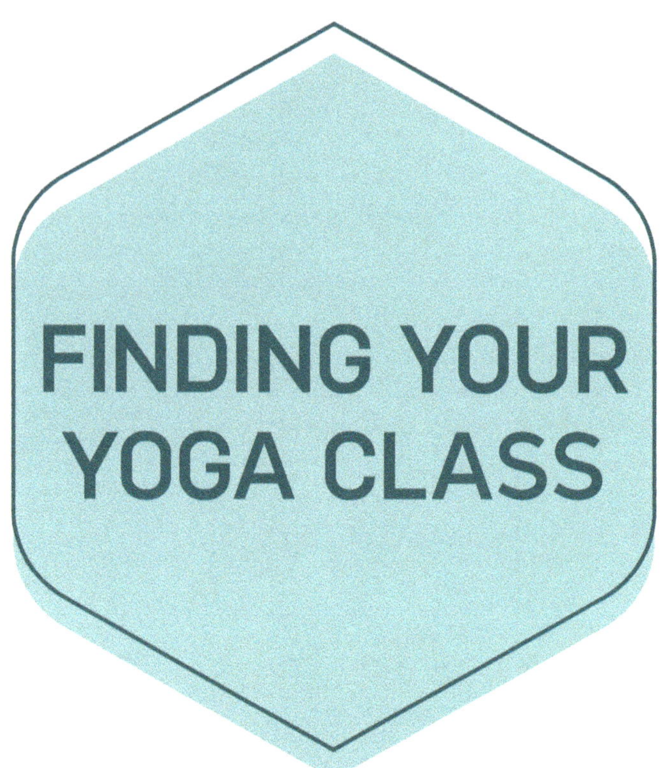

FINDING YOUR YOGA CLASS

Everyone starts practicing yoga for different reasons—to stay fit, to become more flexible, to de-stress after work. And it doesn't really matter why you start. What matters is figuring out how to stick with it, by establishing a sustainable, long-term practice. The first step in creating that type of yoga practice for yourself is to find a class that you'll want to keep coming back to.

Everybody, and every body, can benefit from regularly doing some yoga. But how do you find a class that's a good fit for your personality, body, and goals? This is an important question. Because if you start with a class that's too physically demanding, moves too fast, or is too esoteric and philosophical, you can get turned off and think, *That yoga stuff is definitely not for me.*

The good news is, you *can* find a yoga class that matches your needs. If you don't land on something right away, don't give up. There's never been so many different types of yoga classes available, both online and in person. It just may take a little trial and error to find your best fit.

Yoga is different from other types of exercise classes. It takes time to figure out how to move from pose to pose safely and efficiently. If you're taking up yoga for the first time, start with a slow-moving class even if you are physically fit. Starting in a slower-moving class will help you avoid frustration and injury. Be aware, though, moving slowly in yoga can be much more difficult than moving quickly. A *slow* class is not necessarily an *easy* class.

Yoga is not one-size-fits-all. Don't settle: Shop around until you find an instructor whose tone, skills, and experience best fit your needs. Here are some other factors to consider.

Tone Matters

For a long-lasting yoga practice, it's vital to find an instructor you connect with, and whose personal style fits your own.

My background is in health and medicine, and I don't like long discussions of philosophy during class. For me, the more anatomical and physical the instruction is, the better. On the other hand, you may like a class that includes more philosophical discussion. So try out different instructors until you find someone with a teaching style you like.

Most places have several instructors, and one instructor might teach several different types of classes. Even after you zero in on your go-to class, sampling other options can help you adjust your practice as needed. Over time, you'll figure out where you can get what you need on a particular day. For example, sometimes I'm looking for a raucous room full of people to practice with, so I'll pick a class with loud music and an encouraging instructor with a good sense of humor. Other times, I need a quiet class where I can gather my thoughts and restore my sense of well-being and balance. On those days I'll opt for the class and instructor that offers a more meditative vibe.

FIND THE RIGHT CLASS IN FOUR EASY STEPS

1 **Ask around.** Word of mouth can be helpful. Ask people you know what yoga classes they like, and why. Can they recommend somewhere for you to start?

2 **Consider training and experience.** Look for a venue with instructors who have RYT-200 certification (meaning registered yoga teacher, 200 hours), or a higher level of training. And seek out instructors who've been teaching for several years—the longer the better.

3 **Check it out.** Visit the facility and speak to the staff. Tell them you'd like to start doing yoga, and ask what classes they recommend. Notice the vibe. Do you feel welcome?

4 **Test drive a class or two.** Most places offer a drop-in rate so you can try out one class at a time before committing. Ask if there's a special rate for new students, or a beginner package that may be less expensive.

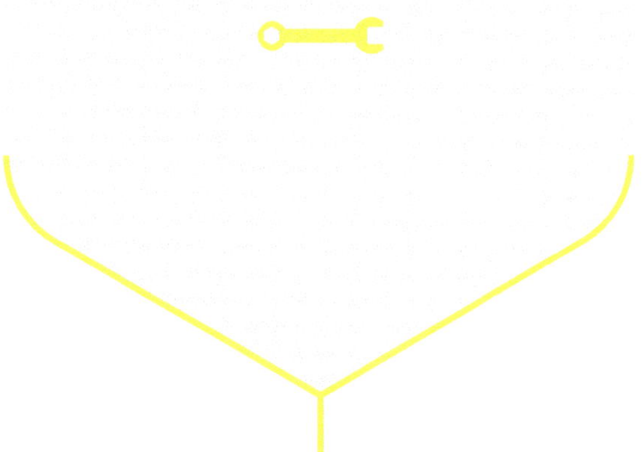

Good Instructors Teach Everyone in the Room

As you evaluate your options, look for an instructor who provides alternatives to difficult poses, and explains how to use tools like blocks, straps, and bolsters in class.

Remember, just because a yoga instructor doesn't *mean* any harm, doesn't mean they can't *do* any harm. A good instructor will be sure that what they say in class is anatomically correct, encouraging, and useful to all of the people in the room, not just the most experienced or most fit.

It is the instructor's job to guide you safely into and out of each pose, in a way that challenges your strength and flexibility without pushing you too far. It's your job to learn when you've reached the level of physical and mental challenge that you can handle today, and stop there–but developing that judgment takes time and experience. Because the instructor has been trained to teach yoga, theirs is the bigger responsibility.

A good instructor won't treat everyone in the class as if they're physically identical. There are important body-type, gender-based, and age-based anatomical differences that come into play. Biological characteristics of your bones and muscles will affect your ability to do particular yoga poses.

For example:

- **Women are generally more flexible than men,** because higher estrogen levels make their connective tissues more elastic. This is evident even among post-menopausal women, who are usually more flexible than men of the same age. Women should also understand that they will be more or less flexible depending on the stage of their menstrual cycle.
- **Women have a wider pelvic bowl than men.** This changes the angle of their muscle attachments at the pelvis, which in turn puts different forces on their joints.
- **Men have less angle in their forearms than women** (called the *carrying angle*), which makes it easier for men to rotate the lower arm and support safe shoulder alignment in poses like Plank and Downward Facing Dog. This greater carrying angle also makes women's elbows appear bent in some poses when, in fact, they are (skeletally-speaking) as straight as possible.

Our bodies change as we age. Our tissues become less flexible and our bones and joints have less cushioning over time, because there's less muscle mass, collagen, and inter-joint cartilage. Sadly, the culture of youth worship tells us to dislike these changes in our bodies, when in fact they're natural, normal, and unavoidable.

If you and your instructor take your age and gender into consideration as you practice yoga, it will go a long way in helping you avoid frustration, negative self-talk, and injuries. One of the biggest advantages to taking classes from the same instructor is that they'll get to know your practice—your physical and mental challenges as well as the poses that you enjoy. For example, among the students who have come to my classes for years, I know who's had a knee replacement, who struggles to get their elbows straight, and who has a cranky neck. They trust me to recommend pose variations that will be safe and effective for them.

Be realistic: Understand yourself. Your age, gender, fitness level, life experience, and biology are unique. All of these factors influence what type of yoga class is most useful for you.

So look for instructors who give clear, verbal guidance to everyone in the room, and who walk around the space to help individual students with tools like blocks, bolsters, or straps. I often have a co-teacher with me, who also knows the regular, long-time students and how they practice. Look for instructors who get off their own mats and walk around the room, and who seem to have a rapport with their students and know them well.

Your Instructor Should Connect the Dots

Although we usually teach the physical poses, regulated breathing, and meditation separately, doing yoga means doing all three of these things together at once.

Many people who practice yoga, both experienced students and beginners alike, misunderstand what a yoga practice actually is. And this is partly due to how yoga is usually taught. For a lot of valid reasons, most places break up the practice of yoga into its three component pieces: physical poses (*asanas*), regulated breathing (*pranayama*), and meditation. This gives the false impression that these three practices should be done in isolation from each other.

In fact, your yoga practice should pull all three together so that, eventually, you do them all at the same time. Doing yoga means doing the physical poses while simultaneously regulating your breath and maintaining a steady mental focus. I know! It sounds impossible, but it's not.

Unfortunately, it's easy to get hung up on practicing one of those elements at a time, dipping into one and then another as your interest rises and falls—doing only the physical poses, doing only the breathing exercises, doing only the meditation. This can lead to boredom, injury, and frustration which can make you stop practicing. A good instructor will cue you to do all three things during class. They will remind you to hold your eyes still to help focus your mind: Don't look all over the room; find one thing to focus on and keep your gaze softly on that. They will tell you to inhale and exhale deeply, especially in poses that challenge the respiratory muscles like back-bends and twists.

Don't miss the memo: Practicing all three elements at once is what yoga is about. Learning to do this is a long process, so your instructors should encourage it from day one. People think yoga is only physically difficult, but it's mentally challenging, too. At the end of class–no matter what type of class it is–you should feel physically tired and mentally focused, clear, and calm.

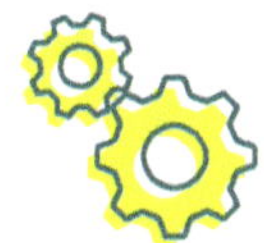

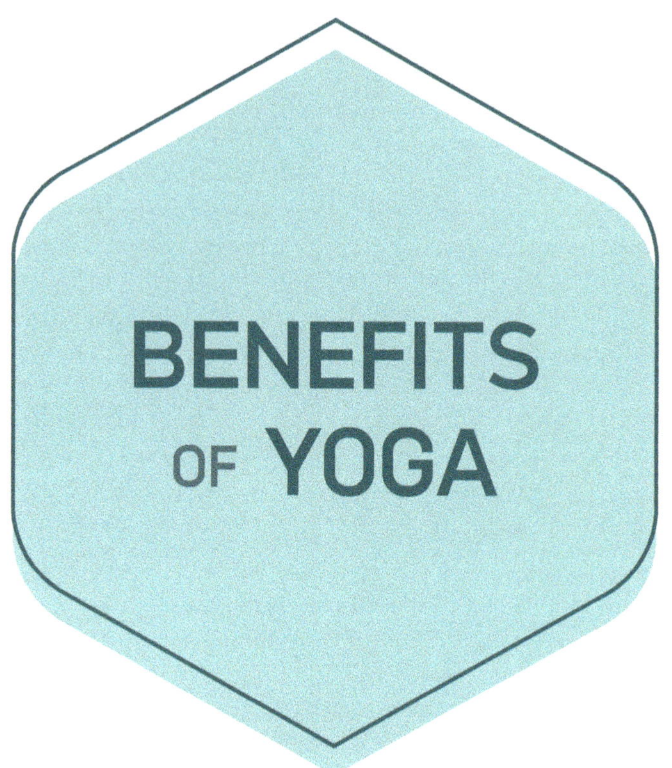

BENEFITS OF YOGA

The physical benefits of yoga are well documented, and the most common reason most people start doing yoga. Some positive physical changes are easy to perceive. You will feel stronger and more flexible. You might lose a few inches around your waist. Other changes are more subtle. You may notice you're less reactive to stressful events, and less anxious or depressed, or that you sleep better. Because your yoga practice is a moving meditation, it shifts your internal biochemistry from being dominated by the sympathetic nervous system (stress hormones like adrenalin and cortisol) to being dominated by the parasympathetic nervous system ("feel good" hormones like serotonin and dopamine). This is a fundamental biological change that has immense mental and physical benefits. In time, you may be able to shift your biochemistry when you're not even doing yoga.

Yoga Helps You Balance

Doing yoga helps you maintain your health as you age. And one important way it does that is to a sharpen your sense of balance, which

It's Never Too Late: No matter your age or level of fitness, yoga helps make you healthier by improving your balance, bone density, circulation, respiration, and muscle mass.

naturally deteriorates as you get older, leading to falls and injuries. There are three biological components of balance: your eyesight (vision), your inner-ear mechanisms which help you tell which way you're moving (vestibular system), and your ability to sense your body's position in space (proprioception). There's little you can do to prevent the first two factors from degrading over time. But you can always practice and improve your proprioception.

Proprioceptors are specialized nerve endings throughout your body that tell your brain about your body's position (am I upright, tilted, bent over?) and muscle tension (which of my muscles are working, which are relaxed?). Doing yoga stimulates and strengthens this nerve network, so you can better keep your balance in stillness and movement. In addition, weight-bearing movements in yoga help maintain bone density and muscle mass, and the wide range of upright and upside-down positions help maintain blood vessel responsiveness and circulatory health. All of which can help prevent dizziness in day-to-day life, like when you stand up from sitting. All of these benefits support a quick, firm reaction to catch your balance if you stumble.

Yoga Preserves Your Range of Motion

The biggest physical benefit of doing yoga poses is that they help maintain normal, full range of motion in all the joints of your body. The two most important words in that sentence are *normal* and *range*. Each of your joints is designed to move only in certain directions, and within certain limits. All joints can flex (move towards the center of your body–flexing at the hips brings your chest closer your thighs), and extend (move away from the center of your body–extending at the hips moves your chest backward away from your thighs). Some joints also have other, more complex movements like side-bending and rotation.

And everyone is built a little differently—that's why there's a *range* of normal movement at each joint. Where you are in that range depends on the unique shape of your bones and how they fit together. Forcing a joint to move in a way that it's not designed to move damages the joint. However, most of us lose some of our normal range of movement over time, and sometimes we become too stiff to move certain joints normally. When a joint can't move in its normal range, it can be damaged by uneven or excess wear to the cartilage—the tissue that protects your bone surfaces inside the joint. Losing range of movement at one joint also puts abnormal stresses on nearby joints and wears them out faster.

Inactivity, poor posture, scarring, and tissue adhesions from an injury or surgery are just a few of reasons we lose range of motion. People who are very sedentary (do more sitting than standing) often develop contractures at their elbows, hips, and knees because they rarely straighten (extend) their arms and legs. A contracture means that a joint gets stuck in a slightly flexed position and can't extend fully.

For very sedentary or inactive people, fully extending their limbs gets harder over time as the muscles that move them get weaker from lack of use. At the same time, the muscles that bend (flex) the limbs get tighter, reinforcing a bend at the joint. Contractures used to primarily be a concern among elderly people. However, as our society does more and more sitting, they're now a common problem for people of all ages. They affect those of us who spend a

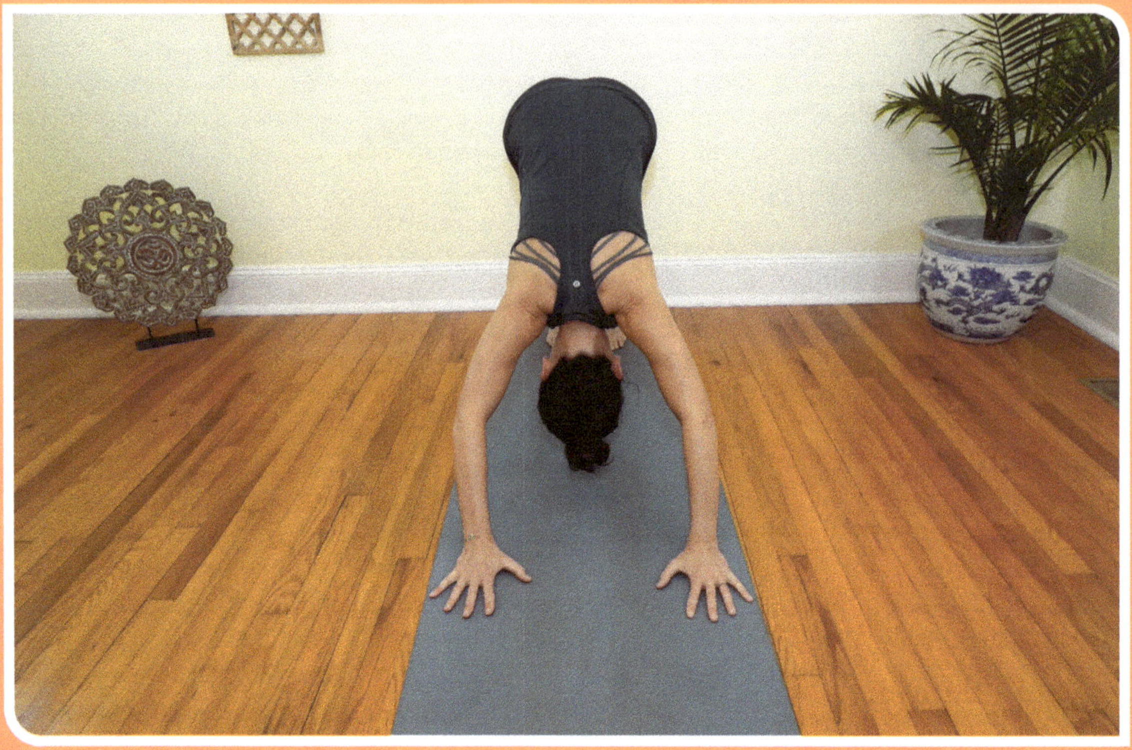

Weakness and inflexibility can keep your elbows bent in Downward Facing Dog Pose.

MECHANIC'S NOTE: Getting Your Elbows Straight

Downward Facing Dog Pose (Adho Mukha Svanasana) is a good opportunity to see whether you have trouble straightening your elbows. This is a common challenge for people who are new to yoga, and is usually caused by a combination of weakness in the upper back and arm muscles that straighten your elbows, and tightness (contractures) in the muscles that bend your elbows.

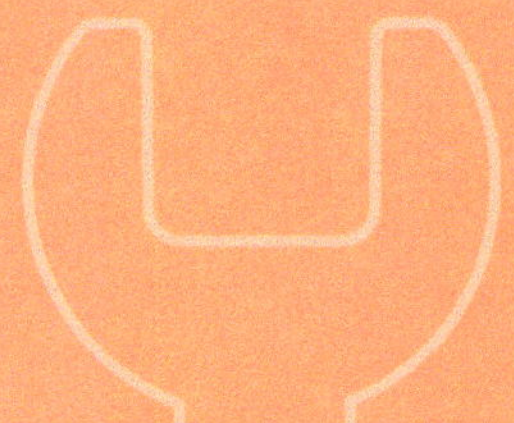

lot of time slumped over a keyboard or a game controller, curled up on the couch watching TV, or hunched behind the wheel of a car for hours, day after day. Yoga poses can help restore this lost strength and flexibility, and keep all of your body parts moving more normally.

Another way that yoga supports your range of motion is by keeping your *fascia* elastic and mobile. Fascia is the specialized, slippery tissue found throughout your body that helps your muscles, nerves, and blood vessels slide past each other. When your fascia doesn't get regularly stretched, it becomes hard and stiff, restricting your ability to move.

Your body is incredibly adaptable. Over time, you develop unconscious movement patterns that shift work away from your weaker muscles and into your stronger muscles. Doing yoga helps you become more conscious of these muscular patterns, and begin building more balanced strength and flexibility. It's a gradual process. Slowly but surely, weak muscles get stronger, and tight muscles get longer.

Yoga Supports Correct Alignment

If you've taken classes, you may have heard a yoga instructor say something about the importance of "correct alignment." Unfortunately, they often fail to explain what this actually means. That explanation is important, because a large part of your instructor's job is to help you find correct alignment while you practice. Correct alignment is essential to effectively stretch and strengthen your muscles without getting injured.

Correct alignment means this: Your weight or the force of movement goes through the centers of the bones and joints involved. You should centrally transfer your weight when you're moving, and centrally distribute your weight when you're holding still.

Stretching Dos and Don'ts: Some parts of your body should not be stretched. Do stretch your muscles. Don't stretch your ligaments and tendon attachments.

Not sure what that means? Look at the wear pattern on the soles of your shoes. Is it uneven? Does the outer sole or heel wear down before the arch and toe area? If so, you have a misaligned walking pattern that puts more weight on the outer foot or heel. In yoga, you'll learn to spread your weight out more evenly across all of the bones in your feet. In this case, by pressing your big toes down and lifting your outer ankles up.

A misaligned habit of walking on your outer feet and heels will also show up as you transfer your weight to move from pose to pose. You may tend to turn your knee outward when you step forward, or let your big toes pop up off the floor when you lift your hips into a back-bend. Over time, as you get better at centering your weight in your feet, you may notice less knee, hip, or low-back pain because that uneven weight pattern was affecting many other joints.

One of the most common alignment problems is forward head carriage and, luckily, yoga can help fix that too. This is caused by too much sitting and walking around with your ears in front of your shoulders, instead of over them. You see, your head is heavy. In fact, the average person's head weighs eight to twelve pounds. (For reference, a full gallon jug of water weighs eight pounds.) Your body is designed to carry the weight of your head directly above your spinal column. When your head gets in front of your shoulders, other parts of your body have to compensate for that abnormal weight distribution. So that forward head carriage sets the stage for problems in your neck, shoulders, back, and hips.

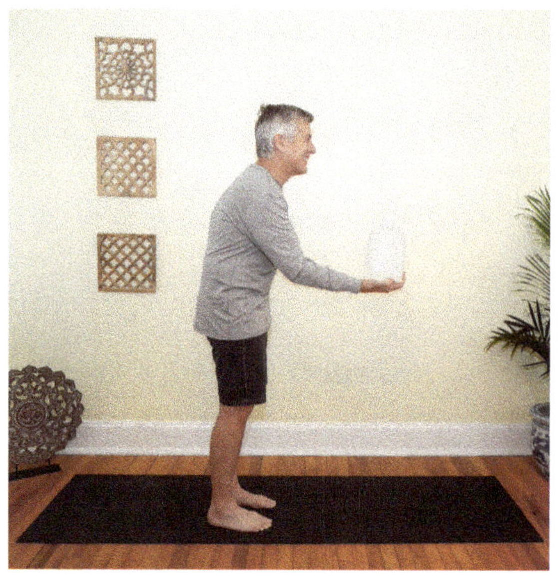

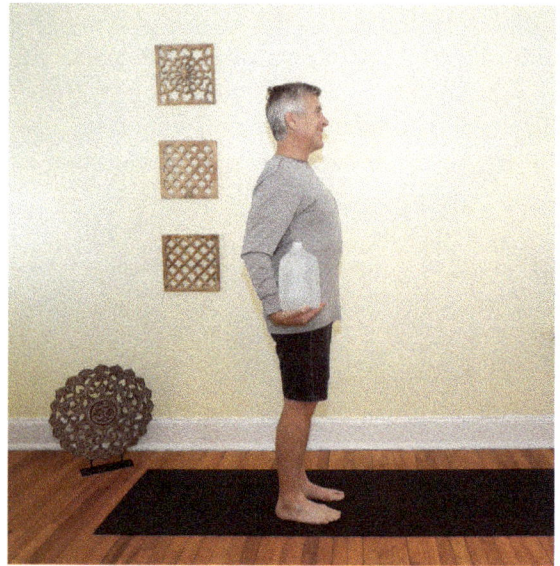

Forward head carriage

Correct head alignment

If this stooped posture goes on for a long time, it can become very difficult or impossible to reverse. You can actually lose the ability to stand up straight.

Habitual, abnormal patterns of weight-bearing—in other words, alignment problems—also cause cellular changes in your connective tissue, muscles, bones, and joints. Eventually those changes can harden, becoming permanent deformities that yoga can help improve but which may never be fully reversed. In yoga, people with a long-term pattern of forward head carriage will find it uncomfortable or impossible to lie flat on their backs, or draw their shouldblades back and down. A steady yoga practice can help unwind this pattern over time, but change is slow. If your yoga practice reveals stubborn alignment problems, just keep practicing, and stick with it. Things will gradually get better. I promise.

Am I Doing It Right? The key to a safe, effective yoga practice is learning how to center your weight when you're holding still, and how to keep it centered when you transition from one pose to another.

Yoga Helps with Hypermobility

While many people come to yoga having lost some range of motion in one or more joints, for other people the opposite is true. Their joints are *too* mobile. In fact, it's harder to fix a joint that's hypermobile (too loose) than a joint that's contracted (too tight).

Hypermobility is most often due to slack ligaments and other supporting structures that have been damaged by overstretching. (Some people have slack ligaments from birth due to genetic anomalies, but misusing a joint is a much more common cause.)

Ligaments and other joint-stabilizing structures can't be re-tightened once they're overstretched. Hypermobility is dangerous, because

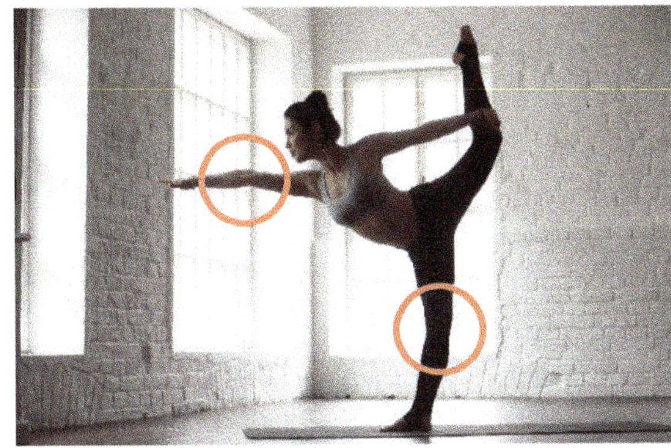

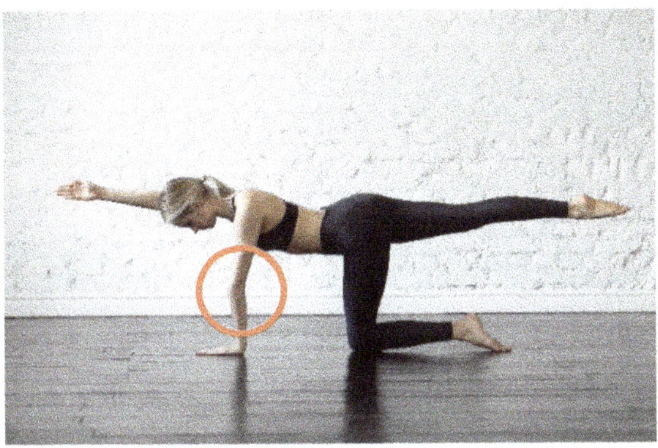

Hypermobile joints are unstable, and move beyond their normal range of motion.

unstable joints move easily beyond their normal range of motion, causing more and more damage to the bones and cartilage. People with hypermobile joints ("double-jointed" elbows or knees, for example) should focus on doing yoga poses that strengthen muscles around that joint (above and below it), to help stabilize it and prevent further damage.

Yoga Trains Your Whole Body, Together

Think of your body like a community, rather than a collection of individuals. Your body is not a collection of parts operating in isolation from one another. Yoga takes the point of view that your whole body works together—each

MECHANIC'S NOTE: BE CAREFUL WHAT YOU STRETCH

You want to stretch and strengthen your muscle tissue in yoga, but it's important to avoid directly stretching or stressing the tendons and ligaments that attach those muscles to your bones, and the bones to each other. Your ligaments and tendons are supporting, connective structures that should not be put under intense stress. Unlike muscle tissue, they don't have good blood supply, and do not heal easily if injured. The job of your muscles is to carry the weight and force of movement out of your joints, so they need to be strong and flexible. But the job of your ligaments and tendons is to stabilize your joints within their normal range of movement, so they need to stay firm and strong. A good general rule is to never force, crank, haul, or push your body into a pose. Use your muscular strength and flexibility to get into position as best you can, and breathe there. As your muscles get stronger and more flexible, you'll be able to go further.

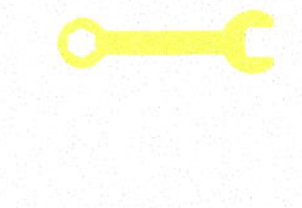

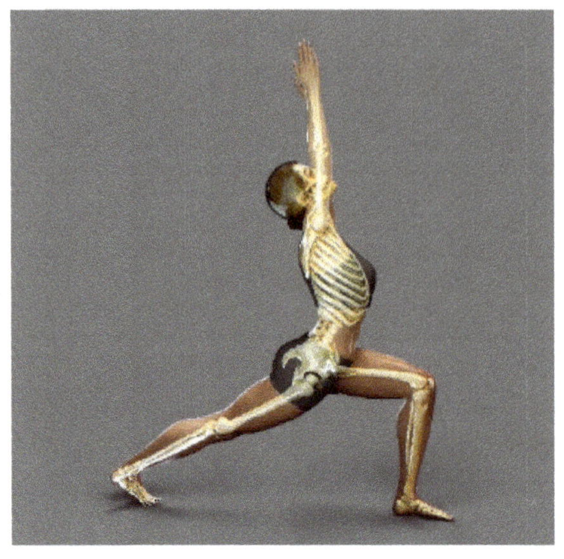
Yoga teaches you to become aware of the kinetic chain created by your movement.

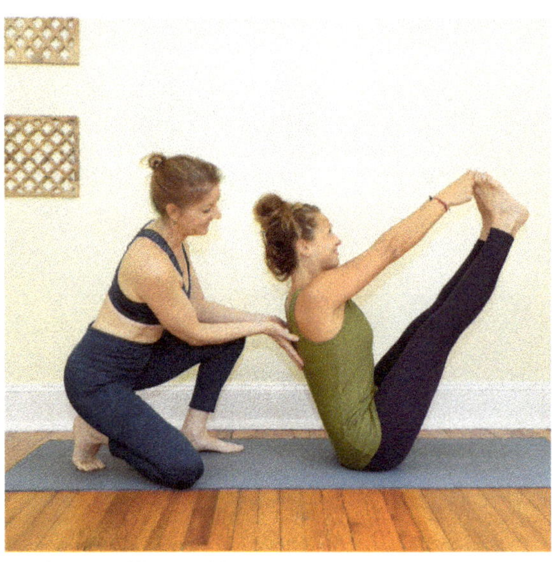
Hard work pays off: Difficult asanas like Both Big Toes Pose become easier as you learn proper alignment, and to recruit the correct muscle groups.

part is like one player on a big biological team. Movement in one section affects the entire system. And when one area can't move normally, others compensate and have to handle a heavier load. So abnormal (too much or too little) movement in one area of your body puts additional force on other muscles and joints, especially its immediate neighbors, leading to problems in other areas.

When you move one part of your body—raise an arm, step a foot forward—a kinetic chain of forces ripples through you, cuing muscles from your feet to the top of your head to help distribute and balance the effort. Over time, you'll become sensitive to this muscular activity, and notice whether it's hindering or helping you to maintain central alignment. As you sharpen your sense of various muscle groups engaging or disengaging, you'll get better at correcting your own alignment during yoga practice and in your everyday life.

It's important to understand that when you use muscles in one part of your body, muscles in another (sometimes distant) part automatically engage or relax. Doing yoga teaches you to recruit many different muscle groups to help establish and maintain correct alignment in the poses. Your muscles move your bones and joints into optimal, central alignment, and then work to hold them there. At first, recruiting the right muscle groups takes a lot of thought. After a while, it becomes second nature—especially in the poses you do most often. You'll notice that various poses get easier as you become stronger and more flexible. After a longer while, you'll find poses that used to be difficult aren't so bad anymore. Your hard work is paying off.

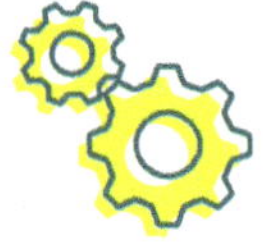

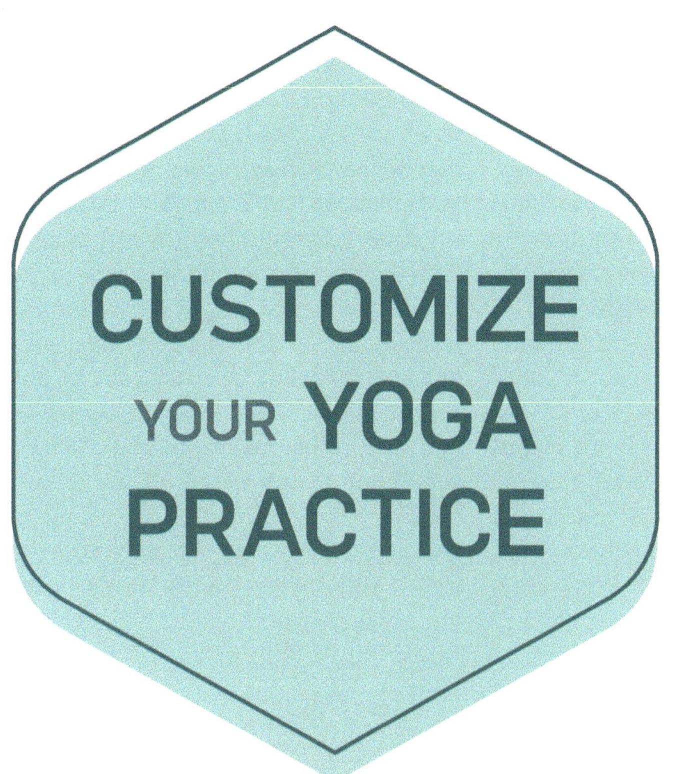
CUSTOMIZE
YOUR YOGA
PRACTICE

When you first start doing yoga, you'll rely on the instructor to help you find the poses and variations that are most appropriate for your body. In each pose, work hard enough to build some strength where you are weak, and flexibility where you've lost range of movement. Over time, you'll know how to adjust certain positions so that you can make progress without getting injured. Don't worry about what anyone else is doing. You do you. I promise, you'll make the most progress if you keep your mind on your own mat, and notice how your body needs different adjustments on different days.

Pose Variations

The pictures in this book show many variations of the poses we're discussing, each requiring different levels of strength and flexibility. Please understand, one variation is not *better*, more *advanced,* or more *real* than the others—some just require more strength and flexibility. I advise playing the long game. That means choosing the pose variations during class that will help you build a little more strength and flexibility without pushing your body too far, too fast.

It's hard to tell how advanced someone's practice is from outside observation. Sure, that guy over there may be doing some physically intense, crazy-looking arm balance. But if he's thinking about how many people are watching and how impressed they must be—he's not a very advanced yogi. He's just a strong, flexible, insecure guy who wants to impress people.

Instead of chasing more and more difficult poses, the goal of an intelligent yoga practice is to *get deeper* in whatever pose you're doing. Please understand, getting deeper is an inside job. Regardless of what variation you're doing with your body, the depth of your practice is measured by how smooth you can keep your breathing, how focused you can keep your mind, and how steady you can keep your gaze.

All pose variations build the strength and flexibility you'll need to eventually do another, more intense, variation. Your task is to find the variation that works best for you today, and physically and mentally apply yourself to it. Sometimes I choose a less intense variation than I normally would, because it feels right for my body that day. This is the joy and responsibility of developing your own personal practice. So follow the sequence of poses being taught in class, but learn to adjust as you go and apply the variations that work best for your body and energy level. Focus on building a little strength and flexibility each time you practice. Remember, Rome wasn't built in a day. If you have an injury or a special physical

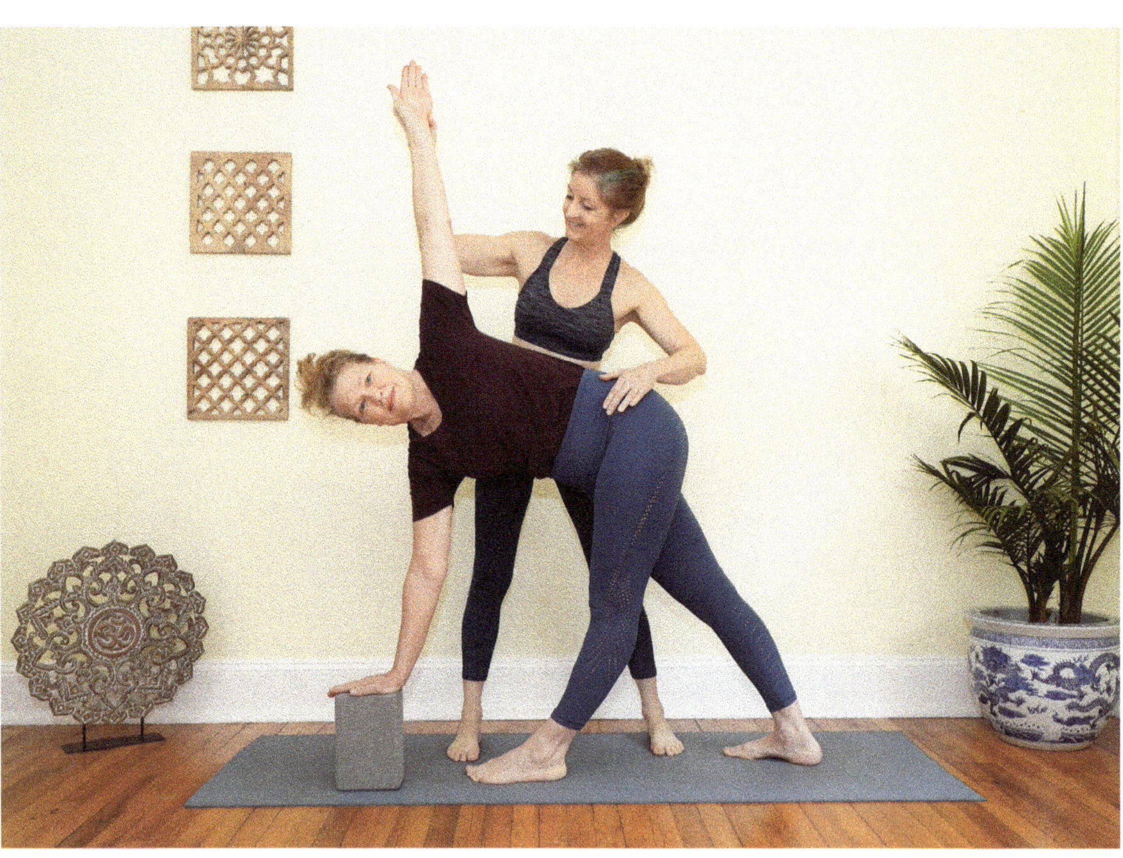

Revolved Triangle Pose, variation with block

circumstance (like scoliosis or arthritis), choose a variation that attends to that need.

Practicing this way means that your choices about how to do a particular pose will change over time. Six months from now, you'll be a little stronger and more flexible, so more options will be available to you in each pose.

All of the above is why it's important to seek out trained, experienced instructors who can help you find the right variation for your body. Beware of instructors who use a one size fits all approach. How can one variation of a pose be right for all twenty people in the room? Impossible! Find an instructor who is willing and able to help you discern the best variation for your body in a particular pose. If there's time and class is small, they might be able to help you during class. In most cases, it's best to ask for highly personalized instruction before or after class, or in a private session.

Pose Sequences

The sequence of poses in a yoga class should be logical and carefully planned, so each pose prepares your body for what will come after. Traditionally, yoga classes follow this classic formula: sun salutations and standing poses; forward folds; twists; backbends; inversions; and a final resting pose.

All classes should begin by slowing down and deepening your breathing, and steadying your gaze (drishti) to clear your mind. Then, you'll start some larger physical movements to gently warm up, waking up your muscle memory and nerve communication pathways. As class goes along, you'll become more focused and steady, so you're ready for any new or complicated poses that come later. Remember, difficult poses don't just challenge your muscles, they also challenge your ability to breathe steadily and keep your mind calm.

Every yoga session should include simple poses that take little physical effort, as well as complex poses that require much more. It takes time and regular practice to not only train your body, but also to train your mind. Arguably, the greatest benefit of a steady yoga practice is that when the going gets tough in your daily life, you're able to stay calm and focused. In this way, your yoga practice might help you to make better decisions under stress, not get derailed as easily when plans go awry, not fall apart when the rug gets yanked out from under your feet. In my opinion, those skills are a lot more useful than being able to stand on your head.

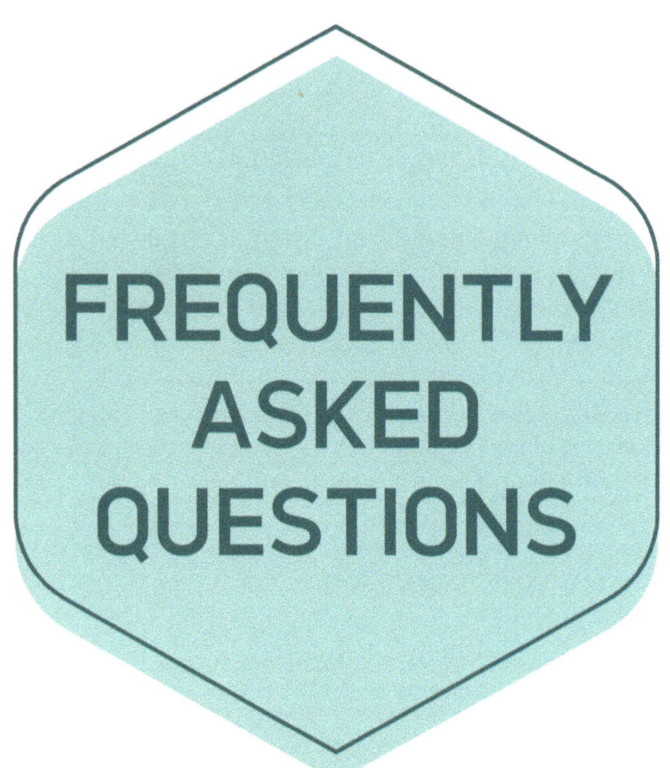

FREQUENTLY ASKED QUESTIONS

Is yoga a cardio work out?

Yoga strengthens your cardiovascular system by increasing your heart rate, lowering blood pressure, and challenging blood vessel reactivity. But most classes don't exceed the aerobic threshold long enough to improve your cardiovascular endurance. That said, doing yoga will help you get better results from any aerobic exercise you do like running, swimming, or cycling.

How can yoga help me?

Physically, yoga helps preserve the normal full range of motion throughout your entire body and makes you stronger. Mentally, yoga helps you focus by clearing your mind and calming you down.

Contrary to what many people think, flexibility is not the primary goal of yoga, and it's not the most important thing to focus on in class. In fact, too much flexibility without enough strength to support your joints can lead to injuries. Yoga practice should make you stronger, so your muscles can protect your bones and joints. After all, your muscles' job is to support your weight and the forces of movement out of your joints, so they don't get damaged or wear out too early.

Yoga poses balance strength against flexibility to help you maintain optimal mobility. Classes are put together (sequenced) in a way that makes different muscle groups take turns working hard—right side, left side, lower body, torso, upper body, front, and back. You learn to resist letting weight sag into your joints while you practice by recruiting more muscle groups to support and stabilize each pose. You'll find that regularly doing some yoga will help you develop a balanced combination of strength and flexibility throughout your body.

How do I keep from getting injured if I'm just starting out?

The safest way to start doing yoga is to practice slowly. Speeding through the poses before you can control your breath and stay mentally focused is a great recipe for getting hurt, building bad habits (that eventually lead to injuries), and getting frustrated. Believe me, moving slowly and holding each pose a little longer is much harder than flinging yourself from one position to the next. Slow and steady wins the race, as they say. Slowing down is hard. Be patient. It'll pay off. I promise. (We'll talk more about injury prevention and management in chapter 6.)

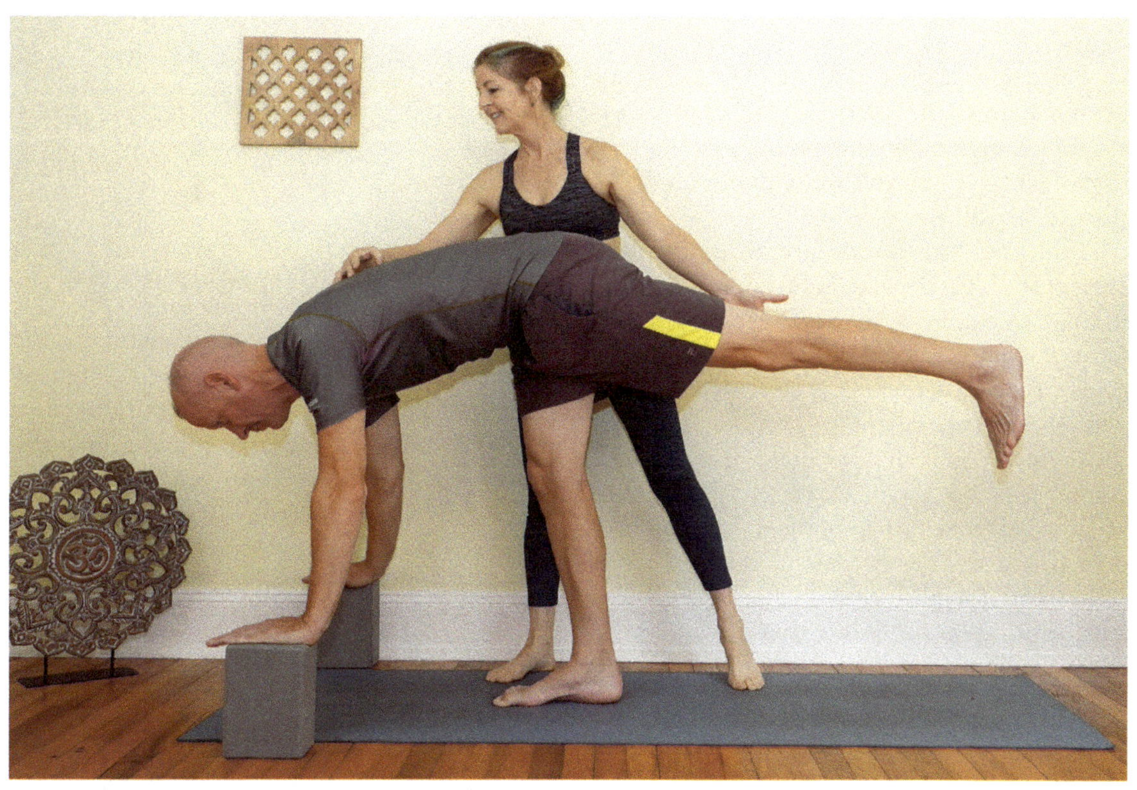

Warrior Three Pose, variation with blocks. Pose variations, often using a tool like a block or strap, help you build the strength and flexibility for more intense poses.

What does it mean to "find my edge?"

A lot of instructors use the phrase "find your edge" during class. Your edge is the limit of your ability to hold correct alignment in a pose. It changes from day to day, depending on your energy, strength, and flexibility.

The limit of your ability to hold proper alignment depends on your energy level, strength, and flexibility at that moment. Encouraging students to find their edge in a pose can be an instructor's way of helping them stay focused and engaged. But some instructors use this phrase to exhort students to push themselves to the point of extreme discomfort or pain, and then tell them to back out of the pose a little from there. This is a dangerously misguided way of instructing and practicing yoga that leads to injuries. Pain is *always* a warning sign that you are being injured right now—not later, not maybe, not almost. The injury may be a micro-tear, a strain, a sprain, or more subtle cellular-level tissue damage, but you must understand that pain equals injury.

That said, you must learn to differentiate true pain from the uncomfortable sensations that are caused by stretching and strengthening tight or weak muscles. I avoid saying "find your edge" in class, because it is so widely misused and misunderstood.

To find your limits in a pose, first, establish correct (central) alignment in a basic variation or stage (called a krama) of the pose. It is a mistake to attempt the hardest possible variation right away. Establish central alignment in your legs, hips, spine, shoulders, head, and neck. Then maintain this correct alignment as you gradually increase the challenge to your strength and flexibility. Exactly how you increase the muscle work and stretch loads depends on what pose you're doing. It may involve bending your knees a little deeper, raising your arms, or pressing your palms together.

Be alert as you increase the stretching and strengthening challenges. When you sense your alignment (the central distribution of weight and force) starting to fall apart, stop increasing the challenge. You've found your "edge" in that pose for today. Hold still, steady your breath, and focus your eyes on one point. Feel the movement of your breath and the sensations of stretching and strengthening in various muscles. If you can't breathe, back out of the pose until you can. You should be working hard—mentally and physically—but not injuring yourself.

Be patient. Changing muscular patterns in your body is a gradual process. During a difficult pose, your mind will certainly jump around and struggle against it like a cat caught in a pillowcase. Focus on calming down and breathing deeply. Changing your mind's reaction to discomfort takes much longer than changing your body, but it's a very useful skill.

What is a "line of energy"?

You hear this phrase a lot on planet yoga, but what does it mean? Recruiting enough muscle groups to support central (correct) alignment in a pose requires engaging muscles throughout your entire body—from your feet to your head. The force of these muscle groups working together creates a unique energy signature for each pose. This is the "line of energy." You'll eventually learn to feel this line of energy inside your body, but it's also visible from the outside. An experienced instructor can look at you during class, and see which muscle groups are working and, to some extent, how hard. He or she can see where your line of energy is strong and where it is weak, and guide you to use some muscles a bit more and others a little less.

To me, the line of energy often feels like a push-me/pull-you type of action inside my body, as one part reaches in one direction while another part reaches in the opposite direction. For example, my arms may reach up while my knees bend to sink my hips down.

Muscle recruitment, consciously activating particular muscle groups, is how you begin to find the line of energy in each pose. By stretching some muscles upward or outward while opposing groups press down or inward, you counterbalance the extending (pranic) actions in one part of your body against the contracting (apanic) actions in another. This balancing of upward and downward muscular actions occurs in every position, even if you're simply standing in Mountain Pose (Tadasana) with your hands by your sides. Working one internal force against another is how you build strength and flexibility in yoga.

Over time, you'll be able to sense which muscles are working too hard, and which ones could work harder to help you maintain alignment during practice. You'll learn to recruit smaller muscle groups deep inside your body, and begin to feel the subtle energy that comes from stimulating your nervous system while you calm your mind. It takes a lot of practice to sense this. Be patient.

How do I "go deeper" in a pose?

Going deeper is another term, like *finding your edge*, that I avoid using in my classes, because the phrase is so commonly misused and misunderstood. Some instructors encourage students to *go deeper* in a pose when they really just mean *push harder* or *bend over further*. The result is that many people think going deeper means getting lower, grasping a bind, touching the floor, or turning yourself further around in a twist. This is incorrect. First, nirvana is not waiting down there on the floor, or somewhere behind you. And second, if you don't have the strength and flexibility to bend lower, twist further, grasp a bind, or touch the floor, you'll injure yourself by forcing your body to do it.

I always say that it's hard to tell how deep someone is in a yoga pose because, as I mentioned earlier, going deeper is an inside job. You go deeper by extending your breath (especially the inhales), holding your eyes still, and focusing your mind on experiencing the present moment. If it feels good—great! If it's uncomfortable—don't worry! This too shall pass. You'll be in the next pose soon. Be here now, then let it go.

To go deeper, establish correct alignment and then slowly increase the weight and flexibility challenge until you feel your alignment falter. Stop. Back up a little to re-center your alignment and hold the pose. Find one point to look at, and establish a slow, steady breathing pattern. It's the same for every pose—easy ones and hard ones alike.

You go deeper by:

- **Connecting** each movement of your practice with a full inhale or exhale.
- **Maintaining** full steady breathing when holding poses, especially the difficult ones.
- **Focusing** your eyes on a single gazing point in each pose (called maintaining your drishti).

Many people who do yoga mistakenly think that steady breathing and eye focus (drishti) are not as important as achieving the physical pose positions. In fact, these are the skills you need to go deeper in your yoga practice. Maintaining your breath and drishti are the hardest parts of any yoga pose.

Try it next time you practice: Establish a steady, full breathing pattern and fix your eyes

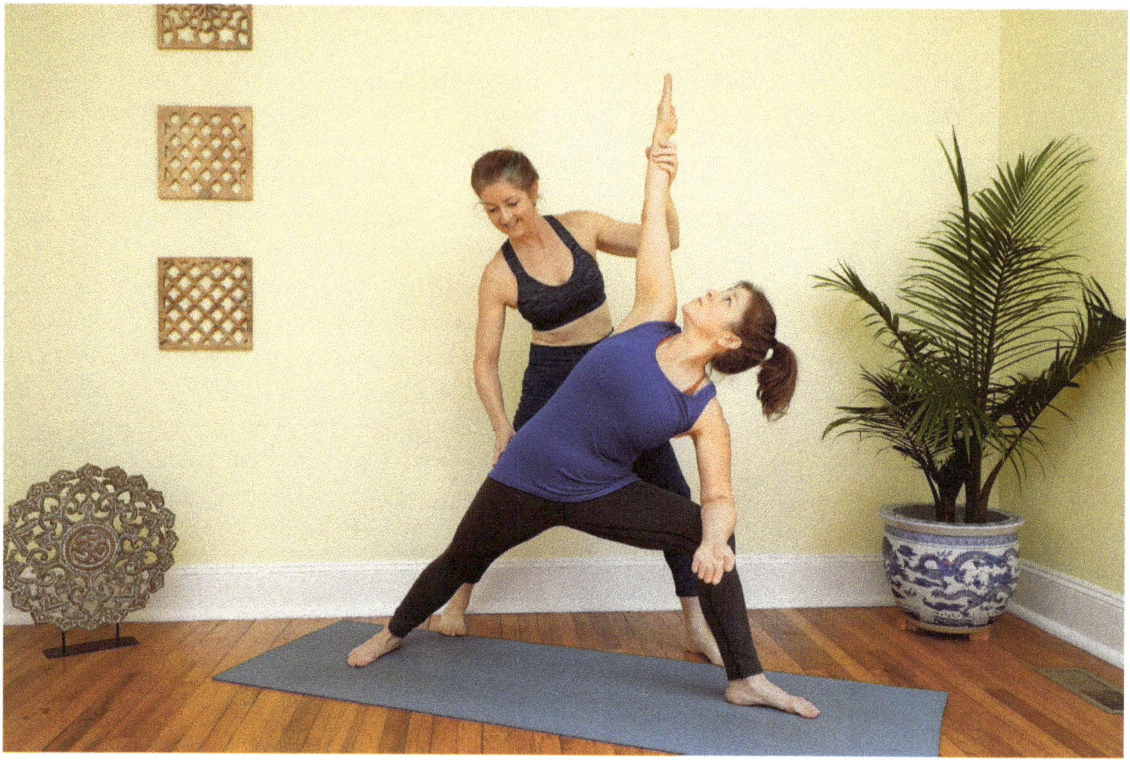

Extended Side Angle Pose, variation. Can you tell how deep in the pose she is, just by looking?

on a single gazing point during each pose. This is astonishingly difficult, but you will notice a big difference in how you feel during class. In terms of physical effort, challenge yourself but don't strain. Treat your body with respect and care while you practice. Set up your alignment and then move your focus inward. I promise, it will pay off.

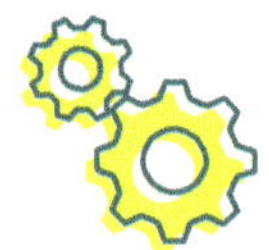

CHAPTER 2

BREATHING

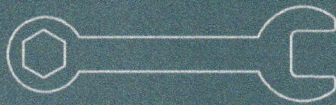

Even though we all breathe—all day and all night, every minute of every day—we're usually not aware that it's happening. But in yoga, we deliberately pay attention to each breath we take, as a tool for keeping our mind focused on what we're doing. Each inhale and exhale only happens in the present moment. We can't revisit a past breath. We can only notice the breath that's happening right now. Every yoga class—no matter what kind—starts with a few moments of stillness, for you to become aware of your breath as it moves in and out of your body.

Besides helping to keep your mind on what you're doing, breathing is a fantastic tool for getting more stretch and strength out of your yoga poses. After you get your body parts into position, hold still and focus on making your inhales and exhales deeper. It takes a lot of different muscles throughout your entire torso to breathe—from your low belly to your neck and jaw; from your waist and chest to your back. Learning to take bigger inhales and fuller exhales is the absolute best way to build core strength from the inside-out. It's like doing internal crunches while you hold a pose. Who knew!?

How Your Lungs Work

Did you know that your lungs are the second-largest organ of elimination in your body, after your skin? You might also be interested to know that your left and right lung are quite different. Your right lung has three lobes, but your left lung has only two, to make room for your heart underneath it. In fact, the best way to feel your heartbeat is to put your right hand on your ribcage, underneath your left breast. Try it. You'll feel your heartbeat much more clearly than when your hand is in the traditional spot up higher on your chest. That's because your heart is tucked up under your left lung, not between your two lungs in the top of your chest.

The upper section of your respiratory system is comprised of your nasal cavity, pharynx, larynx, and trachea (those are the first passageways where air enters your body). The lower section consists of the lungs themselves, and your diaphragm (the main muscle of respiration). This system has two primary functions. First, it brings air into your lungs so oxygen can be absorbed into your bloodstream (the inhale). And second, it removes carbon-dioxide from your bloodstream, and expels it from your body (the exhale). Among other things, your respiratory system helps maintain the acid-base (pH) balance of your bloodstream.

We tend to imagine our lungs filling up like balloons as we breathe in. But actually, as you inhale the lobes of your lungs expand and spiral outward, moving away from the center of your chest. They turn in a corkscrew-like motion, with the upper lobes filling first and rotating over the lower ones. When you exhale, the lobes of your lungs rotate inward, moving toward the center of your chest. On deep exhalations, your left lung gives your heart a gentle hug.

Your lungs are hollow organs, and are largely made of muscle tissue (technically speaking, it's called "smooth" muscle, as opposed to the striped or "striated" muscles that move your

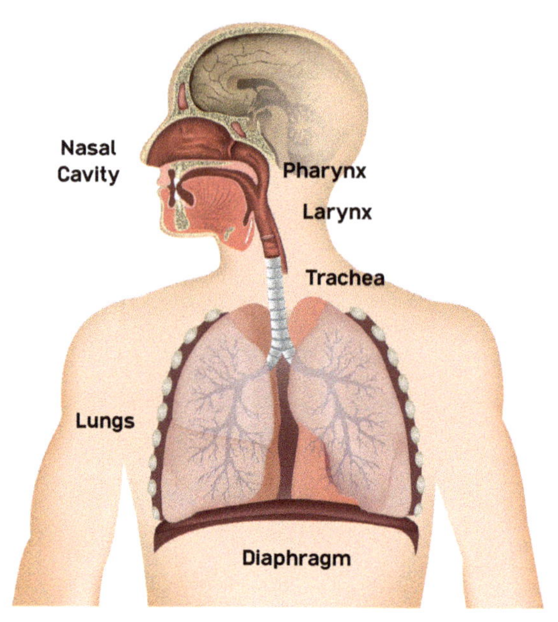

Your respiratory system

bones). So, as with other muscle tissue, it's possible to make the muscle fibers in your lungs work better by exercising them. In yoga we do that by practicing long deep inhalations and slow complete exhalations. Conversely, if this tissue is damaged by disease or pollution, your lungs lose some of their function and elasticity. Along with the diaphragm, many muscle groups in your torso are involved in creating your inhales and exhales, and they also get stronger and more flexible as you practice deep, slow breathing in yoga class.

It Takes Time: Training your mind and breath to stay steady in difficult poses can be harder than training your physical body to hold the pose.

Your diaphragm is the primary muscle of respiration, the engine that moves your breathing. This large, mushroom-shaped muscle has its "cap" attached along the bottom edge of your rib-cage, and its "stem" attached to your

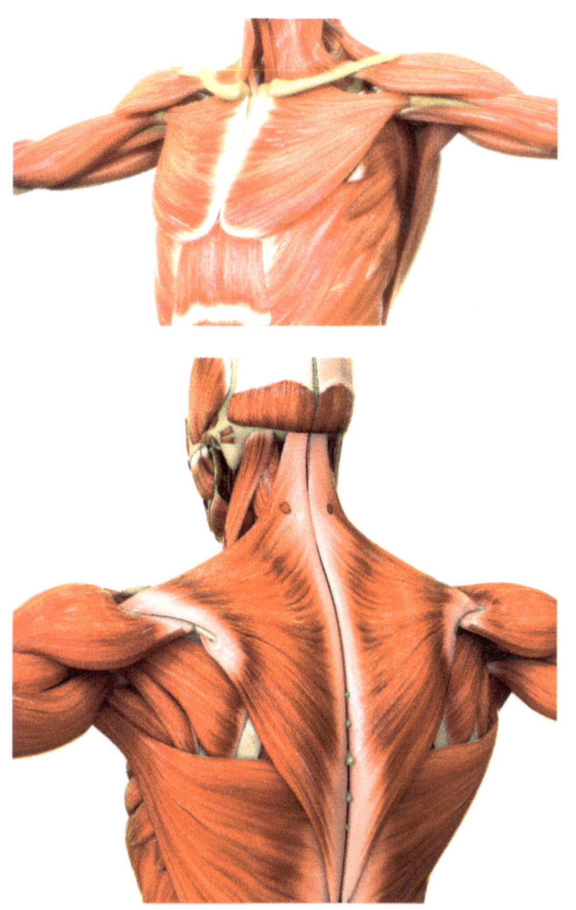

Auxiliary respiratory muscles. Though your diaphragm does most of the work, your breathing is assisted by muscles in your chest, rib cage, neck, and back.

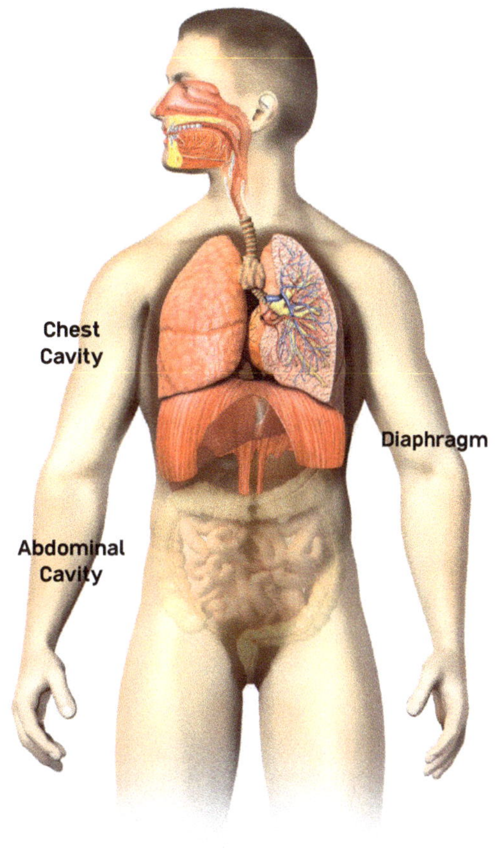

The two cavities of your torso

mid-spine. The many other muscles that help you breathe are called auxiliary respiratory muscles. They include the muscles between your ribs (your intercostals), in your chest (your pectorals), in front of your neck (your sternocleidomastoids), and in your back (your serratus, latissimus dorsi, rhomboids, and trapezius).

When you deepen and lengthen your breath, you make your diaphragm and all of those auxiliary muscles stronger, too. The stronger your auxiliary muscles of breathing are, the easier it is to breathe.

To understand how your breathing works, you should know that your torso (also called your thorax) is divided into two compartments, stacked on top of each other. Your chest cavity holds your lungs and heart, and beneath it, your abdominal cavity contains your stomach, lower digestive tract, and other internal organs. Your chest and your abdomen are separated from one another by a special membrane (called the pleura), as well as by the diaphragm muscle itself.

To create an inhale, your chest cavity changes shape. It becoming larger as your diaphragm drops down, your ribs move out, and your chest lifts up. This increase in size creates a vacuum, and air gets sucked into your lungs through your nose and mouth to fill that unoccupied space, the vacuum in your chest.

To see how this works, try an experiment. Get a kitchen sponge and a bowl filled with water. Squeeze the sponge in your hand and put it underwater, still squeezing. Then let go. You'll see that water rushes in to fill up the empty space inside the sponge as it expands. This is exactly how your inhale works. You create empty space by expanding the size of your chest cavity, and air rushes in to fill it.

On the exhale, all of the muscles that created the inhale relax, and your chest cavity goes back to its original size and shape. Your diaphragm rises back up to its normal "mushroom cap" position, your ribs move inward, and your chest falls. Any air that doesn't fit in this smaller space gets pushed out of your nose and mouth.

Although it may seem like you are "pulling" air into your lungs when you inhale, this is an incorrect understanding. How forcefully air comes into your lungs is determined by how far and how fast you change the shape of your chest cavity. The more empty space that's created, the bigger the vacuum, and the stronger and deeper your inhale.

So generally speaking, your exhale is passive. It's a relaxing of the muscular effort of the inhale. Inhaling makes your muscles of respiration work hard; exhaling releases this work. In yoga, we purposefully deepen the exhale by pressing the chest cavity smaller, which also makes the auxiliary muscles of respiration work hard.

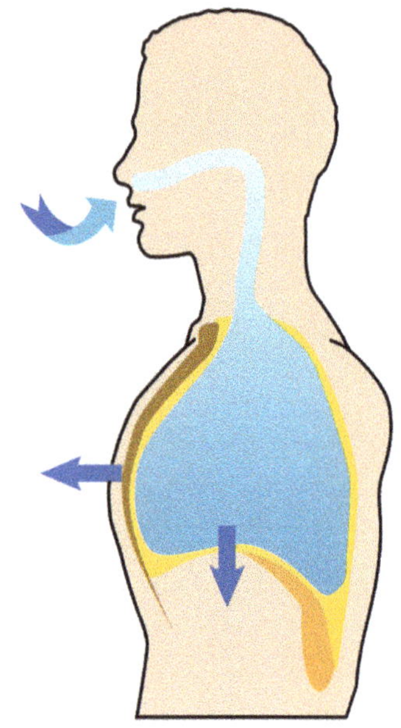
Inhale

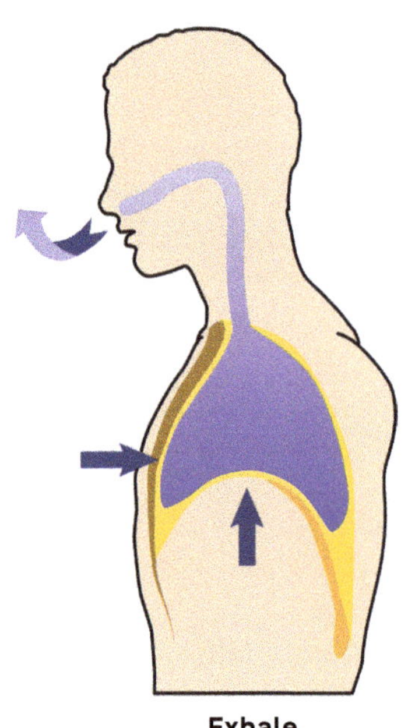
Exhale

Actions of the diaphragm and chest cavity on your inhale and exhale

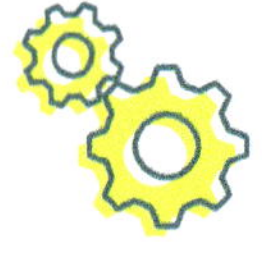

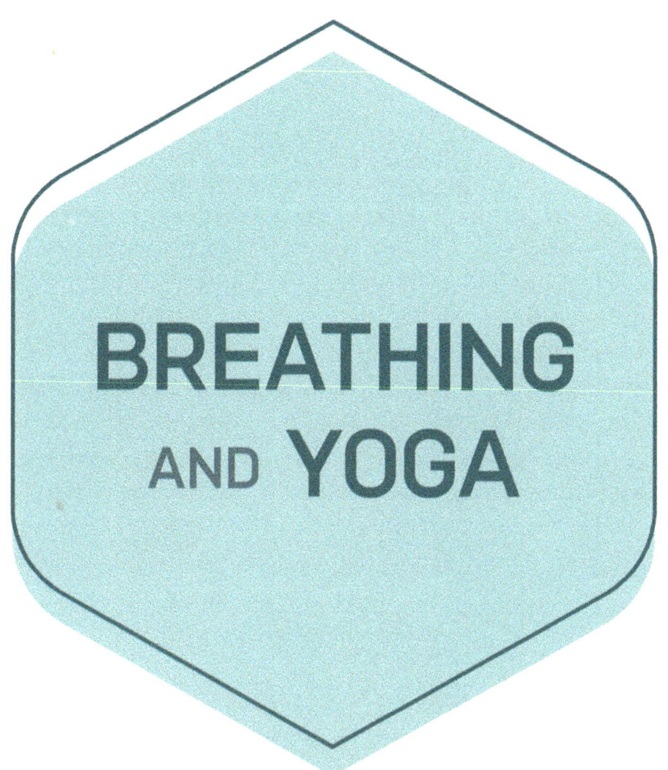

BREATHING AND YOGA

Normally, the act of breathing is unconscious. Most people don't notice how or when they inhale or exhale, unless they're exerting themselves by doing exercise that makes them breathe hard. But even when you do aerobic or cardiovascular exercise and are more aware of your breathing, you probably don't focus on directing or controlling it.

This is where yoga is different. During your yoga practice, you deliberately pay attention to controlling your breath. You bring the act of breathing up into your conscious awareness, and use it as a tool to help focus your thoughts and regulate your practice.

Your breaths and your thoughts have more in common that you realize. I'm sure you've noticed that your mind is always jumping around, from past to present to future. Movement is a natural characteristic of your mind and thoughts. By jumping around, your mind is just doing its job, which is to figure things out: solve problems, calculate risks and rewards, consult with past experiences and apply those lessons to future possibilities. Movement is also a natural characteristic of your breath, which is constantly flowing from inhale to exhale.

When you focus on your breathing during yoga practice, you're not trying to turn your mind off. You're trying to harness your mind to one

> Yoga is different than other types of exercise because you consciously control your breathing, and link it to your movements.

single point of attention that you've chosen. During yoga practice, you learn to direct your thoughts onto a specific thing that you want to focus on, rather than letting your mind leap from one thought to the next at random.

Fortunately, your breath and your mind are natural friends, because both they share this need for constant motion. An inhale leads to the next exhale—over and over—in an unending flow. During your yoga practice, imagine that you're teaching your breath and your thoughts to hold hands and walk along side-by-side. When your mind races ahead or goes off the path, draw it back to your breathing pattern. When your breath stops or gets panicky and gasping, slow down until it's back on track.

As you practice, try to take long, slow, deep breaths, and equalize the length and intensity of your inhales and exhales (this is a technique called Sama Vritti). Most people tend to exhale harder than they inhale. This is partly because more muscular effort is required for the inhale, and our muscles of respiration are often weak and tight. Since the exhale is the "release" side of the breath, it's easier to fall into deeper exhales than to create deeper inhales.

But remember, the inhale is what feeds your cells by bringing fresh oxygen into your body. The exhale is the garbage truck that removes gases from your body that it can't use. By falling into the exhale more heavily than the inhale, you can deplete your oxygen supply during practice and become exhausted. I recommend starting to equalize the two sides of your breath by easing off on your exhales, and focusing on making your inhales a little stronger and longer.

Breathing Practices

A technique called victorious breathing (Ujjayi Pranayama) can be very helpful for evening out your breathing pattern, because it makes your breathing more audible so you can hear it while you practice.

To do victorious breathing, gently narrow the base of your throat so that your breath starts to sound like a distant ocean. Most people find it's easier to make this ocean sound on the exhale at first. After you get the hang of it on the exhale, try making this ocean sound on your inhales. Note: If you sound like Darth Vader, you're doing it too hard; ease up a little. Your victorious breathing should be audible to yourself and the person right next to you. But people across the room should not be able to hear it. Aim for the distant gentle ocean sound you hear when you hold a sea shell to your ear.

Listening to your own breathing pattern helps keep your mind focused, and tells you right away when you start to struggle during practice. Doing yoga poses is really about coordinating your physical movements with your inhales and exhales. When you connect your thoughts to your breathing pattern, and your breathing to your movements, you start really doing yoga—not just exercising.

"Oh, Yogi, do not practice asana without vinyasa."

K. Pattabhi Jois (26 July 1915–18 May 2009), founder of the Ashtanga Vinyasa Yoga practice lineage

Connecting your breath to your movements is called *Vinyasa*. This means that you link your breath to every muscular action during practice—the large ones and the small ones, the flowing sequences, and the moments of stillness. The idea is to connect your inhales and exhales very specifically to every part of your physical yoga practice. Eventually Vinyasa—this linking of your physical movements and your breathing—becomes the center of your practice. This awareness of your breath, and learning to consciously extend it as needed, is actually the "yoga part" of your practice.

This is great news, because it means that doing "real yoga" has nothing to do with the physical difficulty—the strength and flexibility—that various poses might call for. It's irrelevant how complicated or challenging the pose you're doing is. As long as you're staying connected to your breathing pattern, you're doing yoga.

You do not have to work your muscles until you drip with sweat. You're doing real yoga when you stand at the top of your mat in Mountain Pose (Tadasana), and draw your attention to evening out the length and intensity of your inhales and exhales. It's fine to work your muscles hard, but you should understand that pushing the extreme limits of your strength and flexibility is *not* required. Choose pose variations that work best for you each day, but always focus on your breathing.

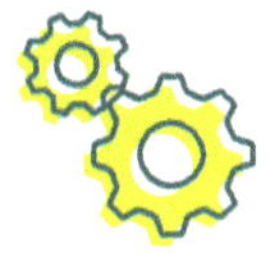

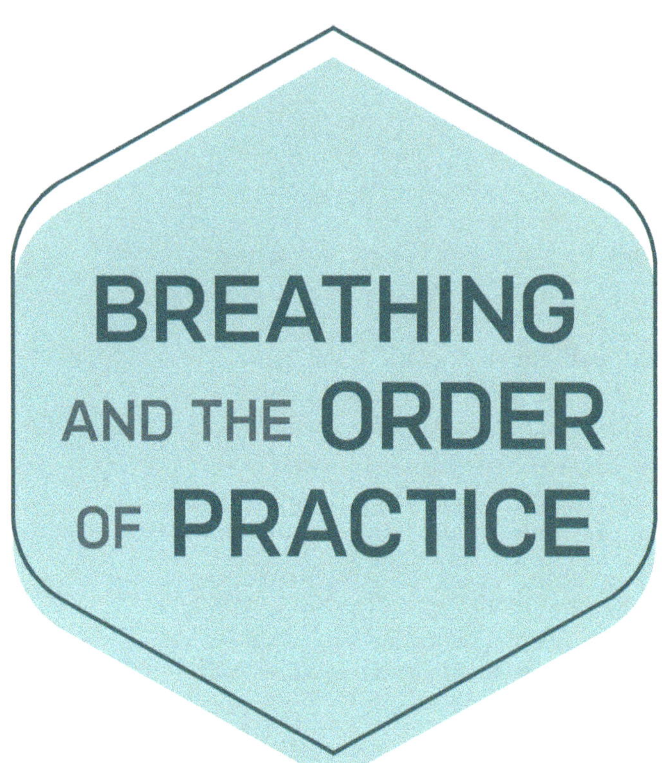

BREATHING AND THE ORDER OF PRACTICE

Although there are many different types of yoga classes, they usually follow a similar pattern, in terms of which poses come first and which ones comes later or at the end (remember the pose sequences mentioned in chapter 1). In the same way that you wouldn't start a run by sprinting a long distance, you don't dive right into the most difficult poses first. You take time to warm up your muscles. What's different about yoga is that you also need time to prepare your mental focus, by sharpening your awareness and control of your breathing. Let's take a look at how the order of a yoga class helps you do this.

Poses early in practice help you get focused on your breathing

It's not easy to stay aware of your breathing throughout a yoga class. I still find my mind wandering sometimes—especially at the beginning. I catch myself thinking about some conversation that happened earlier, or something I'm going to do later, instead of about what I'm doing right now.

That's why yoga classes start with poses that don't present much of a challenge to your ability to breathe deeply and evenly. These early, less challenging poses give you a chance to clear your mind and get it firmly connected to your breath. The poses then get progressively more challenging. Those that make taking a slow, deep breath most difficult—backbends, inversions, arm balances—come nearer to the end of practice.

Examples of early practice poses:

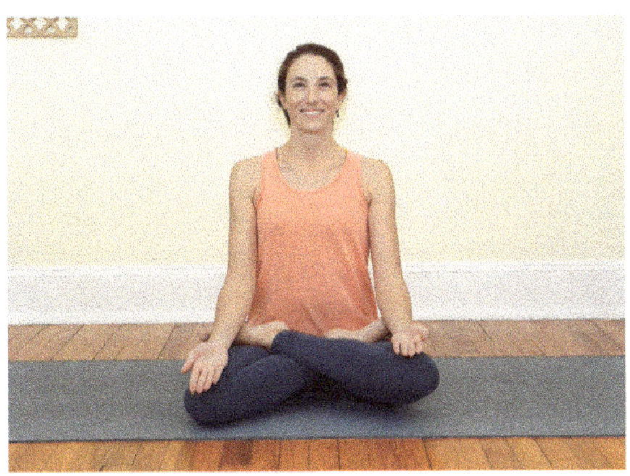

Lotus Pose

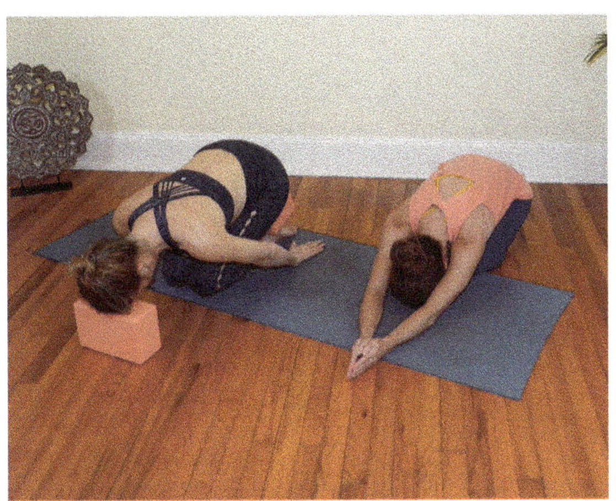

Child's Pose

Comfortable Seated Pose (Sukhasana), Lotus Pose (Padmasana), and Child's Pose (Balasana) are good poses for settling your mind on your breath at the beginning of a class. After a few moments of stillness in these poses, you begin adding some gentle movements to follow your inhales and exhales. Gradually, you come to stand in Mountain Pose (Tadasana), and add familiar sequences like Sun Salutations to further establish Vinyasa, the link between your breath and the movements of your body.

Next time you're practicing these poses, notice how simply establishing a slow, deep breathing pattern starts raising your body temperature, and helps warm up your body from the inside out. The muscle work needed to do the physical poses creates heat inside your body, but the very act of breathing deeply also requires a lot of muscle work in and of itself. You can think of deep, conscious breathing like pumping a bellows to fan your internal furnace.

Poses in the middle of practice call for more oxygen

As a yoga session continues, poses in the middle of the practice demand more strength and flexibility, so you'll need more oxygen to fuel your muscles. Your heart beats harder in these more challenging poses, and it's important to stay very mindful of drawing deep, full inhales. There's a common tendency in difficult poses to exhale harder than you inhale. But the exhales don't bring in the oxygen your body needs. Focus on your inhales to fuel your muscles to do this work.

Examples of middle practice poses:

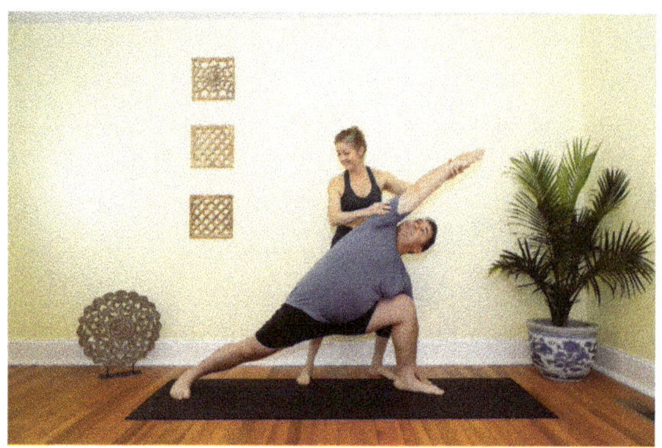

Extended Side Angle Pose

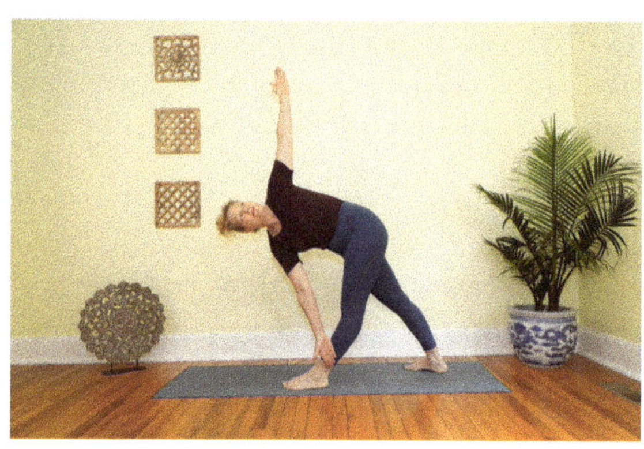

Revolved Triangle Pose

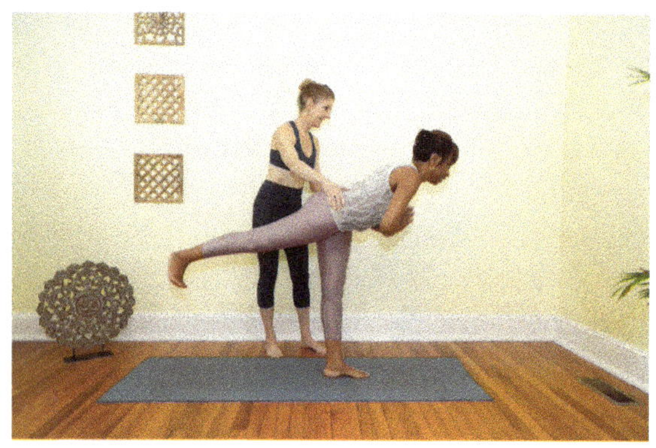

Warrior Three Pose

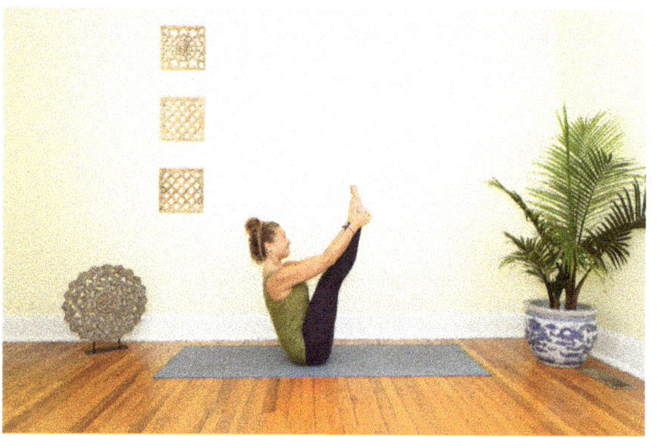

Upward Facing Intense Stretch Pose

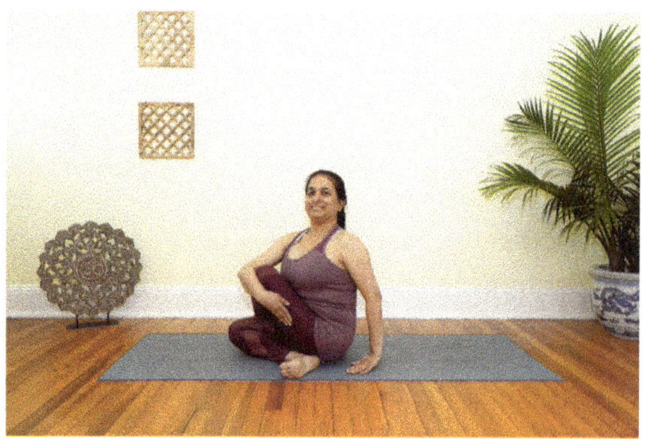

Seated Spinal Twist Pose

If you're panting or gasping for air through your mouth, slow down and take a break in Downward Dog, Mountain, or Child's Pose. Even out your breathing and steady your mind. Then, join back into the practice. Do not keep barreling forward when you lose your breath. Pause. Regroup. Join back in. Resist the ego-driven urge to press ahead when you've lost the ability to focus your mind on the movement of your inhales and exhales. This is when injuries happen.

Poses late in practice challenge your breathing the most

Poses that most challenge your ability to breathe will come near the end of practice. The last third of a class typically includes back bends, standing balances, and inversions. These poses not only require a lot of strength and flexibility, they also put your body in positions that make drawing deep breaths very difficult. By this point your muscles are warm and flexible, and you've had time to really get focused on your breathing, and connect it to your movements. Now you're ready to take on these challenging poses.

Examples of late practice poses:

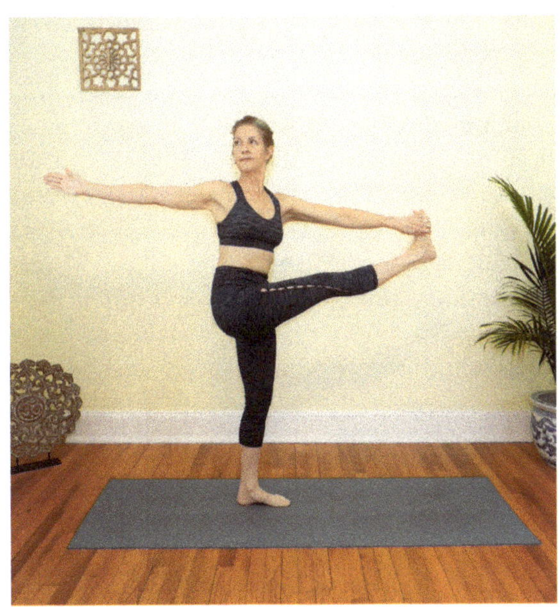

Standing Revolved Hand to Big Toe Pose

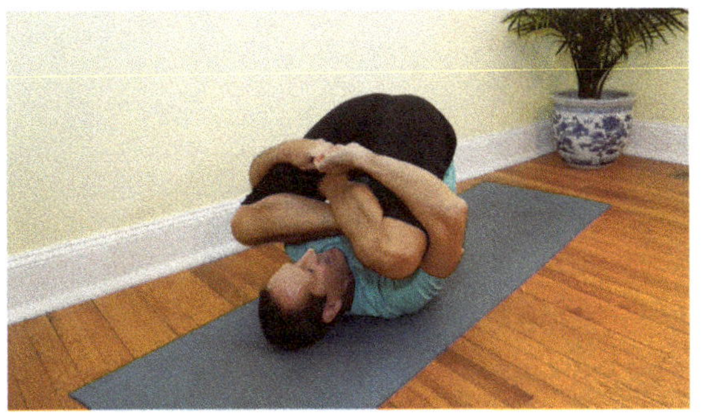

Embryo Pose

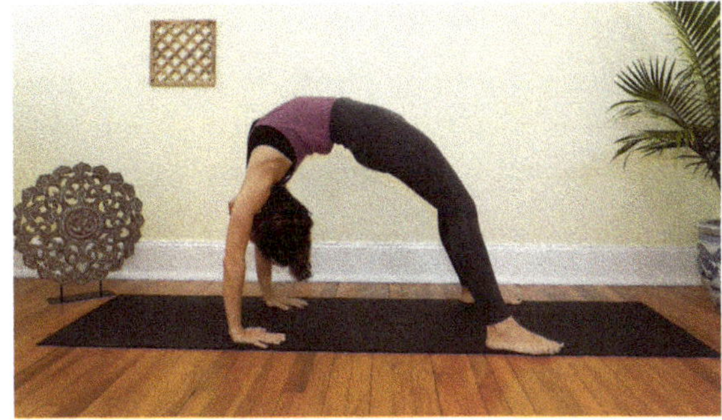

Upward Facing Bow Pose

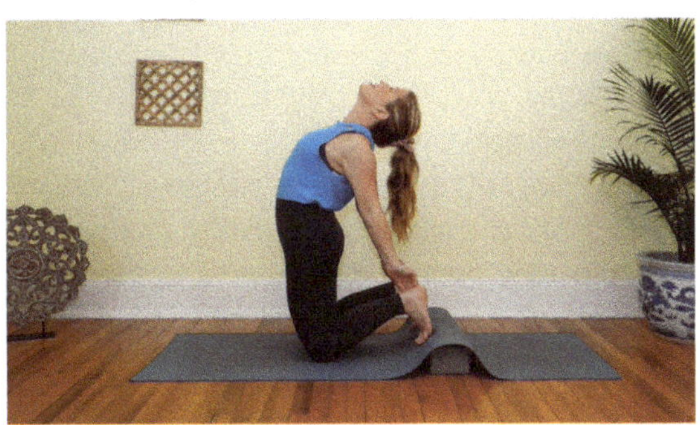

Camel Pose, variation

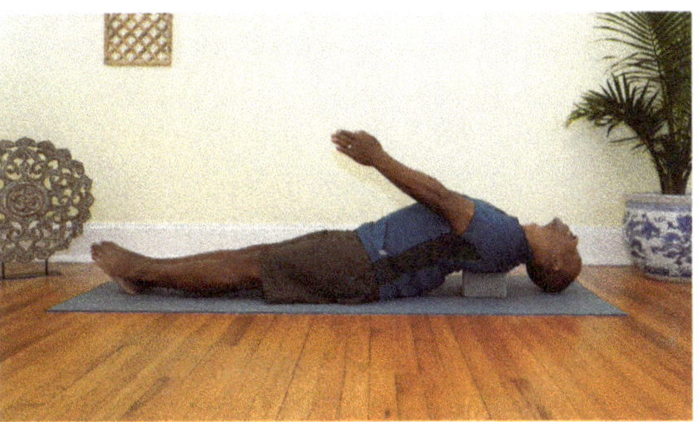

Fish Pose, variation

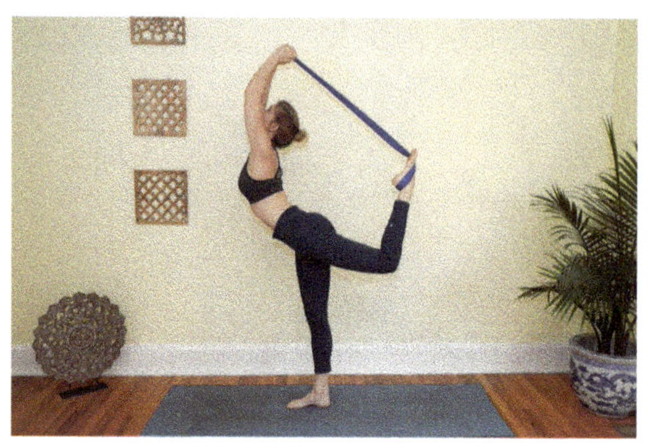

King Dancer Pose, variation

It's common for your breath to shut off completely in difficult or anxiety-provoking positions. Remember, holding your breath is not helpful. If you notice you've stopped breathing, back off the physical intensity, and refocus on your inhales to feed your body the oxygen it needs. When your body realizes that it has enough air coming in, your mind will automatically become calm and steady again, even though you're still working hard.

Doing difficult poses requires keeping your mind calm. Your first thought may well be, "I can't do Wheel Pose!" or "I'm afraid of trying Headstand!" or "I hate Shoulder Stand!" When you hear your own panicky or negative thoughts in practice, you have an opportunity to direct your mind toward remedy thoughts like "I can at least try," or "I can do a variation that suits my body," or "It will be over before I know it."

Physically, it's hard to get air into your lungs when you're upside down or in a backbend. When your upper body's upside down, your diaphragm has to push the organs in your abdominal cavity upwards, against gravity, to create space in your chest for an inhale. It's like your diaphragm muscle has to bench-press the weight of your stomach, liver, and other abdominal organs to expand your lungs. And when your spine is fully extended, as in a backbend, it's very difficult to move your rib cage outward to make that extra chest space for a little sip of air.

Putting the most challenging poses late in practice helps you develop an unwavering mental focus. And this underscores the reason that yoga is more than just a way to train your body. While your ability to do, say, Head Stand Pose will never help you get through a tough situation at home or at work, your ability to stay calm and focused is a great skill to have when life gets crazy.

Take comfort; it's not just you who sometimes has trouble maintaining control of your breathing during certain yoga poses. No matter how long someone has been practicing yoga, upside down poses (inversions) and back bends will always be the hardest ones to breathe in. Go slowly when you learn these poses. Take them one step at a time, and keep alert for the moment you lose touch with your breath and can't find it again. That's your signal to come out of the pose.

One day, you'll notice that you can follow your breath (Vinyasa) through an entire practice. You'll automatically inhale when you lift your body, and naturally exhale when you fold forward or press down. Moving with the rise and fall of your breath will begin to feel organic and natural. This takes time. Focus on building a safe, sustainable, regular practice and these skills will emerge. I promise. You'll see.

Ending poses help you release control of your breathing

At the end of every yoga practice, it's time to let go of this awareness of your breath, and let the act of breathing subside back down into your unconscious where it usually lives. If you've become very acutely aware of your breathing during practice, it might take a few minutes to separate your conscious awareness from your breath. That's where the ending poses come in for a few minutes of final rest.

Examples of ending practice poses:

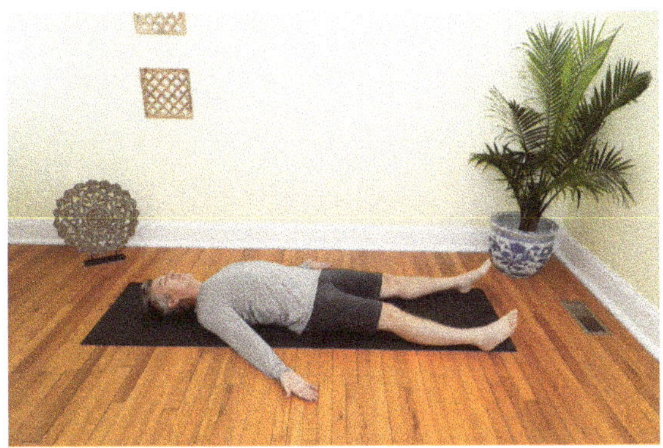

Corpse Pose

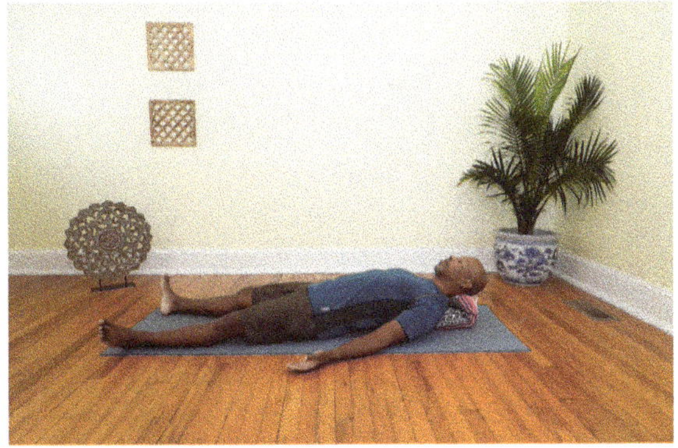

Corpse Pose, variation

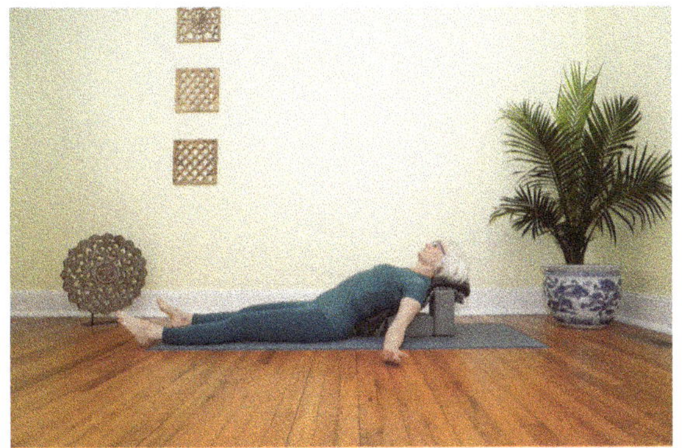

Corpse Pose, variation

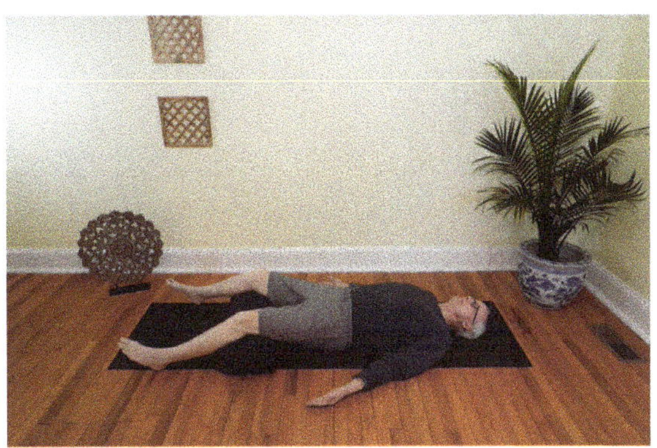

Corpse Pose, variation

Lie down in Corpse Pose (Savasana), and commit to being absolutely physically still. As with every yoga pose, there are many variations of Corpse Pose. Choose one that you can be comfortably still in for three to five minutes.

Close your eyes, and let go of the intense mental focus that you developed during practice. Here, in complete physical stillness, notice the deep effects of your yoga practice. How do your mind and body feel? Your mind may be more clear, more open, or less worried. Your thoughts may be moving more slowly and serenely. Many people experience a deep sense of calm and peace at the end of practice.

You may feel less anxious after practice because Vinyasa (moving consciously with deep breathing) can stimulate your brain to produce comforting, "feel-good" biochemicals called endorphins. Please know that it is not uncommon to get a little tearful in Savasana—especially if you've had some emotional challenges in your life lately. Don't worry. Tears are a normal response to releasing stress. Sometimes, just lying still in an environment where you feel safe, protected, and loved can bring up a few tears.

However you feel, don't fret. Just relax and rest for a few minutes. The world with all its troubles and joys is waiting right outside the door. Hopefully, you're a little more prepared to face them after doing your practice.

CHAPTER 3

LEGS

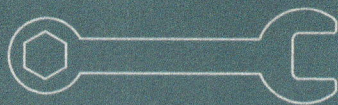

Okay, now let's get down to the physical nuts and bolts. In chapter 1, we looked at some of the key principles of a strong yoga practice, things you need to know whether you're just starting out or you're an old hand. In chapter 2, we explored the how awareness of your breathing is a fundamental yoga tool. The take home message: your yoga practice is about more than just doing the exercises. With that established, let's move from concepts and breath to muscles and bones.

Beginning in this chapter, we'll deepen your understanding of how to do yoga by exploring how your body actually works—how the components of your musculoskeletal system interact to move you in space. When you know why your bones and muscles move the way they do, you'll find it easier to develop a yoga practice that works best for your particular body. We'll start by taking a close look at the nuts and bolts—the anatomy that makes it all possible. Then we'll review how specific poses stretch and strengthen different parts of your body, starting with your feet and working our way up.

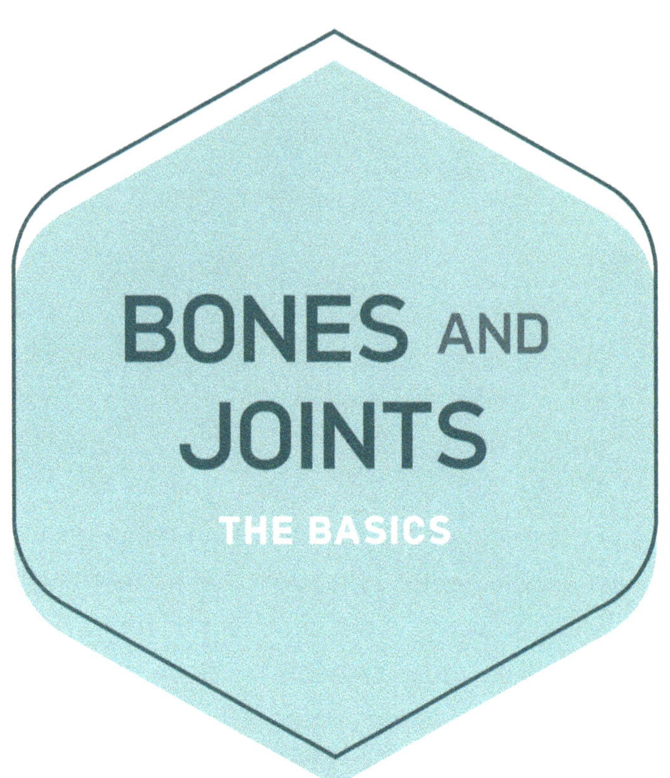

BONES AND JOINTS

THE BASICS

Since this is our first deep dive into anatomy, let's begin with a few important general points about your bones, joints, and muscles, and how they work together. These principles apply to your entire body, but we'll use your leg anatomy as examples here.

The shape of a bone reflects its function.

Blocky, square bones are built to handle impact and weight, while long, thinner bones are made to provide leverage and mobility. This difference is clear if you consider the bones of your feet. Your lower ankle bone (talus) sits between the bottom of your shin bone (your tibia) and your heel bone (calcaneus, see page 55). Your lower ankle and heel bones are thick and boxy because when you stand, walk, run, and jump, they're at the end of the chain of impact.

What this means for your yoga practice: It's OK to bear weight on the larger, thicker bones, but you must learn to use your muscles to lift weight off of the smaller bones. That's why it's important to gradually build up to doing poses like arm balances and headstands. Spend time doing the preparatory stages (called kramas) to be sure you have enough strength and body-awareness to protect small bones (like in your wrist and neck) during intense poses.

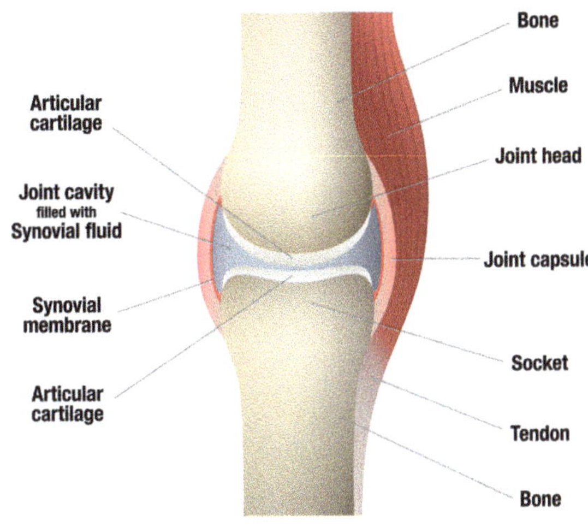

A synovial joint is enclosed in a fluid-filled capsule.

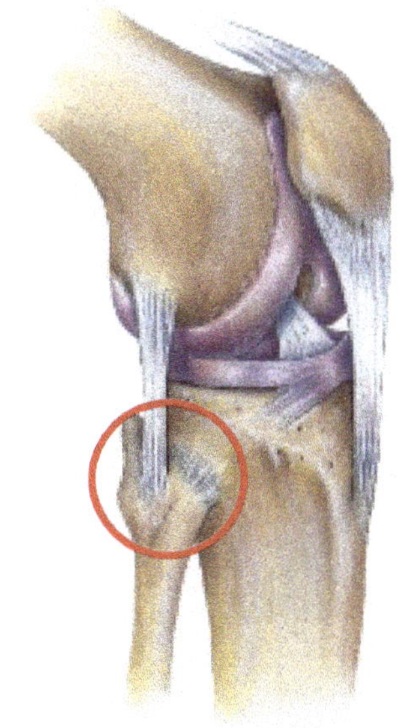

A cartilaginous joint connects the tibia and fibula.

Joints come in two types.

Joints connect the ends of two bones in a single mobile structure. The two main types are *synovial* joints and *cartilaginous* (or *fibrous*) joints. Your ankles, knees, and hips are some of the synovial joints in your legs. Each is sealed inside a joint capsule that's filled with synovial fluid (a mixture of water, sugars, and proteins). Synovial joints are lubricated and freely mobile within their normal range of motion, meaning they glide easily through a relatively wide range of movement. For example, your knee moves easily from being deeply bent to fully straight as you squat and stand back up.

By contrast, the joint where your shin bone (tibia) meets the smaller, secondary bone of your lower leg (your fibula) is a cartilaginous joint. These joints are not sealed inside a fluid-filled capsule. They're held together by ligaments (more about those later) and are designed for structural support, not for mobility. Most cartilaginous joints move only a few centimeters; they can slightly shift position to accommodate movements and forces at nearby synovial joints. Other examples include the pubic symphysis joining the front of your pelvis, the sacroiliac joints (SI joints) at the back of your pelvis, and the suture joints connecting the bones of your skull.

What it means for your yoga practice: Take care during practice not to make your cartilaginous joints too mobile. For example, you're at risk of overstretching your SI joints whenever you force your way into twists or forward folds using your arms and hands to "crank" your way in. Unfortunately this is such a common mistake that hypermobile SI joints have been called an "epidemic injury" in yoga.

Cartilage keeps things covered.

The ends of your bones, at both synovial and cartilaginous joints, are covered with a layer of cartilage to help cushion and lubricate joint movement. In other words, cartilage keeps bone from rubbing against bone. Cartilage is the only tissue in your body that is not fed by blood. So when it gets torn, worn down, or otherwise damaged, your cartilage cannot grow back like your muscle fibers can. Cartilage naturally thins with age, but take care not to wear it down faster with unnecessary wear and tear.

What it means for your yoga practice: It's important not to sag your weight down into your joints during your yoga sessions. The job of your muscles is to lift the weight and force of movement off of your joints. Practice using them. For example, in all standing and seated poses, use your waist and back muscles to lift your ribs away from your hips. As we discuss individual poses later in this chapter and throughout this book, you'll find lots of advice on how to recruit and use specific muscle groups to help protect your joints.

Your joints have a normal range of motion.

Each of your joints is designed to move in specific directions, to a particular extent or degree. This range of motion is limited by your *ligaments*, and the shape of your bones. Ligaments are tissues that connect bones to bones, and determine how far each joint can move in any direction. Ligaments act like straps that hold a joint in its correct alignment. Cartilaginous joints, which do not move much, are held together very tightly by ligaments. Also, a single joint can have multiple ligaments stabilizing it. Your knee, for example, has a very complex system of ligaments that prevent abnormal movements like rotation or sideways shearing.

Stretching your ligaments destabilizes your joints, and makes them prone to injury and abnormal wear and tear. Once they get stretched out and loose, ligaments cannot do their job of stabilizing your joint movements. And please understand, your ligaments do not tighten back up if you overstretch them. Ligaments have almost no blood supply, so they can't repair themselves to their pre-stretched state. This is reflected in anatomical drawings: muscles are colored red to indicate that they have good blood supply and are changeable. Ligaments are colored white, indicating that they have poor blood supply, and are mostly stabilizing structures. When your ligaments get too loose, the forces of weight and movement that act on a joint can easily damage the cartilage and bones.

What it means for your yoga practice: To lower the risk of overstretching your ligaments during practice, focus more on building strength and less on gaining flexibility. Enter poses slowly, pausing to engage each muscle group as you go. Use muscle groups throughout your whole body—from your feet to your fingertips. Once you're in a pose, as far into it as is safe for your body, focus on keeping your muscles engaged. Don't worry, flexibility will come. In fact, stretching an activated muscle (active, dynamic stretching) is the most effective way to stretch, and will give you better results faster than stretching a limp, passive muscle.

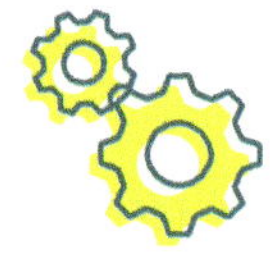

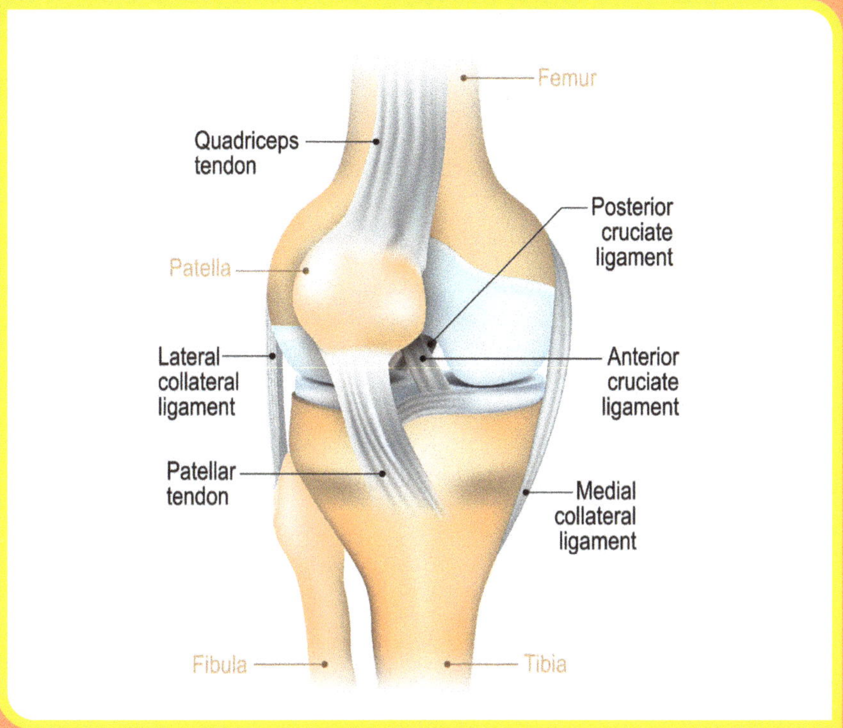

MECHANIC'S NOTE: The Ligaments Inside of Your Knee

Two ligaments cross your knee joint: the anterior cruciate ligament (ACL) in front, and the posterior cruciate ligament (PCL) in back. They form an X ("cruciate" means "cross-shaped") that prevents rotation of the knee joint, and keeps your thigh and shin bone (your femur and tibia) from sliding forward and backward over each other. You may know someone who tore their ACL or PCL while playing a sport like soccer, tennis, or football, where players change direction while running. In the heat of the game, players sometimes plant their weight on one foot and turn their hips and torso. The hip joint can handle this rotation, but the rotating forces can get transferred down into the knee, which is not designed for rotation. If the force is too great, the cruciate ligaments sprain, strain, or tear.

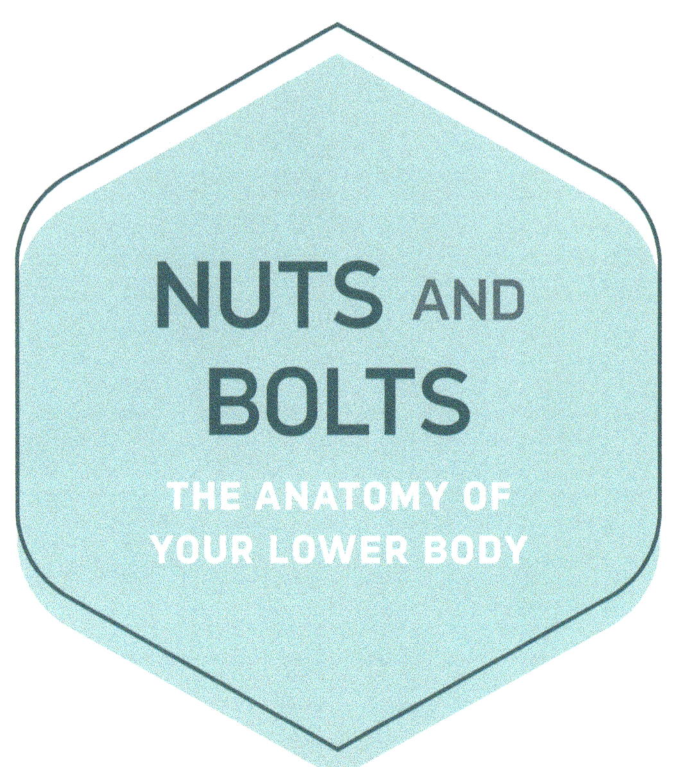
NUTS AND
BOLTS
THE ANATOMY OF
YOUR LOWER BODY

There's a reason that we're starting our anatomical survey from the ground up. Your feet, ankles, knees, and hips are—literally—the foundation of your yoga poses (aka asanas). This is pretty obvious in standing poses, where your legs are supporting the weight and movement of your body. But your leg muscles are also essential for doing seated poses, backbends, arm balances, and inversions safely and effectively. Recruiting the powerful muscles in your legs supports your lower back, and protects your joints from inappropriate force. Learning to use your leg muscles correctly in every pose is an important part of developing a sustainable, safe, and effective yoga practice.

And as a bonus, you'll find that using your legs correctly during your yoga sessions will help you with other physical activities as well. You'll build healthy habits that will support you during all sorts of movement, from to playing tennis to carrying groceries.

Bones and Joints

Before we get into how various poses stretch and strengthen the muscles of your lower body, you need to understand the bones and joints those muscles are attached to. After all, it's the bones and joints that do the movements. When you understand how your lower body's skeleton is put together, it's much easier to figure out why certain poses are easy or difficult for you, and how to start making progress in your practice.

Your feet

The bones of your feet may be small, but they have to be sturdy enough to withstand the force of your entire body weight landing on them with every step you take. So a combination of hinge and gliding joints between the small bones in your feet work together, distributing and directing weight to move your body in a particular direction. When your heel strikes the ground, the impact is transferred forward into the mid-foot and arch, where a series of smaller, cube-shaped bones (your cuneiforms) distribute the force into the ball of your foot (your metatarsals). Finally, the long lever-bones in your toes (your phalanges) propel you forward. Notice how far your heel bone (calcaneus) extends behind your ankle joint. That's because your feet are designed to function like the rockers on a rocking chair, with the most force striking your heel, shifting forward to your arch, and, finally, pushing off from your toes.

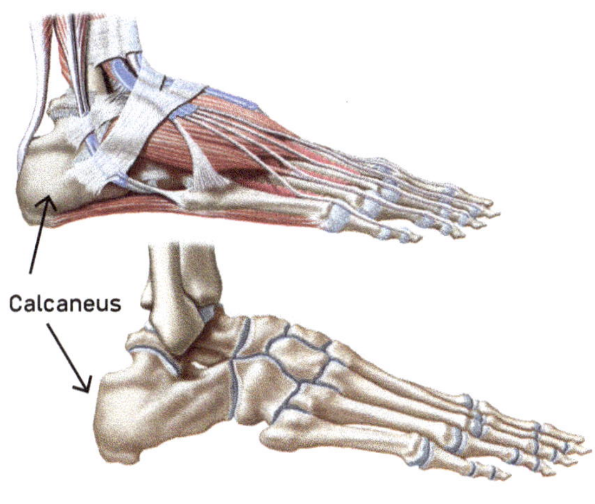

The bones of your foot and ankle

Your ankles

The ankle is a hinge joint, which means that it moves like the hinge on a door: forward and back in one plane. Your ankle does not rotate. It can't, because of the two bones in your lower leg: your shin bone (your tibia) and a smaller, lower-leg bone that runs parallel to it (your fibula). They extend down each side of your ankle bone (talus), capturing it like an open-ended wrench around a nut. Look at your ankle. The two bumps you see on the sides of your ankles are the ends of those two separate lower-leg bones: your tibia on the inside and your fibula on the outside.

I know that some yoga instructors ask students to rotate or circle their ankles, but anatomically speaking that's not possible. It certainly *looks* like you can rotate your ankles. What's really happening is that your ankle joint is nodding up and down, while the smaller bones of your mid-foot (your cuneiforms) are sliding past one another to create a circling movement in your mid-foot. So, technically speaking, you're circling your feet.

Your knees

The knee joint is where your shin bone (tibia) connects to your thigh bone (femur). The smaller fibula connects to your outer shin just below your knee joint. Your knees are hinge joints, like your ankles, and do not rotate. This is important to know for keeping your knee joints healthy during your yoga practice: Always avoid putting any rotational force on your knees.

Your hips

The top of each thigh bone (femur) has an angled neck and a big, ball-shaped head. This ball sits inside a deep, cave-like socket in your pelvis, forming your hip joint. Unlike the hinge joints at your knees and ankles, your hip is a ball-and-socket joint. This allows it to rotate

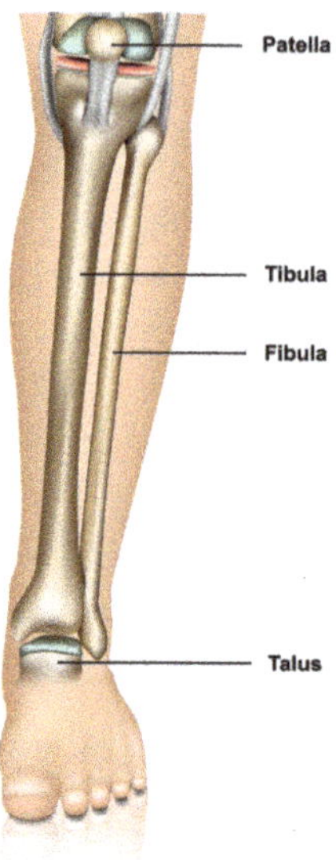

Your knee joint and lower leg bones

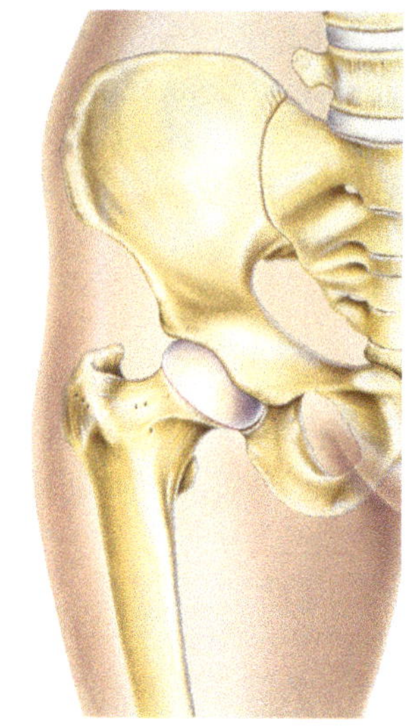

Your hip joint

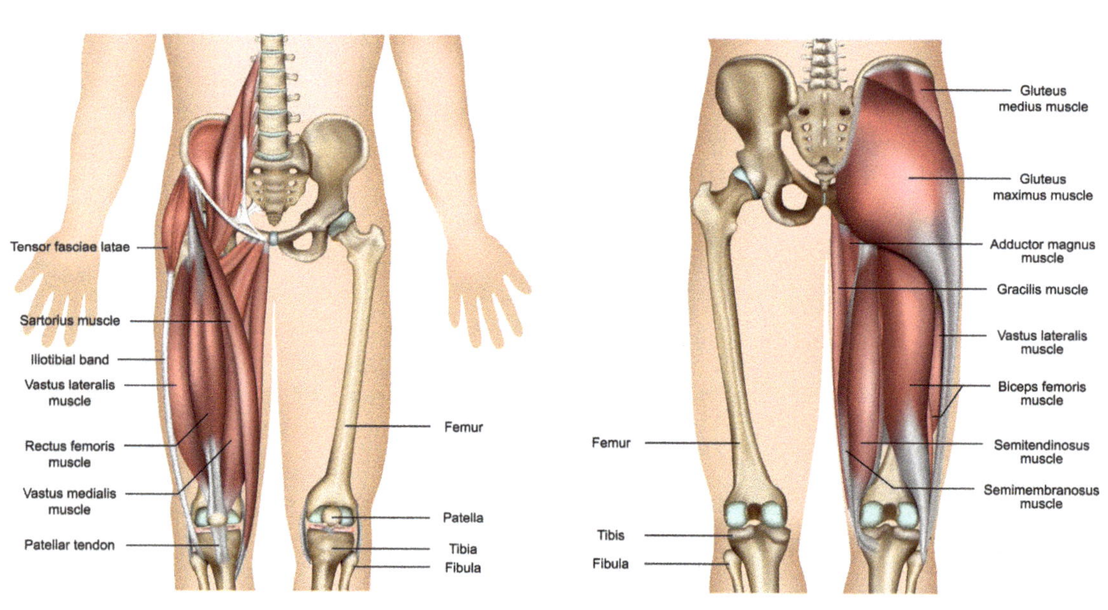

Bones and muscles of the upper legs

both outward (external rotation, i.e. turning away from the center of your body) and inward (internal rotation, i.e. turning toward the center of your body).

I've noticed that many yoga instructors are very diligent about teaching poses focused on outward hip rotation, but say little about the importance of optimal inward hip rotation. As a result, it's common to see yoga students who've developed a lot of outward rotation but have limited internal rotation. This can create muscular imbalances in the hip flexor muscles, glutes (your butt), and low back muscles. What happens is, the muscles that turn the hip outward become much stronger than the ones that turn it inward. This puts uneven tension on the joint, so that it no longer rests in a neutral, centered position. This can cause uneven stress and wear, leading to problems in the ligaments, tendons, and cartilage that support the hip joint.

Everyone has their own unique collection of muscular imbalances from a lifetime of body habits. We tend to stand on one foot more than the other, reach and lift with our dominant hand, hold our shoulders forward or back. In yoga, doing a pose with one side of the body may feel radically different than engaging the other side. That's just your own muscular imbalances coming into play. Work on your "hard side" a little more than your "easy side" and move all of your joints through their full range of motion in every class.

Muscles

Muscles are the workhorses of your body. All of your muscles are attached to your bones, contracting and releasing as needed to move your joints. It's their job to protect your bones and joints from the forces of weight and movement. When muscles get too weak, more weight sags down into your joints, causing more wear-and-tear.

MECHANIC'S NOTE: INJURY PREVENTION PRINCIPLES

Protect your joints in yoga by focusing on stretching and strengthening your muscles rather than straining to reach a pose your body isn't ready for. Keep these principles in mind:

Use correct alignment. That means you must keep your weight in the centers of your bones and joints during movement and stillness.

Don't force your way into poses that require more strength or flexibility than you have. Be patient. Be mindful.

Always remember, yoga should be healing, not harmful. Learn to distinguish between the safe discomfort and tiredness of muscular work, and the dangerous sharp pain of muscular injury.

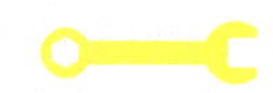

It's important to understand that your muscles work in opposing groups, and react to what their partner groups are doing. For example, when your biceps contract, your triceps release. When muscles in front of your neck pull your chin down, muscles on the back of your neck relax and extend.

Your lower legs

The main muscles of your legs below the knee are your shins (anterior tibialis), outer calves (peroneus longus and peroneus brevis), and calves (gastrocnemius or gastroc, and soleus). Several other smaller muscles, tendons, and ligaments support the bones and joints of your ankles and feet. Wearing shoes all day can weaken these lower leg muscles and affect how you walk. For example, when your front shin muscle gets weak, you start skimming your toes over the floor (a phenomenon called toe drop, or toe drag), instead of flexing at the ankle to lift your forefoot. This walking pattern makes you much more likely to trip and fall. Yoga is done barefoot, which helps strengthen your lower leg muscles and sharpen the nerve signaling between your soles and your brain. In yoga you also flex and point your feet in various poses, and learn to grip the floor for balance, all of which strengthens your lower leg muscles.

Your thighs

The primary muscle group in your thighs is called the quadriceps. Your quads consist of four muscles: rectus femoris, vastus lateralis, vastus medialis, and vastus intermedius. Your central quadricep (rectus femoris) is what we call a *poly-articulated* muscle, because it crosses more than one joint. The upper tendon attaches it to the top of your pelvis. The muscle then crosses your hip joint and fills out the middle of your thigh, before the lower tendon attaches on the front of your shin bone. So your central thigh muscle crosses over both your hip and knee joints. Your quads are one of the biggest,

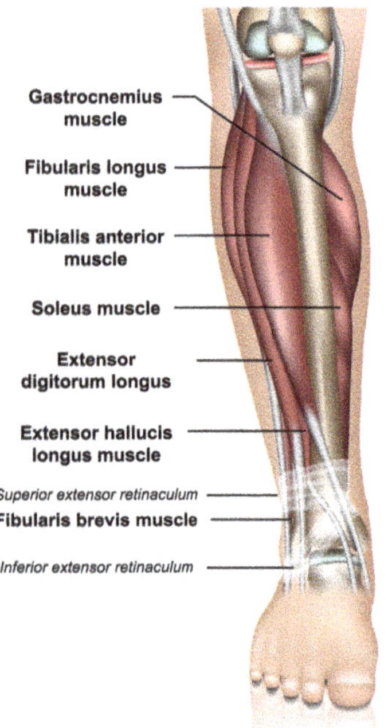

Muscles of the lower leg

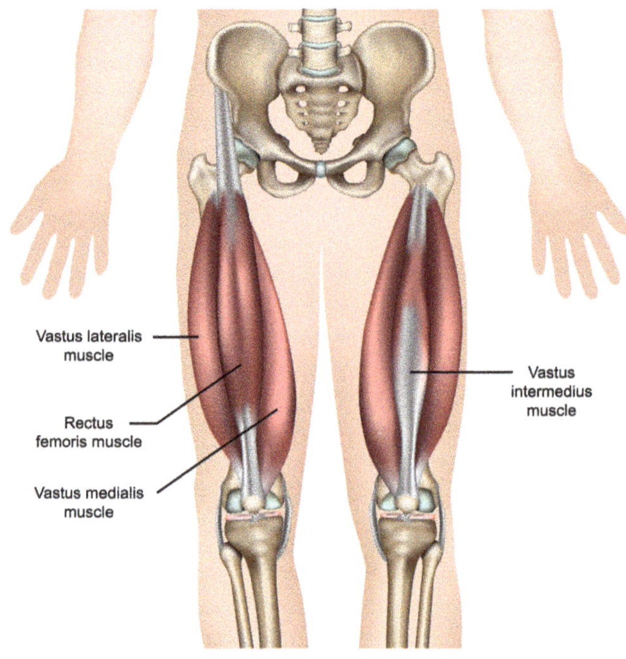

Four muscles make up your quadriceps

strongest muscle groups in your entire body.

When stretching your thigh muscles, bending your knee and pressing your pelvis slightly forward will increase the stretch intensity. Many poses call for these actions, including all back bends such as King Dancer Pose (Natarajansana), Bow Pose (Dhanurasana), Bridge Pose (Setu Bandhasana), Wheel Pose (Urdhva Dhanurasana), and One-Legged, King Pigeon Pose (Eka Pada Rajakapotasana). Most yoga poses that stretch and strengthen your quads will also stretch and strengthen your hip flexors.

Your hips

All of the largest muscle groups in your body attach to your pelvis, and are involved in moving and stabilizing multiple joints. Tightness or weakness in any of these large muscle groups affects both the stability and movement of your hips, but also your legs, low back, and torso.

While the main job of your quadriceps is to handle weight and the forces of impact, your hip flexors' main job is to lift your thigh bone up (like when you're walking). You can locate your hip flexors (ilio-psoas major and minor, and illiacus) by digging your fingertips into the front of each hip joint at your hip creases. To find your hip creases, sit in a chair; your hip crease is the bend-line where your thighs go forward and your torso goes upward. Now, stand up, press your fingertips firmly into your hip creases, and lift one foot off the floor. The muscle that pops up under your fingers is your main hip flexor. Your hip flexors are at work every time you lift your foot, pulling your thigh bone (femur) upwards. Your main hip flexor (ilio-psoas major) is attached to your spine at your lower back (your lumbar spine). From there, it passes through your abdomen, runs along the inner pelvis, and then attaches to the top of your thigh bone.

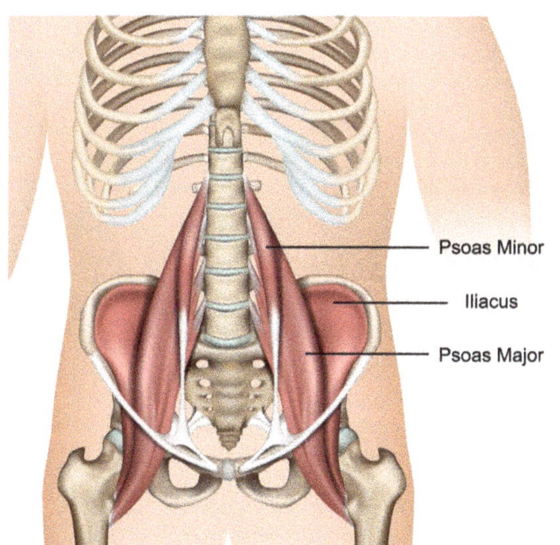

Your hip flexors lift your thigh bones for walking.

Spending a lot of time sitting can lead to tight, weak hip flexors. Because they originate on your low back, tight hip flexors pull your spine slightly forward each time you lift your foot. So tight hip flexors can cause low back pain by constantly tugging your lumbar vertebrae forward, out of alignment and causing abnormal movement of the vertebrae that make up your lower spine. A lot of people have low back pain that's either caused or aggravated by tight hip flexors. So stretching your hip flexors is an important and effective tool to help relieve low back pain. As with any body work, you should stretch and strengthen your hip flexors gradually.

Always stretch and strengthen your muscles gradually. Forcing change before your body is ready causes injuries. Forcing any muscle to stretch or strengthen too quickly can create irritation rather than relief. Patience!

Your hamstrings

A group of three muscles on the back of your thigh, your hamstrings (semi-tendinosus, semi-membranosus, and biceps femoris) work in opposition to your quadriceps; they pull your femur backwards. All three hamstrings connect to the same place on your sitting bones, a spot called the ischeal tuberosity. This is important because forcing a hamstring stretch (for example, in a seated forward fold) can injure all three of your hamstrings where they attach. This type of injury can take months, and even years, to heal. During yoga practice, we tend to overuse and over-stretch the middle hamstring (biceps femoris). The moral of this story: be mindful when stretching your hamstrings.

Slowly stretching and strengthening your hamstrings provides one of the great benefits of doing yoga poses (asanas). A lot of people have weak, tight hamstrings from spending so much time sitting—in chairs, in cars, on the sofa. This contributes to problems like low back pain because your hamstrings attach directly to your pelvis (on your sitting bones). Tight hamstrings can pull the back of your pelvis down, flattening out the natural forward curve in your low back that's meant to act like a shock-absorber. Without it, your low back muscles are at risk for strains and sprains. In addition, without its natural shock-absorbing curve and spring-like action, the forces of impact can gradually damage the cartilage, discs, and other structures in your low back.

Many yoga poses help restore the strength and flexibility of your hamstrings, but you must be patient and change them slowly. Remember, it took years to develop tight, weak hamstrings. Safely stretching and strengthening them can be a long, slow journey. Take it easy.

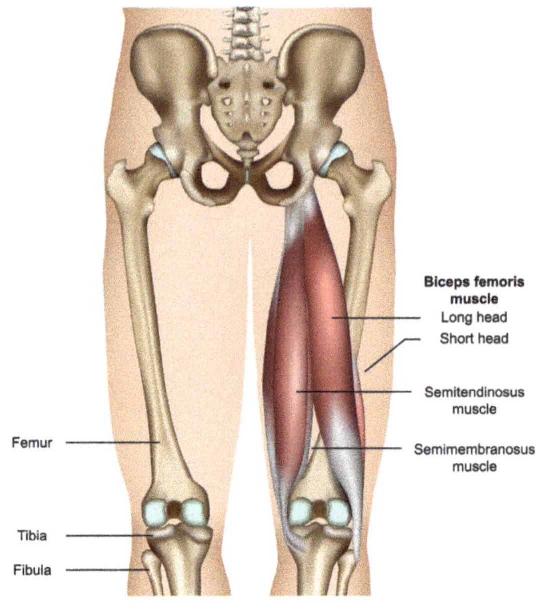

Tight hamstrings can pull on the pelvis and create low back pain.

It's important to understand that your pelvic- and shoulder-girdles are copy-cats. When tight hamstrings cause your pelvis to tuck slightly under, your shoulders will copy that action by rounding or slumping forward, which leads to shoulder and neck problems as well as back pain. So pay close attention to your shoulder alignment while you stretch your hamstrings. Many people round their shoulders forward during a hamstring stretch. This is counter-productive, and won't work very well. When your shoulders hunch forward, your pelvis tucks under and releases the hamstring stretch. It's true!

Your glutes

A group of three muscles covers the back and sides of your pelvis: gluteus maximus, gluteus medius, and gluteus minimus. They handle weight-bearing and stability for the pelvis.

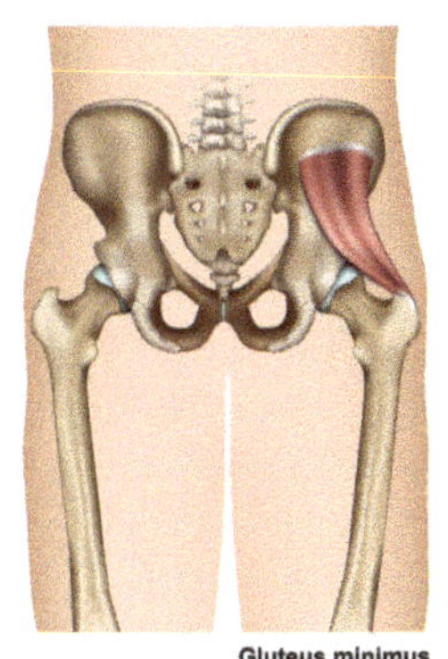

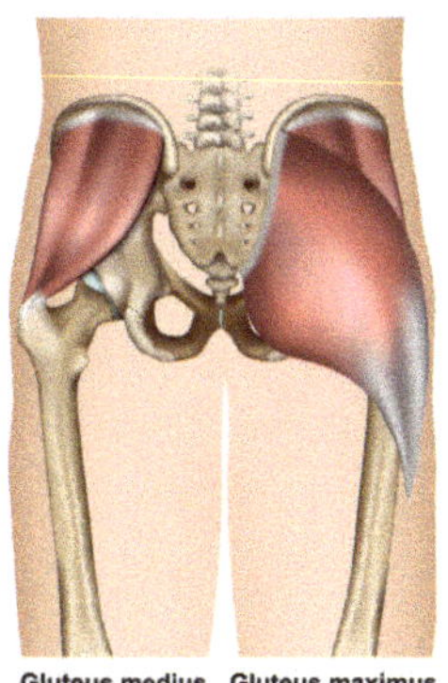

Three muscles make up your gluteals, or glutes.

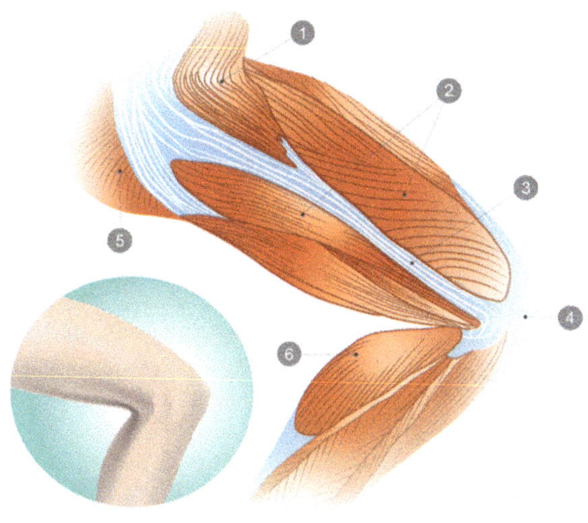

The IT band stabilizes the hip and knee joints.

It may not surprise you to learn that your main glute, gluteus maximus, is the largest muscle in the human body. Interestingly, chronic emotional tension (anxiety, stress, or unexpressed anger) creates certain muscular patterns. Many people who live with a lot of daily stress, habitually clench their jaws, grind their teeth, or squeeze their glutes. These patterns, in turn, often cause other problems. In the case of squeezing your glutes, this action rotates your thigh bones outward, which pushes the two halves of your pelvis in toward your sacrum (the bone at the base of your spine). This constant pressure can cause low back pain, and/or hinder the normal full range of motion in your low back and hip joints.

By contrast, if you spend a lot of time sitting, you can develop weak glutes that cause different mobility problems. Weak glutes make normal, everyday actions–like standing up from a chair or climbing stairs–difficult. Developing a sustainable, effective yoga practice is a great way to stretch and strengthen your gluteal muscles.

Ilio-Tibial Band

Your glutes, and a small muscle at the front of your outer hip called tensor fasciae latae or TFL, attach to a structure called the IT band (for ilio-tibial band). That's a strip of connective tissue which runs from your outer hip, down your outer thigh, to the top of your shin bone (tibia). Your IT band stabilizes your hip and knee joints during weight bearing and rapid movement. This dense strap of connective tissue (fascia) becomes less effective when the muscles that tie into it (your glutes and TFL) are weak or tight. While you don't want to overstretch your IT band (its job is to stabilize your hip and knee), you do want to make sure it's flexible enough to let your knee and hip joints move normally—that is, in their full normal ranges.

Yoga poses that pull your thigh bone across the center of your torso are effective for stretching your glutes, TFL, and IT band. That said, approach these so-called "hip-opening poses" carefully, and with patience. Do not push or force your body.

Groin

You have a group of five groin muscles (your adductors: adductor magnus, adductor longus, adductor brevis, pectineus, and gracilis) that attach to your upper inner pelvis and the tops of your thigh bones. These need to be stretched

MECHANIC'S NOTE: KNOW WHICH WAY TO GO

It's good to understand what "extension" and "flexion" mean anatomically, since we use these terms to describe various body movements. First, you have to locate the center of your body. Think of your navel as your center spot, and an imaginary vertical line running through it from head to toe as your centerline. Extension refers to moving part of the body away from those centers, and flexion refers to moving toward them. For example, tipping your chin up to look at the ceiling puts your neck into extension; dropping your chin toward your chest to look down, puts your neck into flexion. Back bends extend your spine, while forward folds flex it. Bending your legs into a squat flexes your knees, ankles, and hips.

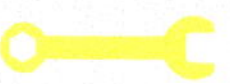

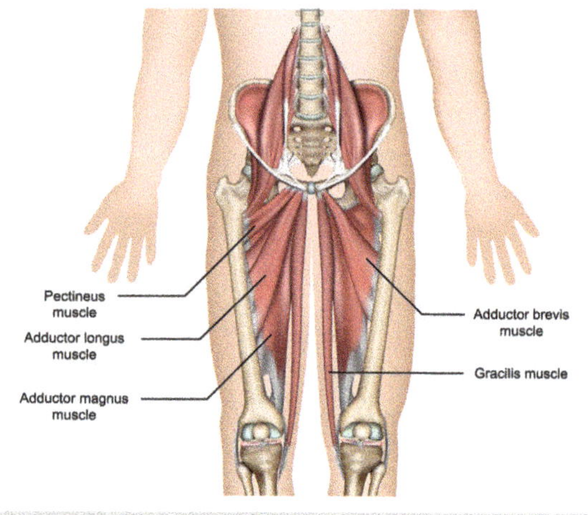

Your groin muscles

and strengthened along with your glutes. Your groin muscles primarily stabilize your pelvis, and draw your thigh bones inward, toward each other. Generally speaking, standing poses that place your feet wide apart and seated poses that turn your thigh bones (femurs) outward will effectively stretch some or all of your groin muscles.

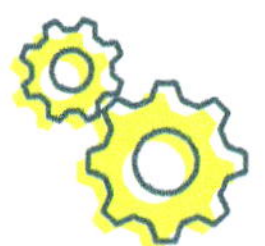

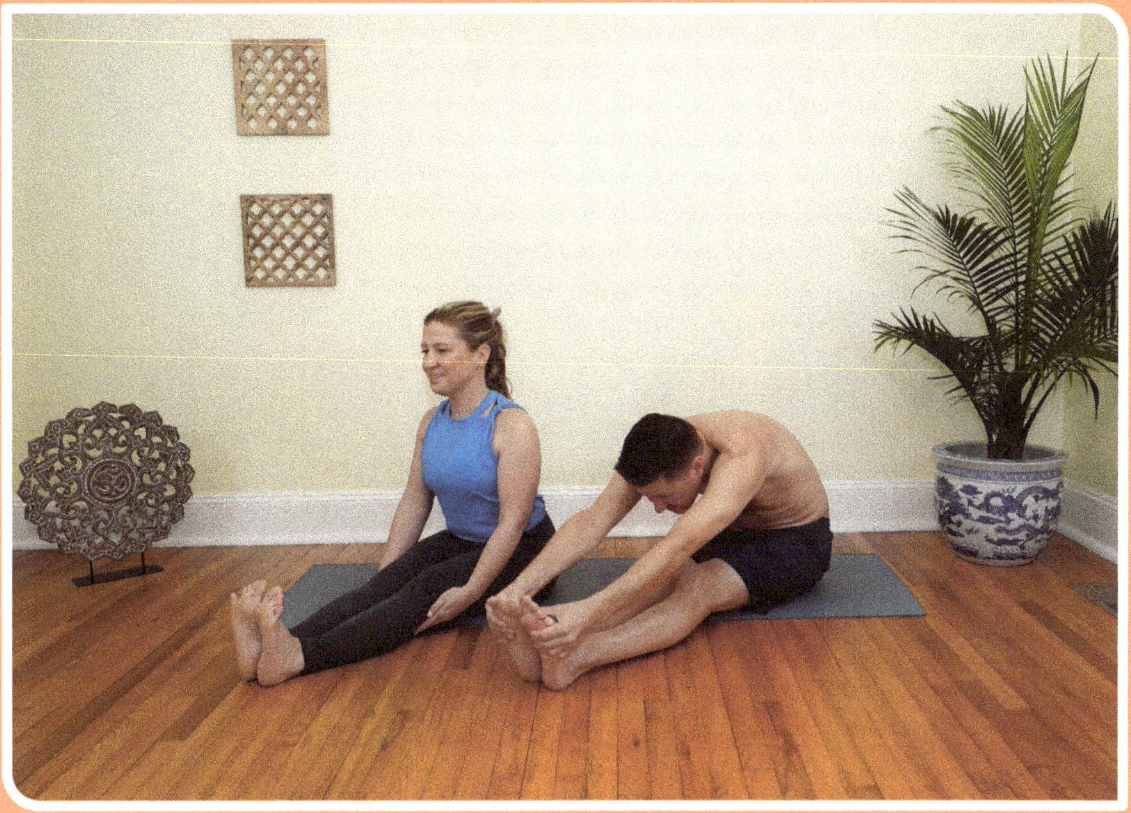

Seated Forward Fold, correct alignment at left. Don't round your shoulders.

MECHANIC'S NOTE: Don't be a downer!

When doing forward-folding poses, like the seated forward fold shown here, don't mistakenly focus on reaching forward to grab hold of your legs or feet to pull yourself down with your arms. Instead, focus on reaching your chest toward your feet. Pulling with your arms is a terrible way to stretch your hamstrings, and an excellent way to injure your back. Rounding your shoulders to grab for your feet also reinforces the slouchy posture that you're trying to avoid by doing yoga in the first place. Don't be a downer; there are lots of forward folding poses in yoga, but there are no downward folds.

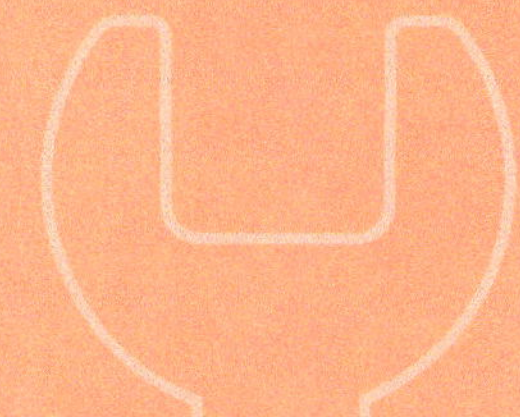

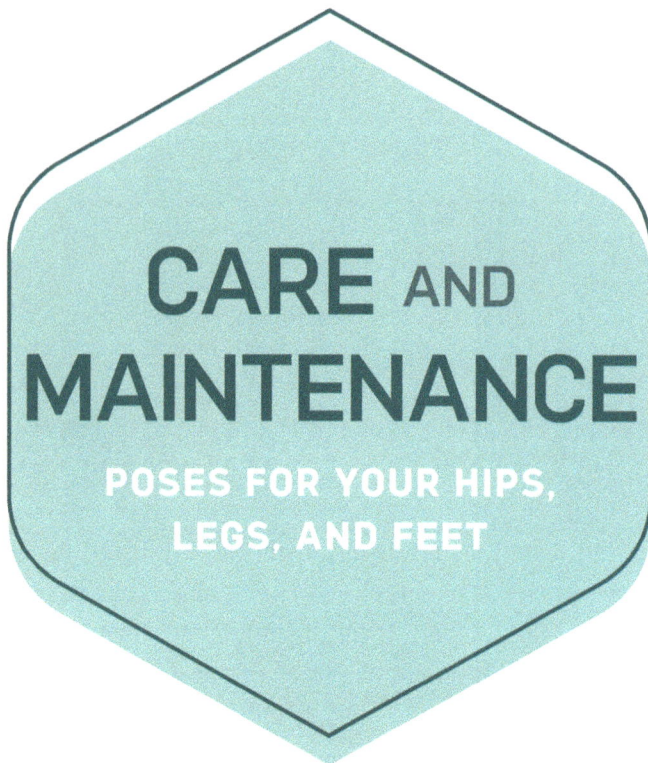

CARE AND MAINTENANCE

POSES FOR YOUR HIPS, LEGS, AND FEET

Now that you have a thorough grounding in how your lower body is put together, let's put those bones, muscles, and joints to work. In this section we'll tune up your practice as we explore a wide variety of poses that stretch and strengthen the muscles of the lower leg. Some of these asanas are physically demanding, while others are not so challenging. No matter what your level of strength and flexibility may be, there are lots of variations of every pose that will help you get the benefits of the position while avoiding injury.

Please understand that yoga poses are complex, so one pose affects multiple muscle groups—stretching some while strengthening others. For this reason, you'll see that a few poses are repeated in different sections of this book. For example, Warrior I stretches the calf muscles on the back leg, and strengthens the quads on the front leg. We'll look at those actions separately, in two different places.

As you work your way through the next chapters, I encourage you to try some new variations of poses you already feel very familiar with. Who knows, maybe you'll find a different sensation you've not felt before. Remember, you have to go down a new path to arrive at a new destination.

Thunderbolt Pose

ALSO CALLED: Diamond Pose, Vajrasana

WHAT IT DOES FOR YOUR LOWER LEGS: Brings your ankles into full extension and your knees into full flexion. Classes often begin with a seated pose like this one to help you get calm and focused.

TUNE IT UP: Place your hands flat on your thighs and lift your chest. Don't slouch. Breathe deeply.

If you have tight muscles in your lower legs, or restricted knee flexion, sitting on a block or two can relieve the intensity of this pose.

If your ankle extension is restricted, roll up a blanket and tuck it under the fronts of your ankles, so they're lifted higher than your toes (not shown).

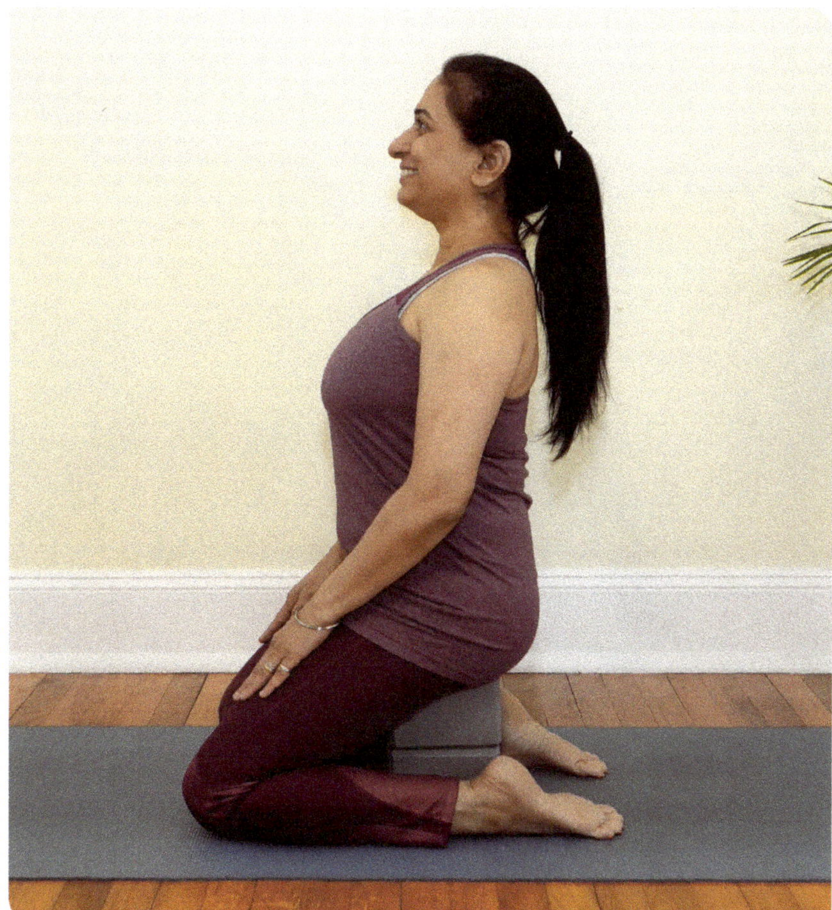

Thunderbolt Pose, variation

Downward Facing Dog Pose

ALSO CALLED: Adho Mukha Svanasana

WHAT IT DOES FOR YOUR LOWER LEGS: This well-known yoga pose is a great stretch for the backs of your lower legs (hamstrings, gastroc, soleus, Achilles tendon) and the soles of your feet. This pose is typically done early in class, and repeated during Sun Salutations (Surya Namaskar), and between sequences of poses.

TUNE IT UP: To increase the stretch for your lower legs and feet, firm up your thigh muscles and press down with your heels. Look back and notice if your feet are turned slightly in or out, or if one foot is turned differently than the other. If so, congratulations! You've found a muscular imbalance you can start fixing. Line your heels up directly behind your ankles (you should not be able to see your heels when you look back). Then lift the arches of your feet a little and press evenly on the big toe and pinky toe sides of your feet. Be aware, these small adjustments might make a big difference in the stretching sensation you feel in your feet and lower legs.

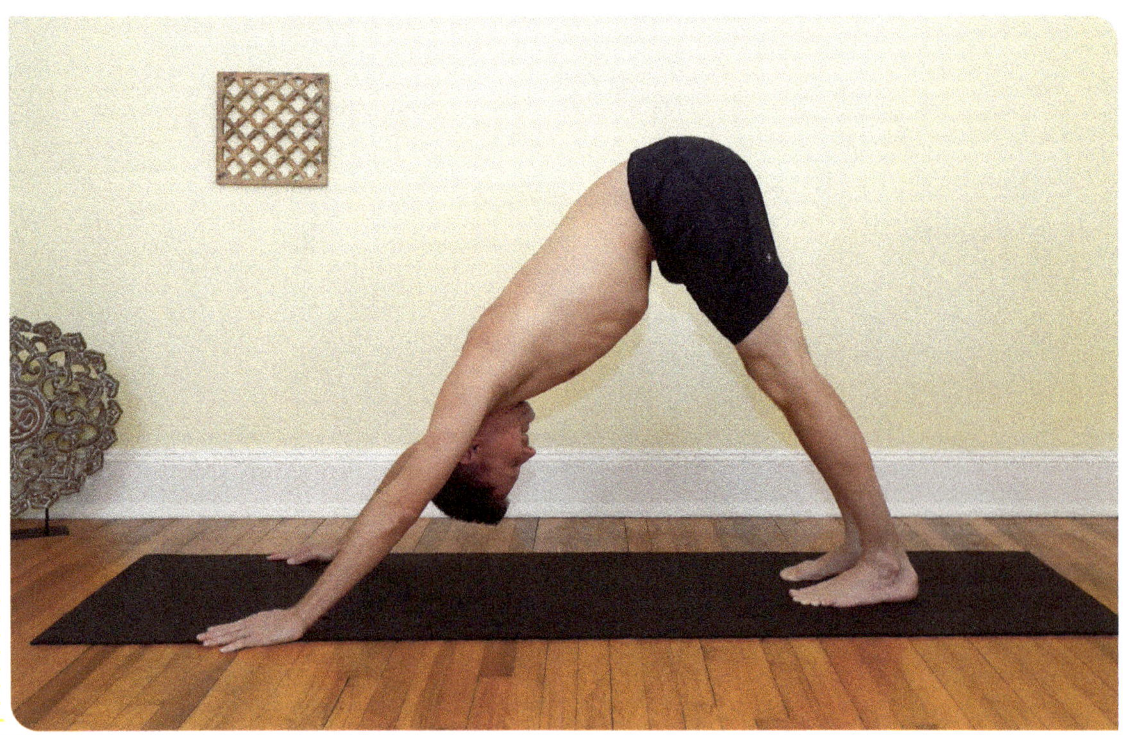

Downward Facing Dog Pose

Three Limbed, One Footed, Seated Forward Fold Pose

ALSO CALLED: Triang Mukhaikapada Paschimottanasana

WHAT IT DOES FOR YOUR LOWER LEGS: Stretches your shin muscle (tibialis anterior) and extends your ankle, and flexes your knee on the bent-leg side, while also stretching the muscles on the back of the straight leg (hamstrings, gastroc, soleus, and achilles tendon).

TUNE IT UP: If you have limited knee mobility or tight muscles on the bent-leg shin, sit up on a block or bolster, and don't reach far forward (see photo).

Raising your hips on a block and keeping your torso upright will help protect your knee joint from rotational force and excess pressure.

In all variations, keep drawing your shoulders up away from the floor. Do not round your back in order to hold your foot. Only hold your foot if it comes relatively easily into your hands.

Sitting up on a block and resisting the urge to grab at your foot will bring you great benefits without risking injury. In this and all forward folds, focus on strengthening your core abdominal muscles and keeping your spine straight. Bend at the hip creases; do not round your back and shoulders to grab for your foot.

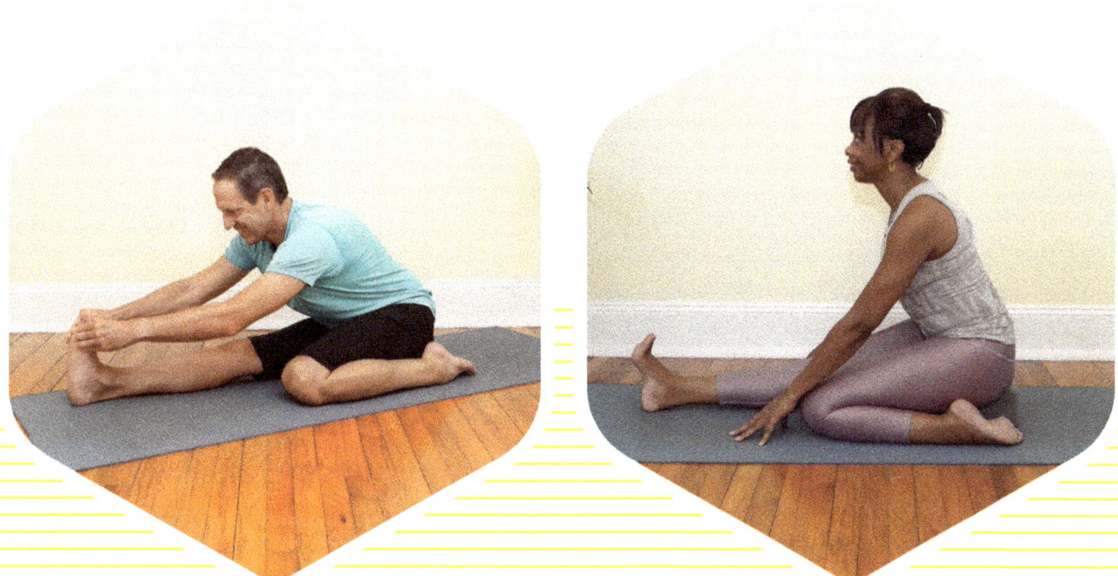

Three Limbed, One Footed, Seated Forward Fold

Variation with block

Warrior One Pose

ALSO CALLED: Virabhadrasana One

WHAT IT DOES FOR YOUR LOWER LEGS: This is a good stretch for the outer shin (peroneus longus and peroneus brevis) and calf (gastroc, soleus, and achilles tendon) of the back leg. Besides what it does for the lower legs, it also stretches your thigh and hip flexor muscles on the back leg.

TUNE IT UP: Be patient with this pose. Many people have challenges straightening the back leg and turning that hip forward due to tight or weak thigh muscles (quadriceps) and hip flexors. It will come, just keep trying. As your lower leg muscles, hip flexors, and thigh muscles become more flexible, your back leg will straighten more, and your back hip will turn further forward. Turning further forward, in turn, increases the stretch on your outer calf and ankle on the back leg. It's a process.

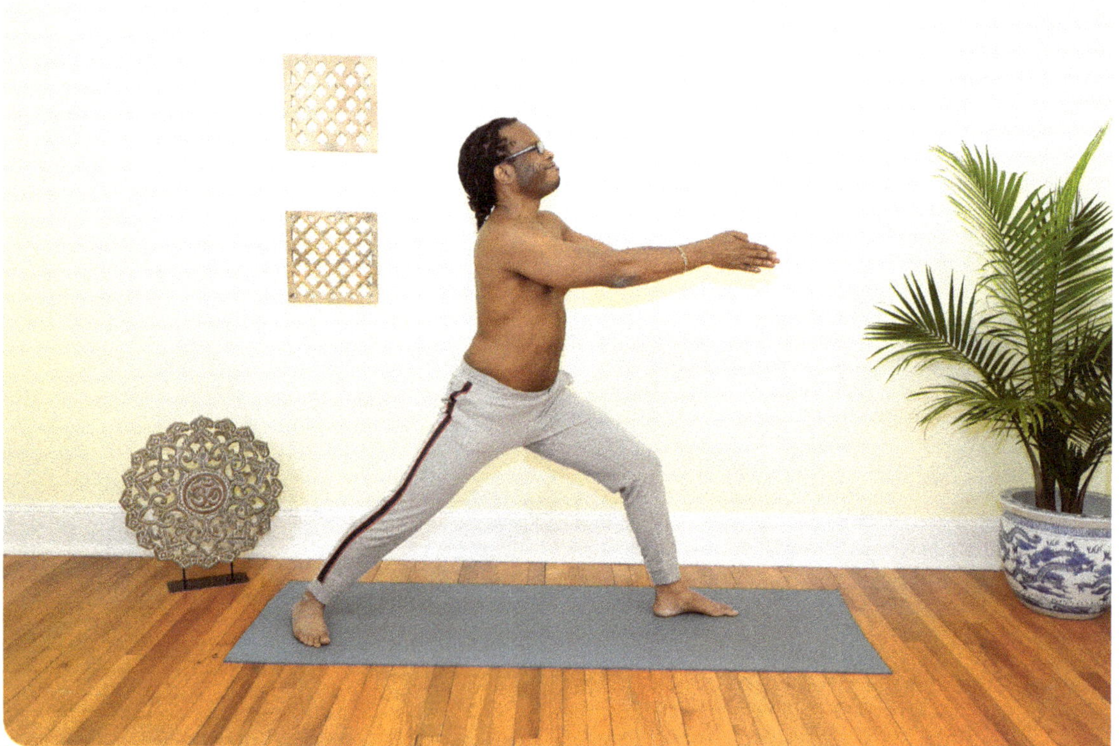

Warrior One, variation with arms forward

Reclined Hero Pose

ALSO CALLED: Supta Virasana

WHAT IT DOES FOR YOUR LOWER LEGS: This is an intense stretch for the tops of the feet, ankles, and shin muscles (as well as the thighs and hip flexors). It's intense for the lower legs because your ankles are in full extension and your knees are in full flexion. Although your feet are outside your hips (not under them), your body weight is still pressing the fronts of your ankles down.

TUNE IT UP: It's common for your knees to pop up off the floor when you start doing this pose; that's OK, as long as your knees stay about hip distance apart and do not move out much wider than your hips.

If you can't keep your knees pointing forward (on or off the floor), raise yourself up onto your elbows, or sit on a block with your hands on a bolster or folded blanket behind you. (See Reclined Hero Pose, variation with block and blanket, page 81.)

It's very important to keep your knees pointing forward, in line with your hips, to protect your knee and low-back joints. Focus on reaching your knee-caps down toward the floor and drawing your shoulder blades together. Don't worry about lying all the way back. Draw your knees toward each other and press them down toward the floor.

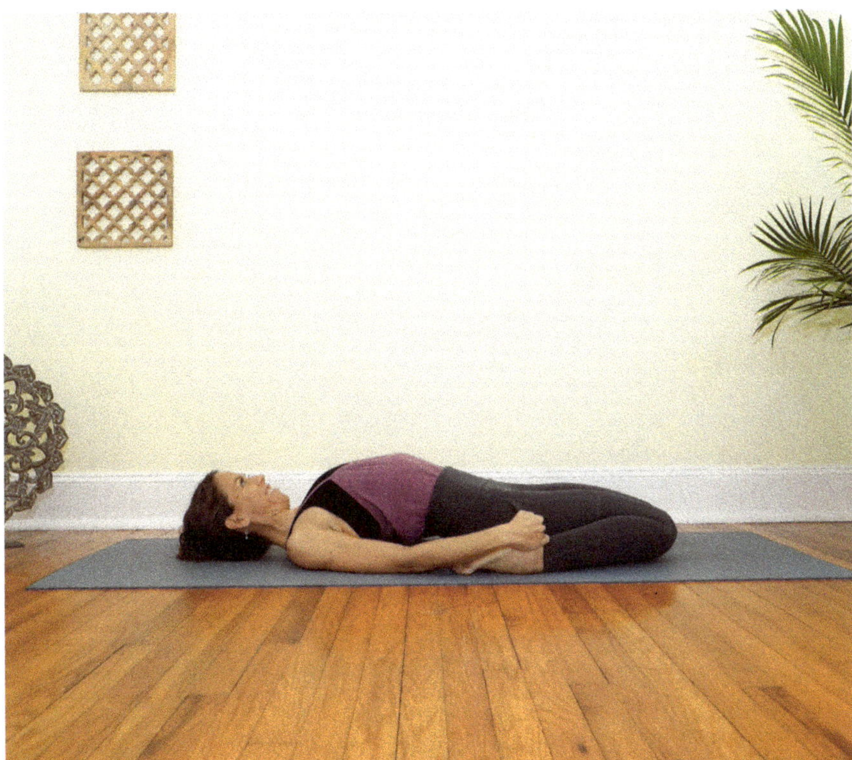

Reclined Hero Pose

Head of Knee Pose, B and C

ALSO CALLED: Janu Sirsansana B and C

WHAT IT DOES FOR YOUR LOWER LEGS (HEAD OF KNEE POSE B): The ankle on the bent-knee side is in full extension while your knee is in full flexion. This is an intense stretch for the top of the ankle and foot of the bent leg, because you're sitting on them. Compared to Janu Sirsansana C, it's also a more intense stretch for the calf muscles and hamstrings on the straight leg, because your hips are raised up off the floor.

WHAT IT DOES FOR YOUR LOWER LEGS (HEAD OF KNEE POSE C): Your ankle, toes, and knee on the bent-knee side are in full flexion. This an intense stretch for the sole of your foot (your plantar fascia), as well as your thigh and groin muscles (your quadriceps and adductors), on the bent leg. It also stretches the hamstrings on the back of the straight leg.

TUNE IT UP: Do not do these poses if they cause pain in the bent knee. Instead, do Janu Sirsasana A, with the foot on the bent-knee side placed flat against the inner thigh of the straight leg. Do not force these poses! Only bend your knee as much as the joint allows without pain.

Approach learning these poses with humility. It's very easy to introduce rotation into the knee joint and injure it when first trying them.

In Janu Sirsasana C, do not tuck your toes so far that you feel pain in the ankle or bent knee. Discomfort in the sole of the tucked foot is normal, but it should not be painful.

These poses take many years of slow, incremental practice. Spend several months sitting fairly upright before trying to fold far forward. Be humble. It's not worth getting injured.

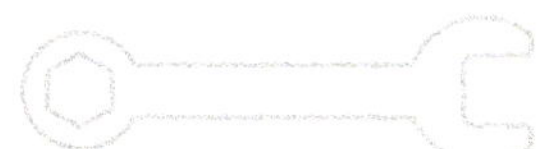

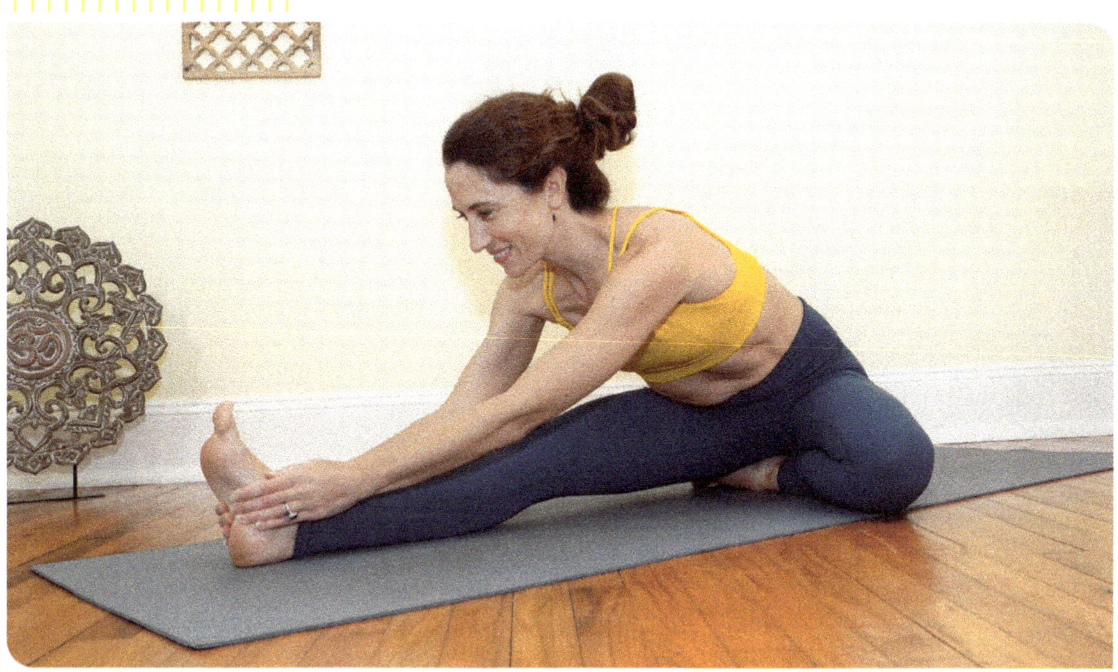

Head of Knee Pose Variation B

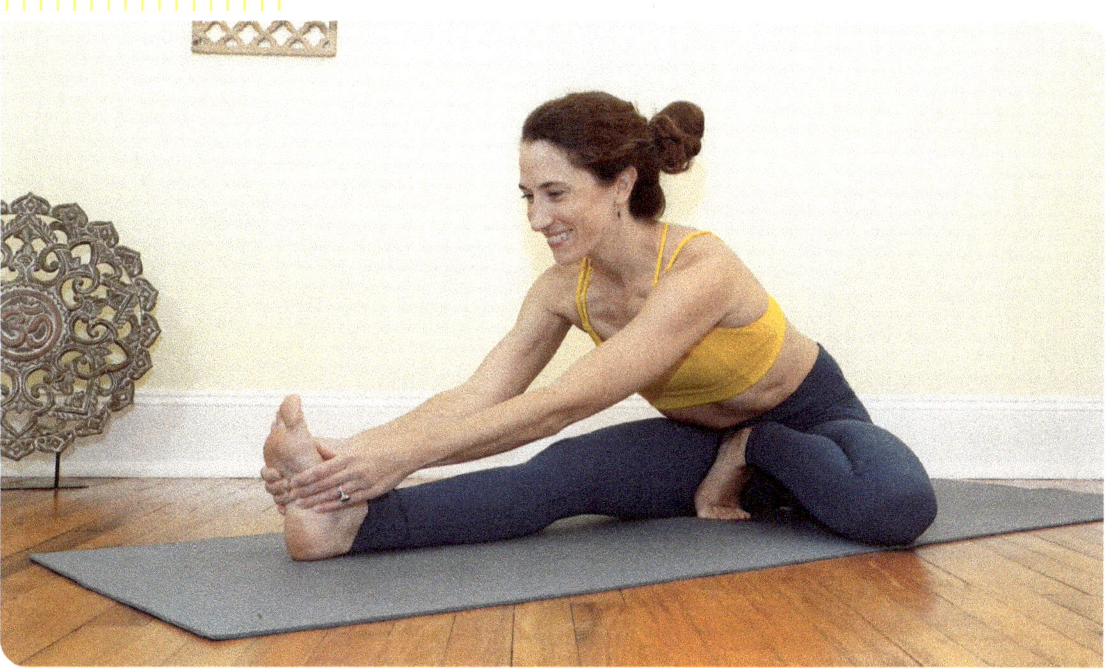

Head of Knee Pose Variation C

Garland Pose

ALSO CALLED: Malasana

WHAT IT DOES FOR YOUR LOWER LEGS: Strengthens the muscles on the fronts of your shins (tibialis anterior) and outer calves (peroneus longus and peroneus brevis). Your knees and ankles are in full flexion.

TUNE IT UP: If you are one of the many people who cannot lower their heels to the floor in this pose, just roll up a blanket, or the end of your mat, and place it under your heels to lift them up (see photo).

You can sit on a block to support your body weight if you have an injury or other health issue (eg, recovering from a surgery) in your low back, knees, or hips. However, I do not recommend habitually sitting on a block in Garland Pose, because that prevents you from activating your belly and back muscles, and reduces or eliminates the strengthening benefits of this pose. Your goal is to use your own muscles to support your torso. To do that, pull the heels of your hands downward to help press your elbows into your knees and lift your chest. Keep lifting your ribs away from your hips. Do not sag your weight down into your hips, knees, and low back. Be patient and breathe.

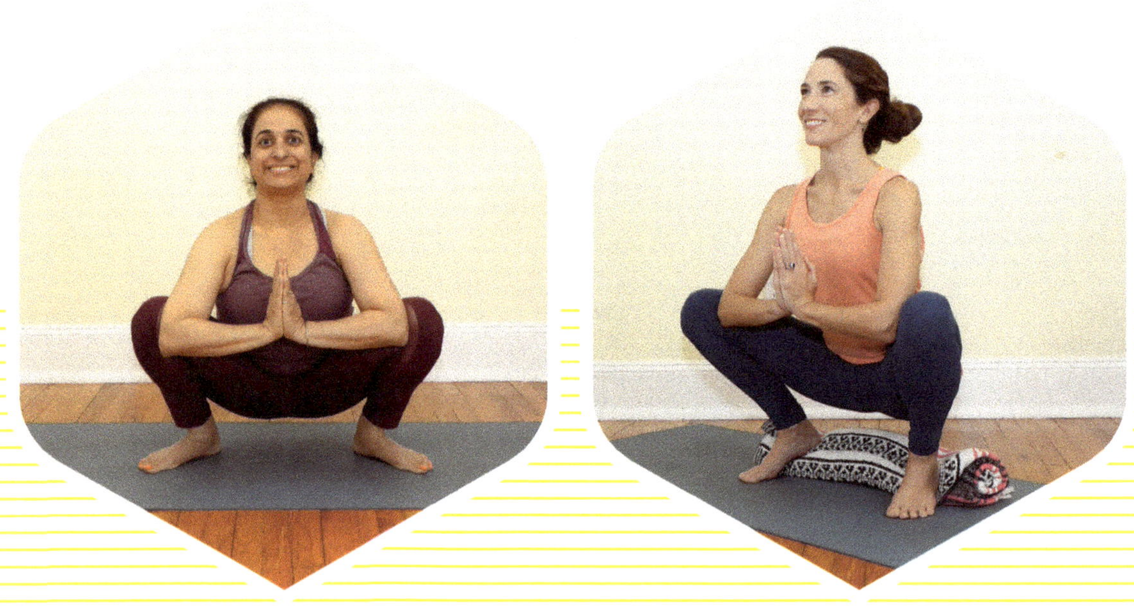

Garland Pose

Variation with blanket

Toe Balance Pose

ALSO CALLED: Utitha Tadasana, Prapadasana

WHAT IT DOES FOR YOUR LOWER LEGS: Seated and standing toe balances strengthen the lower leg muscles and build tremendous mental focus. Standing toe balance extends your ankles while keeping other joints in neutral. Seated toe balance puts the knees and ankles into flexion.

TUNE IT UP: Your balance will feel steadier in all toe balances if you draw your knees toward each other and focus on compacting your outer hips inward to your centerline. If you have limited knee mobility, don't squat all the way down in order to protect your knee joints in the seated version. But beware, it's much more challenging to stop half-way.

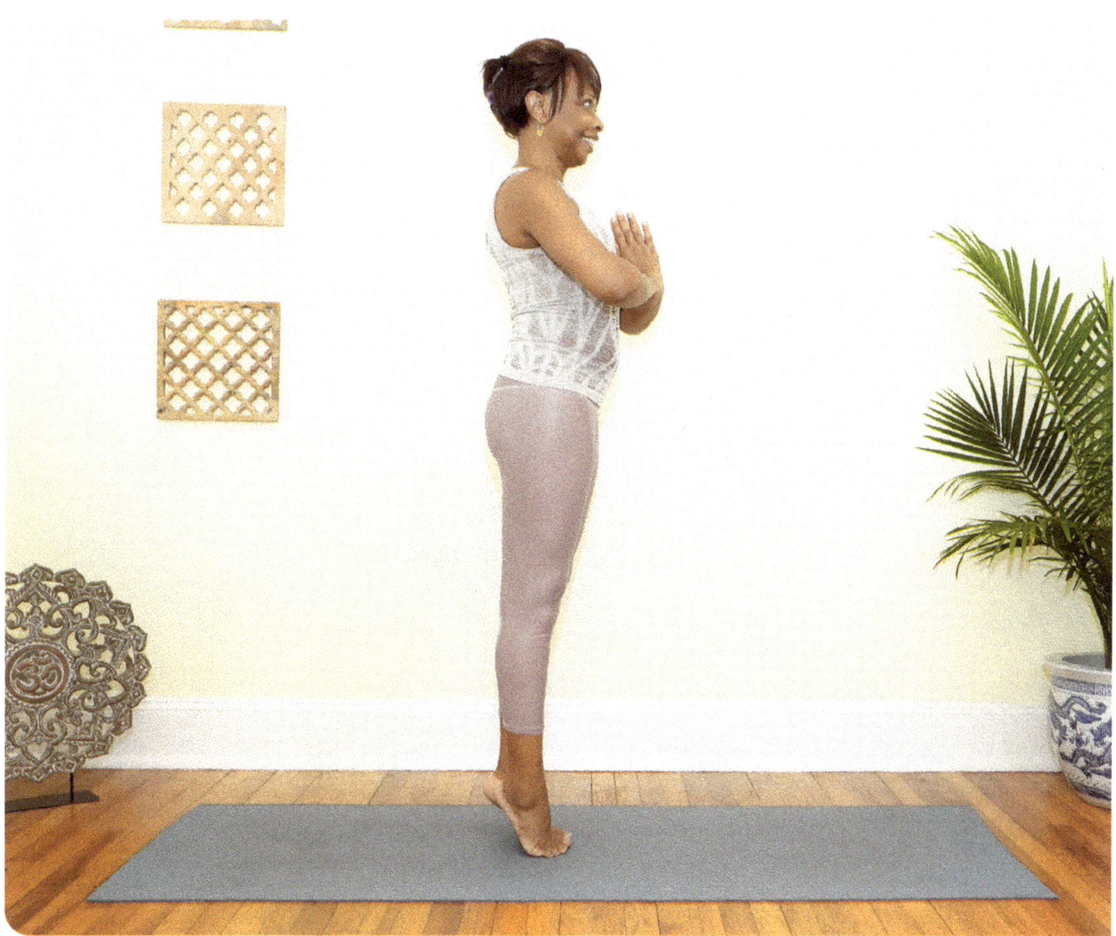

Standing Toe Balance

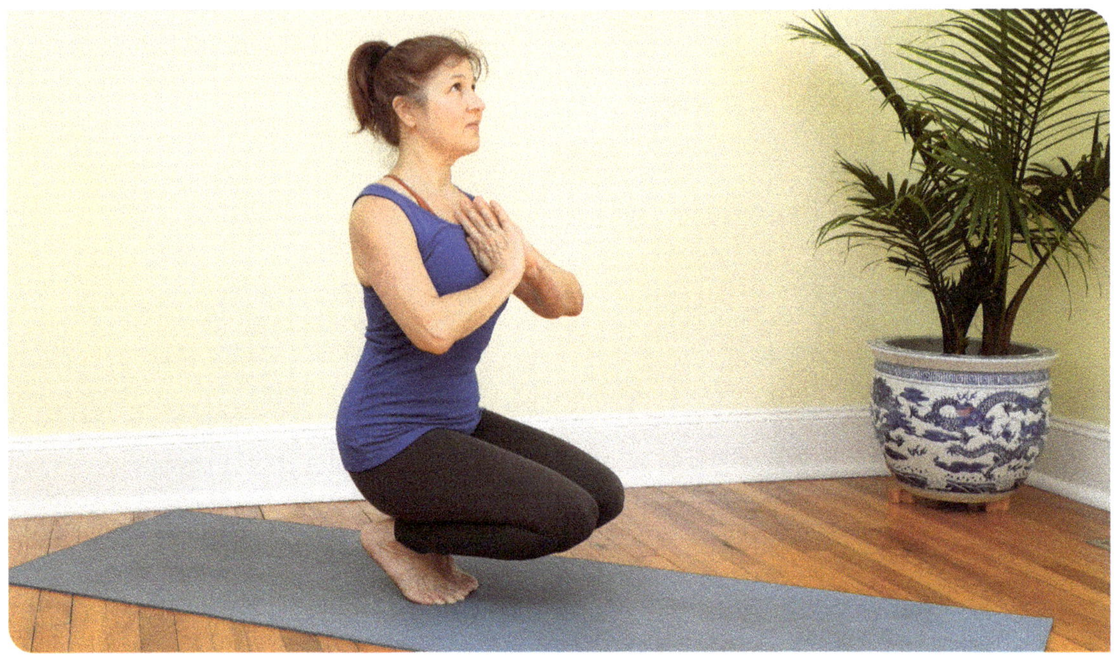

Seated Toe Balance Pose

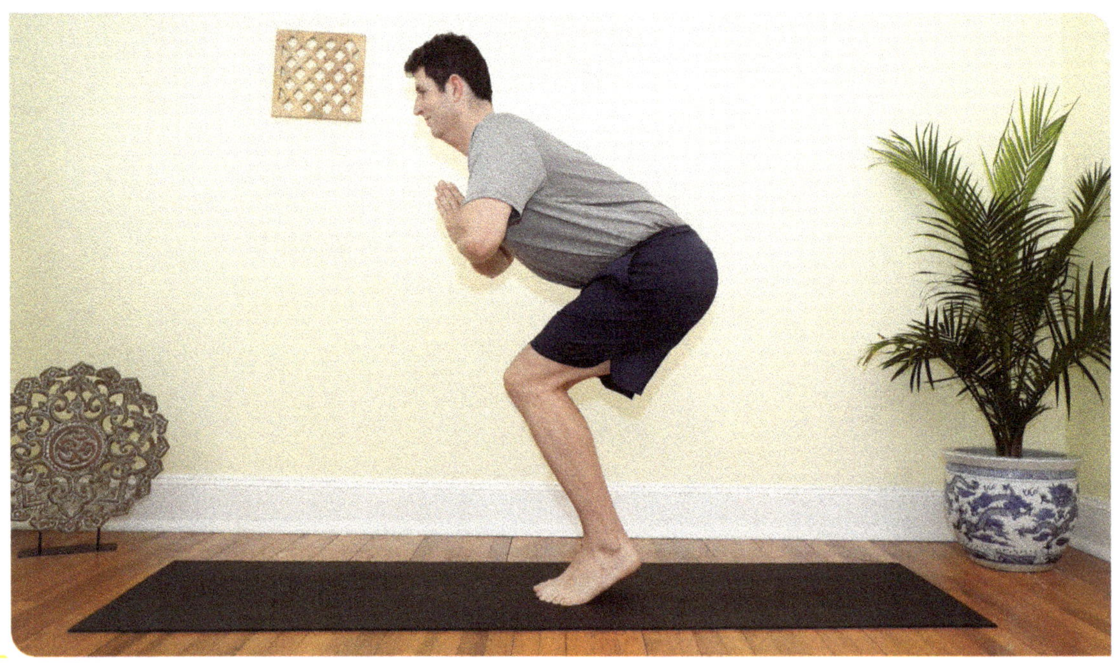

Seated Toe Balance, variation

Low Lunge Pose/High Lunge Pose

ALSO CALLED: Anjaneyasana

WHAT THEY DO FOR YOUR THIGHS AND HIP FLEXORS: Stretch your quads and hip flexors on the back (straight) leg.

TUNE IT UP: If your back knee is sensitive to bearing weight, put a blanket under it in Low Lunge Pose (see picture).

In both, lift your chest and press your hips forward and draw your inner thighs toward each other. Don't sag your hips down toward the floor, because this causes the back hip to turn outward, releasing the stretch.

In High Lunge, focus on keeping the back knee straight while bending the front knee. How far you bend your front knee is determined by how straight you can keep your back knee. If you have tight quads and hip flexors, you will not be able to bend your front knee deeply without also bending the back one. Focus on keeping your back knee firm and straight, while drawing your inner thighs toward each other. Don't worry; as your back thigh and hip flexors get more flexible, your front knee bend will deepen. Don't give up the back leg benefits just to bend your front knee more. That only robs you of the stretching benefit on the back leg. These basic poses are quite difficult when done correctly, so don't be too hard on yourself.

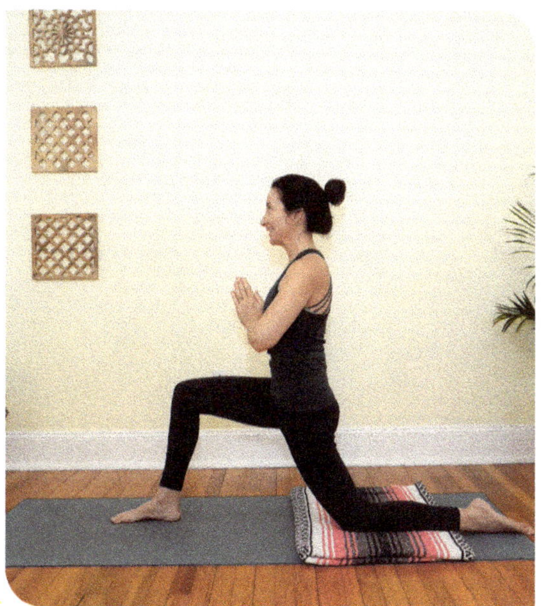

Low Lunge Pose, variation with blanket

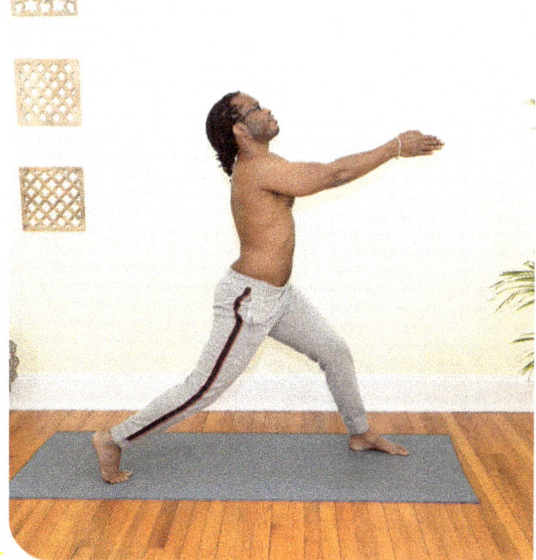

High Lunge Pose, variation with arms forward

King Dancer Pose

ALSO CALLED: Natarajansana

WHAT IT DOES FOR YOUR THIGHS AND HIP FLEXORS: Stretches your quads and hip flexors on the back (lifted) leg. Because you're balanced on one foot, this pose also builds mental focus, and strengthens the standing leg. The ankle is in extension and the bent knee is in deep flexion.

TUNE IT UP: Even if you can do this pose without support, try it near a wall, where you can rest the back of your front (raised) hand to steady your balance. Using the wall to help with the balance allows you to lift your back foot higher and explore the limits of your strength, flexibility, and breathing, without the risk of tipping over on your neighbor. When you start learning this pose, don't rush to extend. Stay standing upright and work on getting comfortable with the balance, and that level of stretching. When you're ready, only move your leg back a little bit (into a partially extended variation). Pause there and re-calibrate your breath and balance. Don't rush into your fullest extension. The thighs tend to move apart, so keep drawing your inner thighs toward your centerline in all variations.

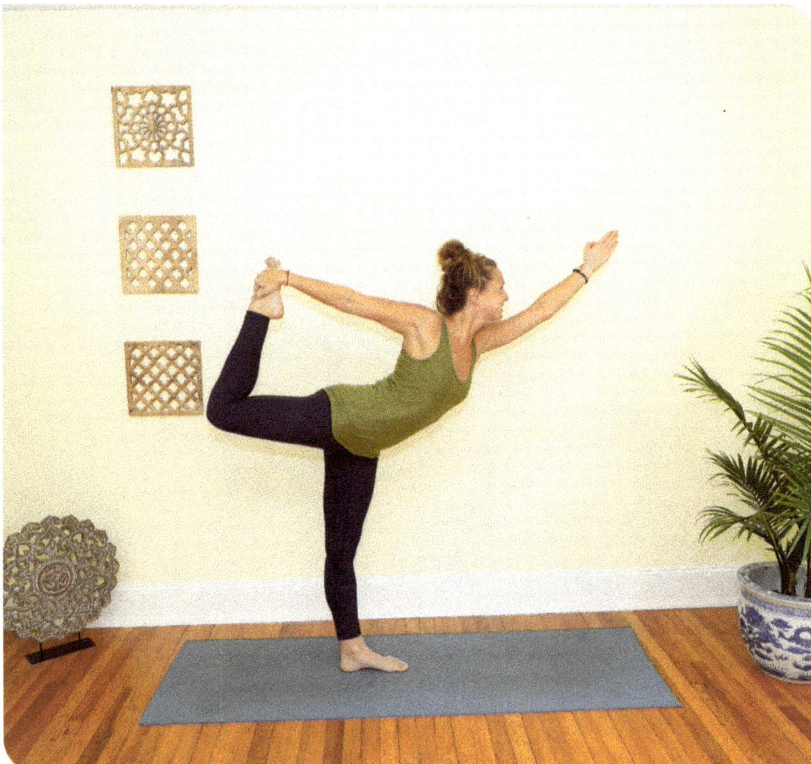

King Dancer Pose

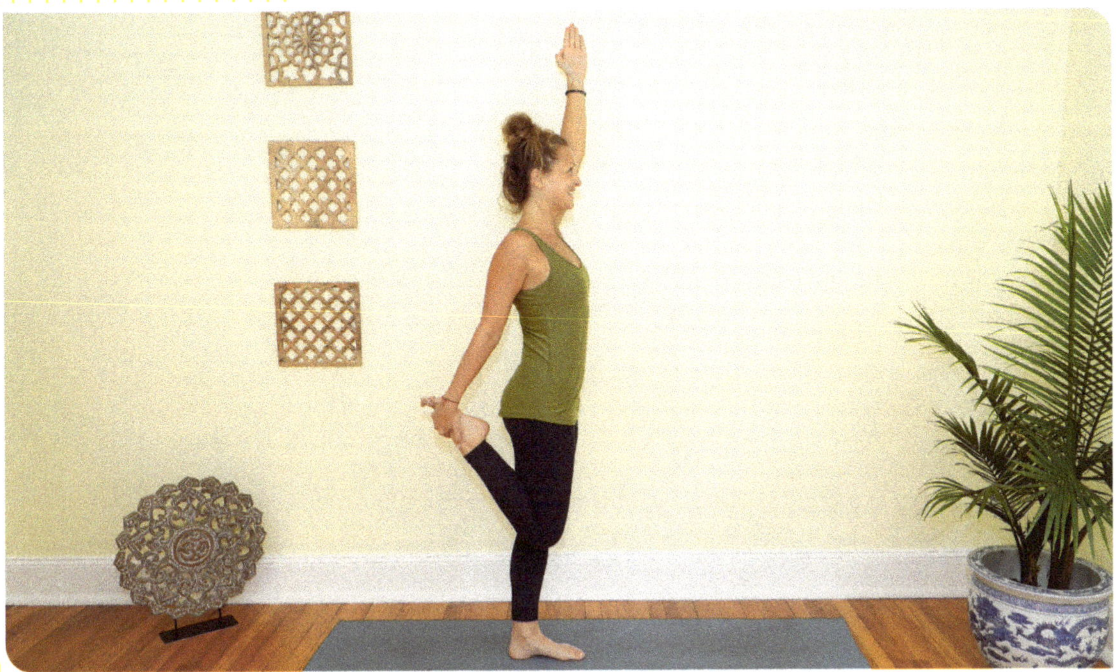

Upright variation

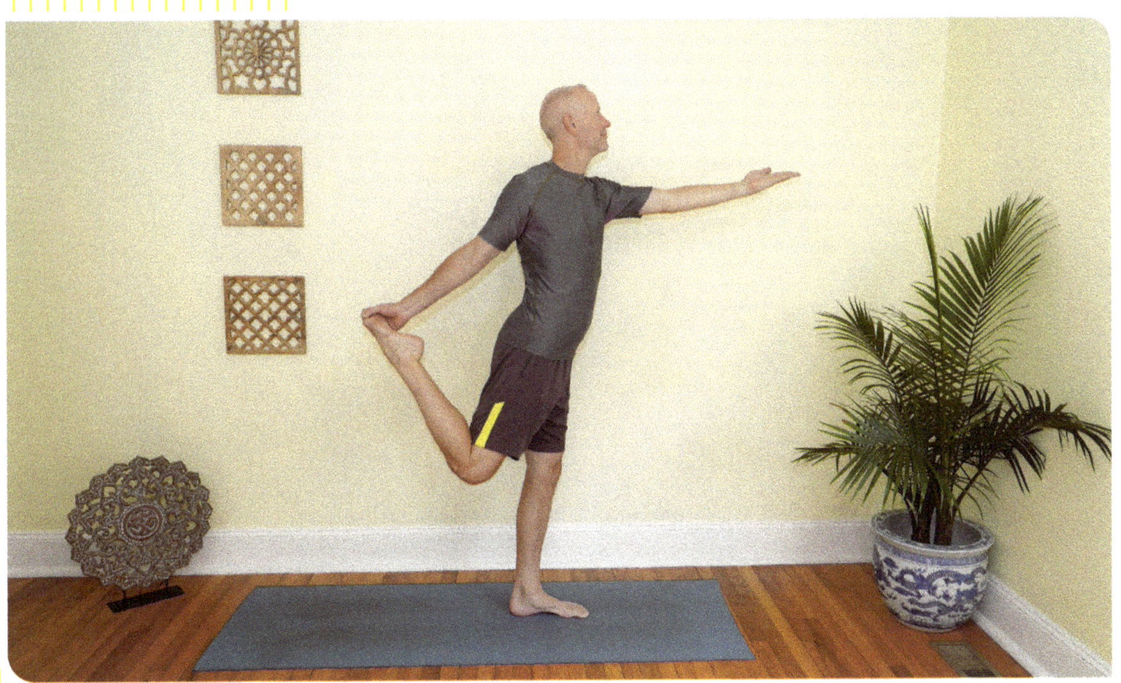

Partially extended variation

Bow Pose

ALSO CALLED: Dhanurasana

WHAT IT DOES FOR YOUR THIGHS AND HIP FLEXORS: Bow Pose is an intense stretch for your quads and hip flexors, which are in full extension.

TUNE IT UP: If you can't reach your feet, hold a strap looped behind your ankles (see picture).

Many people automatically hold their breath in this pose. It's very difficult to keep your breath deep and steady when you're lying on your belly. So focus on taking slow, deep inhales.

Draw your knees slightly inward toward each other, and press your hips into the floor. There's an automatic tendency to thrust your chin forward when you lift up in any prone back bend. It's a common muscular pattern, but it doesn't help you hold the pose, and it creates tension in the back of your neck and shoulders. Do not stick your chin forward. Instead, draw your chin slightly in toward your throat (a tiny bit, not a lot) to lengthen the back of your neck. Look at the floor a foot or two in front of you.

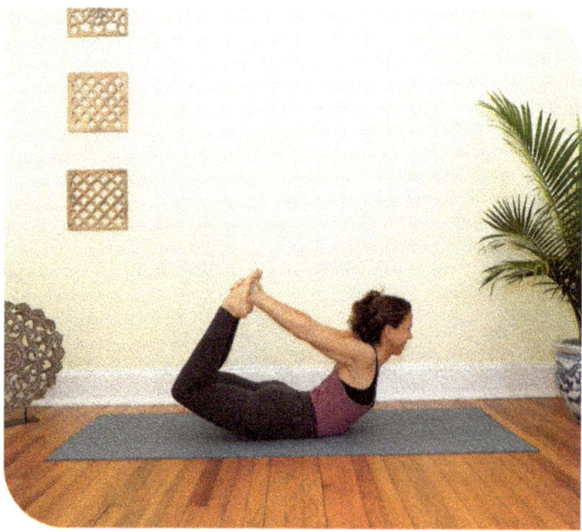

Bow Pose

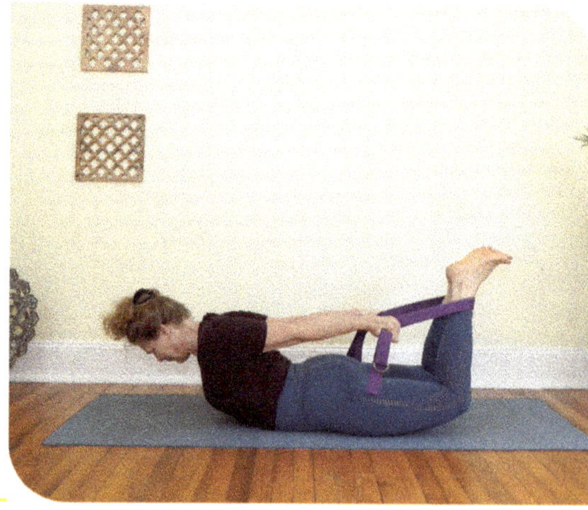

Variation with strap

Bridge Pose

ALSO CALLED: Setu Bandhasana

WHAT IT DOES FOR YOUR THIGHS AND HIP FLEXORS: Stretches your hip flexors and quadriceps. Because your quads are contracting while you stretch them, this pose is a good example of active dynamic stretching, the most effective way to build flexibility.

TUNE IT UP: When learning this pose, start with your hips supported on a single block. Gradually increase the height by adding blocks as your muscles get longer. If your thigh muscles and hip flexors are very tight, you may not be able to put your feet directly under your knees with your hips raised on blocks. Never fear—just move your feet forward of your knees (see picture).

Some people experience irritation behind the kneecaps during this pose, because their tight quads pull the knee caps back against the knee joint. Move your feet forward a bit to ease this. Over time, as your quads and hip flexors get longer, you'll be able to place your feet directly under your knees.

Be patient. Focus on pressing the fronts of your feet down into the floor and forward (as if you are trying to stretch your mat longer) to keep your leg muscles engaged. Keep your knees in front of your hips; don't let them fall outward away from your centerline. Keep your legs active. Do not just sit on the blocks with limp legs.

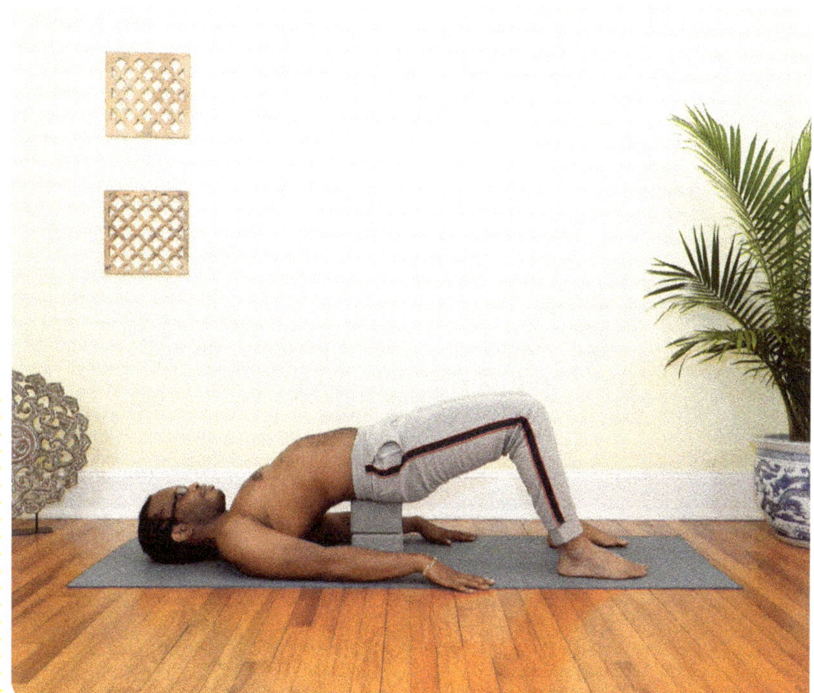

Bridge Pose, variation with blocks and feet forward

Upward Facing Bow Pose

ALSO CALLED: Urdhva Dhanurasana, Wheel Pose

WHAT IT DOES FOR YOUR THIGHS AND HIP FLEXORS: This is an intense stretch for the quads and hip flexors (illio-psoas major and illiacus) and builds a lot of strength in all of the upper leg muscles.

TUNE IT UP: Focus on using your leg muscles in this pose by pushing the fronts of your feet down into the floor and forward (as if you were trying to stretch your mat longer). Do not press into your heels so much that your toes pop up, or shove your low back up towards the ceiling. Think about using your legs to shift your chest backwards toward your wrists.

It's extremely challenging to breathe in this pose, because the muscles on your front are completely extended, leaving little space for your rib cage to move. Concentrate on making your inhales as full and steady as possible.

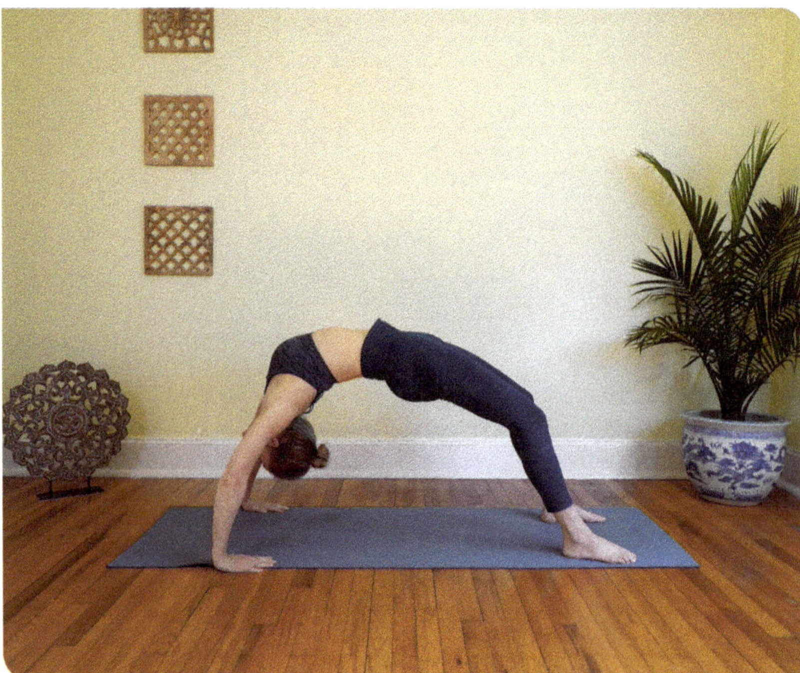

Upward Facing Bow Pose

Reclined Hero Pose

ALSO CALLED: Supta Virasana

WHAT IT DOES FOR YOUR THIGHS AND HIP FLEXORS: This is another intense stretch for the quads and hip flexors.

TUNE IT UP: If your knees are unhappy in a deep bend (full flexion), sitting up on a block will relieve them a bit. If you're sitting on a block, put a rolled-up blanket or a bolster under your elbows to lift them as well (see photo). With your hips on a block, you won't have to lean back very far to feel a strong thigh stretch.

Lift your chest and draw your knees slightly inward toward each other; do not let your knees slide apart into a wide V-shape. When your knees come off the floor, stop there, and focus on reaching them down. Do not keep lying further back after your knees lift up.

Focus on your breathing, especially the inhales.

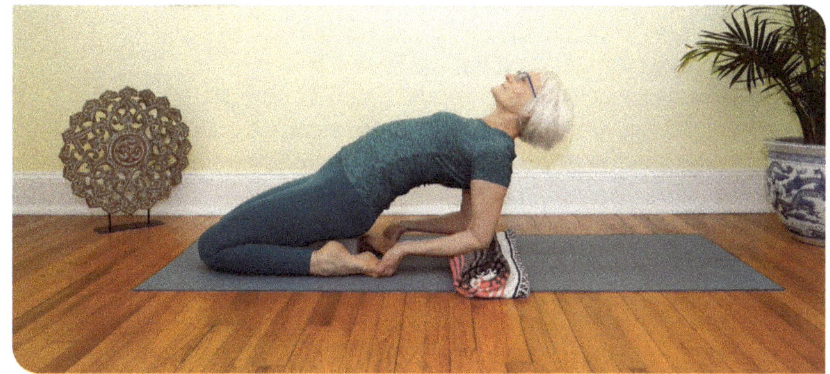

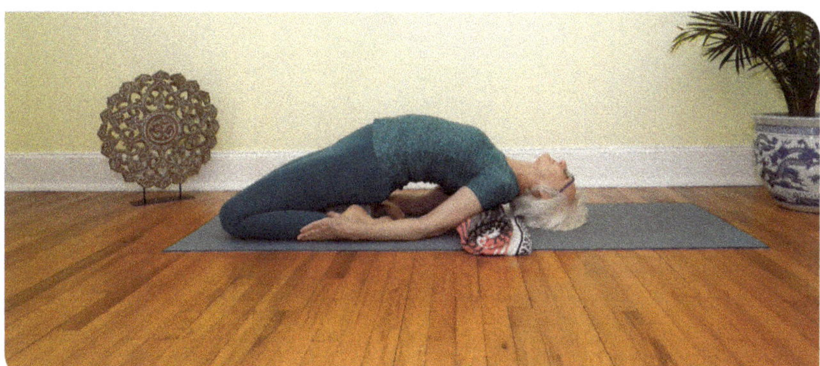

Reclined Hero Pose, variation with block and blanket

One-Legged King Pigeon Pose

ALSO CALLED: Eka Pada Rajakapotasana, or simply Kapotasana

WHAT IT DOES FOR YOUR THIGHS AND HIP FLEXORS: Gives the thigh and hip flexors on the back (straight) leg an intense stretch.

TUNE IT UP: This complex pose requires many years of practice to build the strength and flexibility to do it safely without tools. Almost everyone should start doing this pose with a bolster or rolled up blanket under their front knee and hip, supporting the bent leg.

Until this pose feels very comfortable (which may be never!), keep your front knee elevated higher than your front foot. In other words, elevate both the knee and the hip on the bent leg. Do not raise just the hip, leaving your knee on the floor. Raising your bent knee helps protect your knee joint from the rotational forces in this pose which can injure it—especially if your butt muscles (your glutes) and groins (adductors) are tight.

Keep both the hip and knee raised for this pose until you develop enough rotational flexibility in your hip joint to allow your bent leg (the knee and hip) to sit comfortably on the floor. Also, bending the front knee more to bring the front heel toward your inner groins will help protect your knee joint. Moving the front heel forward, and opening the bend in the front knee, can allow rotational force to enter your knee joint. So be careful—move mindfully a little at a time.

Bring your hands onto blocks so you don't have to sag your chest and shoulders forward to reach the floor. Place your palms flat and firmly press down, straightening your elbows. You may need to move the blocks forward to get your elbows straight. The higher you set the blocks with straight elbows, the deeper your back bend will be. If your back is unhappy in this pose, keep the blocks on the lowest setting (or put your hands on the floor forward of your body) to reduce or eliminate the back bending.

Focus on lifting your chest and drawing your shoulders back. Breathe. Be calm. Be patient.

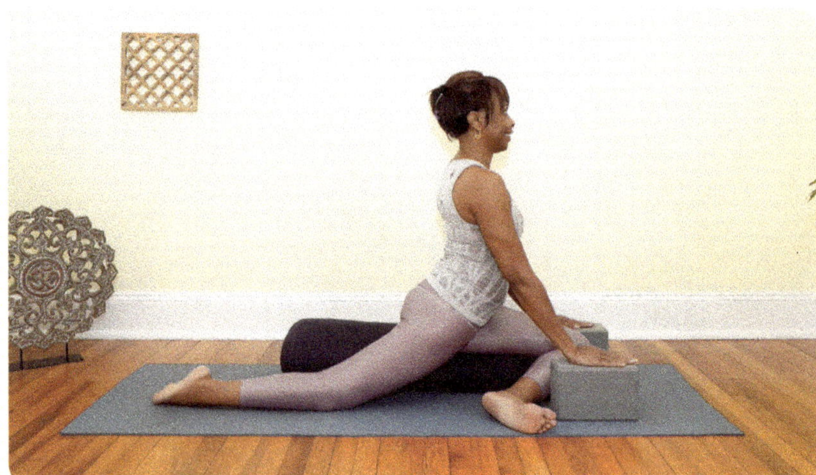

One-Legged King Pigeon Pose, variation with blocks and bolster

Camel Pose

ALSO CALLED: Ustrasana

WHAT IT DOES FOR YOUR THIGHS AND HIP FLEXORS: This pose extends your quads and hip flexors while pressing your pelvis and thigh bones forward for another great stretch.

TUNE IT UP: When learning this pose, start with your toes elevated on a "speed bump" (two blocks end-to-end under your mat). Hook the crease of your toes (where your toes meet the ball of your foot, see photo) on the front edge of the speed bump; do not put your toes flat on top of it. Raising your feet does two things: It increases the thigh stretch by creating a deeper bend in your knees, and brings your heels closer to your fingertips, making it easier to eventually hold them as your flexibility increases.

If your knee caps are sensitive to weight bearing, put a folded blanket under your knees.

At first, most people can't press their hips forward very much, or hold their heels with their hands. Don't worry! Hold a strap behind your back palms facing forward if you can't reach your heels. Pull outward on the strap with straight elbows, and try to turn your palms outward away from your centerline.

In all variations of this pose, focus on pressing your hips forward and lifting your chest and ribs away from your hips. Do not focus on dropping down and backward—this action can hurt your low back. Remember, stretching is a gradual process. Be patient with your body.

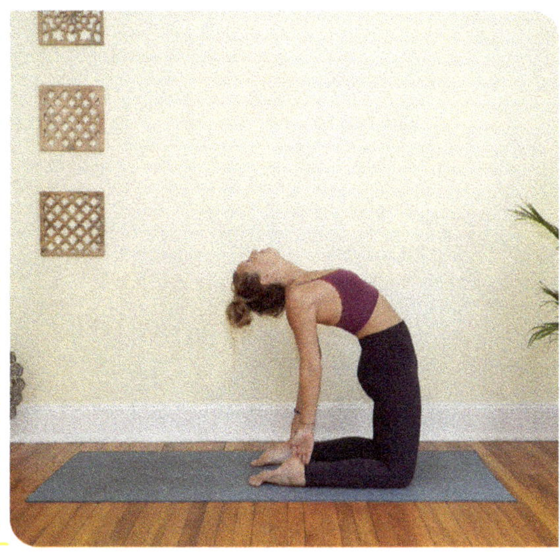

Camel Pose

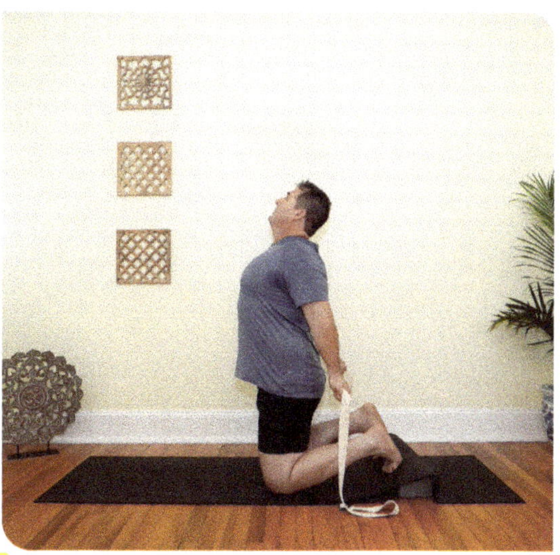

Variation with strap

Chair Pose

ALSO CALLED: Utkatasana, Fierce Pose

WHAT IT DOES FOR YOUR THIGHS AND HIP FLEXORS: This pose is great for strengthening your thigh muscles and hip flexors (as well as the fronts of your shins). It flexes your knees, hips, and ankles.

TUNE IT UP: Press your knees together, and at the same time draw your ankles apart. These two actions activate muscles in both your upper and lower legs.

Lift your chest and elbows if your hands are in front of your chest (see photo). If you raise your arms up with straight elbows, it becomes even harder to breathe so choose your arm position carefully and match it to your level of strength and energy for today's practice. Look forward or slightly up; do not look at the floor.

Many people automatically hold their breath in this pose. Take care to focus on your inhales. Remember, because you're already using many of the auxiliary muscles of breathing in your back and belly to lift your torso, practicing deep inhales will build a lot of strength. So take this chance to breathe deeply and build a lot of core strength.

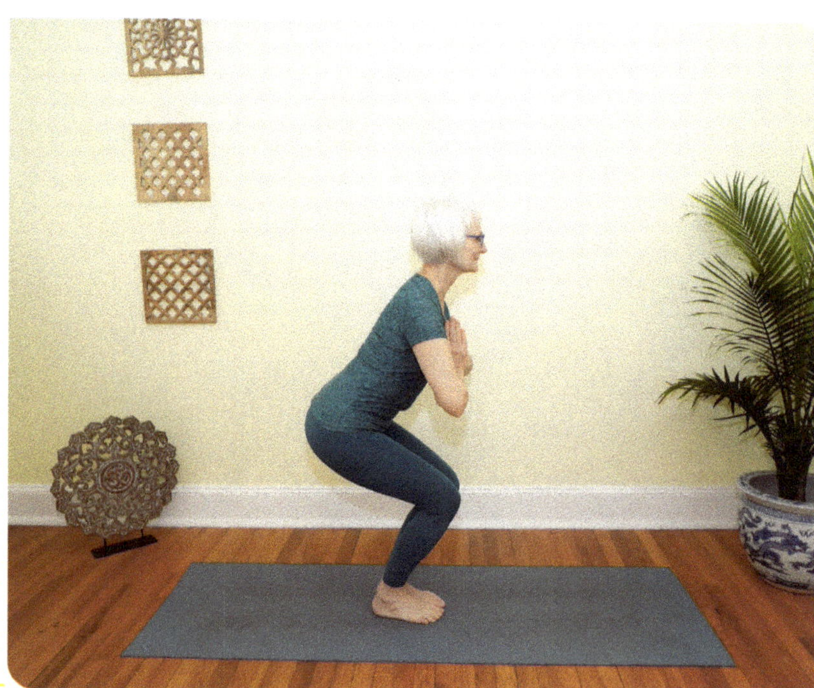

Chair Pose, variation with hands at the chest

Warrior Two Pose

ALSO CALLED: Virabhadrasana Two

WHAT IT DOES FOR YOUR THIGHS AND HIP FLEXORS: Strengthens your thigh muscles on both legs and stretches your hip flexors on the back leg. This pose flexes your front knee and hip while extending your back knee and hip.

TUNE IT UP: Many people lean out over their front leg in this pose, making it work harder than the back leg. This is incorrect. Maintain correct (central) alignment by centering your torso and hips in the middle of your feet. It's also common for the back hip to hike up higher than the forward hip. This is incorrect alignment. Keep your back hip down, level with the front one to ensure you get a good stretch on the hip flexor and groin muscles of your back leg.

Hold your chest upright. This is very difficult; if you can't keep your chest, torso, and hips upright and centered between your feet, just un-bend your front knee a little until you are upright with correct (central) alignment.

The thigh muscles (your quads) on *both* legs should be very firm. Do not let your back leg (the straight leg) get lazy!

It's also common for the back shoulder and ribs to turn slightly forward. That's because the back hip flexor is tight and your waist muscles (your obliques) are weak. Your chest, torso, and hips should all be facing the long edge of your mat.

Use your neck muscles to turn only your head and look at your front fingers. In other words, turn your head, not your body.

Take steady, deep breaths to strengthen your core.

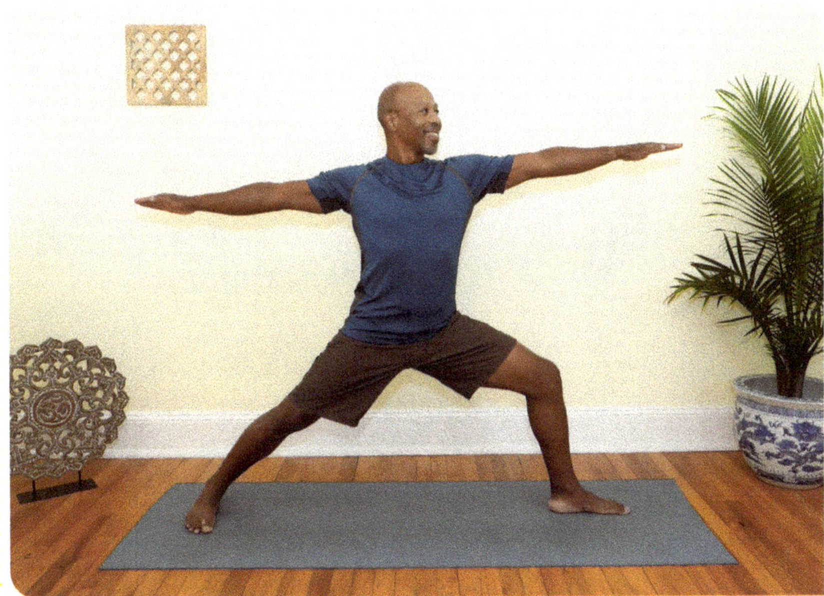

Warrior Two Pose

Extended Side Angle Pose

ALSO CALLED: Utthita Parsvakonasana

WHAT IT DOES FOR YOUR THIGHS AND HIP FLEXORS: This pose requires a great deal of strength in both thighs (quads). Your back leg will get a good hip flexor stretch as you press your back knee straight. It also stretches the outer shin muscles (peroneus longus and brevis) on the back (straight) leg. Like Warrior Two, the front knee and hip are in flexion while the back knee and hip are in extension. So you're getting different benefits in each leg.

TUNE IT UP: If your outer shin and hip flexors are tight, start trying this pose with your back heel lifted, and put a block under your front hand (the lower hand; see photo). If your back heel is lifted and you can't completely straighten your back knee, reach the top arm straight up to the ceiling instead of forward. Reaching your arm forward intensifies the hip flexor and thigh stretch by engaging your side waist muscles (your obliques).

Keep stretching your side-waist and ribs upward, and pressing your heel back. Gradually, as your hip flexors, thigh, and outer shin muscles become more flexible, the back knee will straighten, and your back foot will flatten to the floor.

As your thigh and waist muscles (quads and obliques) get stronger, you can move the bottom hand to the floor, and bring the top arm over your ear. Do not move your bottom hand closer to the floor if that makes your chest and shoulders turn downward. Be patient. Focus on your breathing to build strength from the inside out. It will all happen in time.

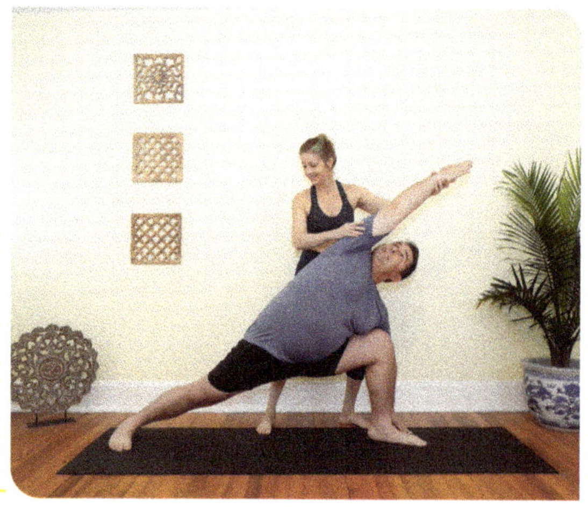
Extended Side Angle Pose

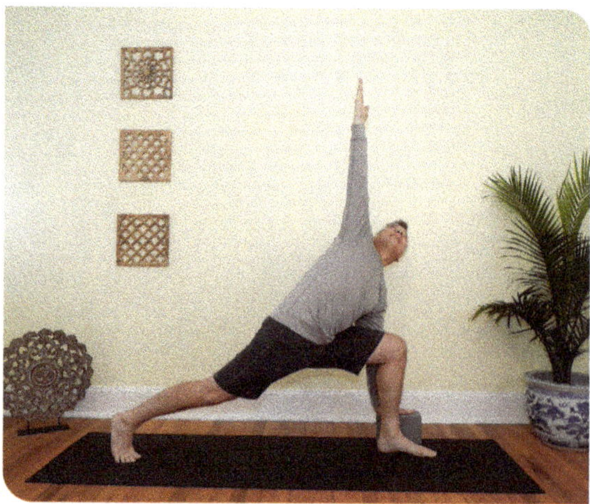
Variation with block and back heel lifted

Boat Pose

ALSO CALLED: Navasana

Extended Hand to Big Toe Pose, D

ALSO CALLED: Utthita Hasta Padangustasana, D

WHAT THEY DO FOR YOUR THIGHS AND HIP FLEXORS: Both poses strengthen the hip flexors and quads because you have to hold your legs up in front of your torso. That's super hard, your legs are heavy! In Boat Pose both hips are flexed while your knees and ankles are extended (in the straight-leg version). In Extended Hand to Big Toe Pose, D, the hip on the lifted leg is flexed. Both poses ask your quads and hip flexors to work very hard.

TUNE IT UP: The tendency with these poses is to lean backward, to try and lift your leg(s) by shifting your torso. Resist that. Focus on lifting your chest and ribs up off your hips and pulling your shoulder blades toward the middle of your back.

If you cannot hold your leg(s) up without leaning far back, bend your knee(s) to relieve some of the challenge. Working with bent knees is better than developing a bad habit of leaning backward that you'll have to break later. Holding your legs up with your knees bent builds flexibility in the hip joint, and gradually strengthens your hip flexor and abdominal muscles. Make your thigh, hip flexor, and abdominal muscles do the work.

Breathing deeply is very difficult because your entire core (back, sides, and front) is already working really hard to hold up your legs and deep breaths make those muscles work even harder. But remember, your muscles need oxygen to do this work, so focus on taking deep inhales.

Everyone finds these poses mentally challenging—they make us grumpy. It's not just you. When you can finally smile a little in Boat Pose or Extended Hand to Big Toe Pose, D, you'll know you've reached an advanced level of practice!

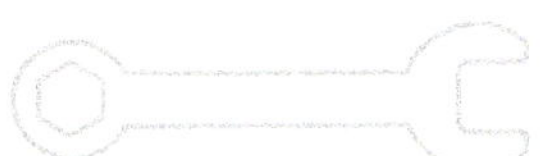

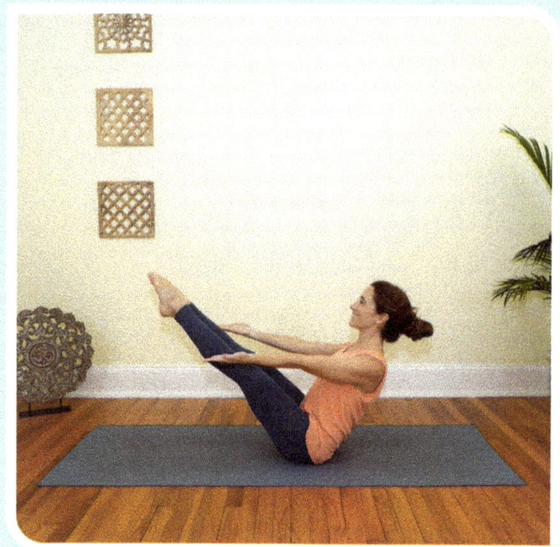
Boat Pose

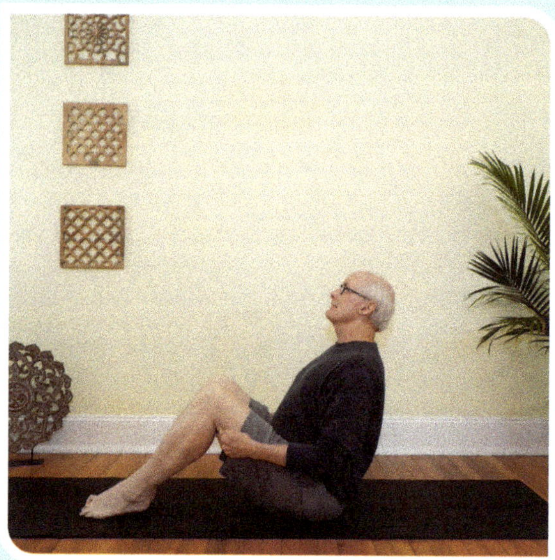
Variation with bent knees

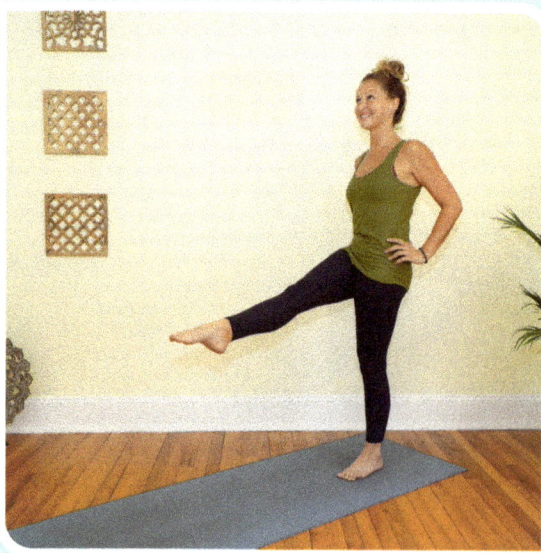
Extended Hand to Big Toe Pose, D

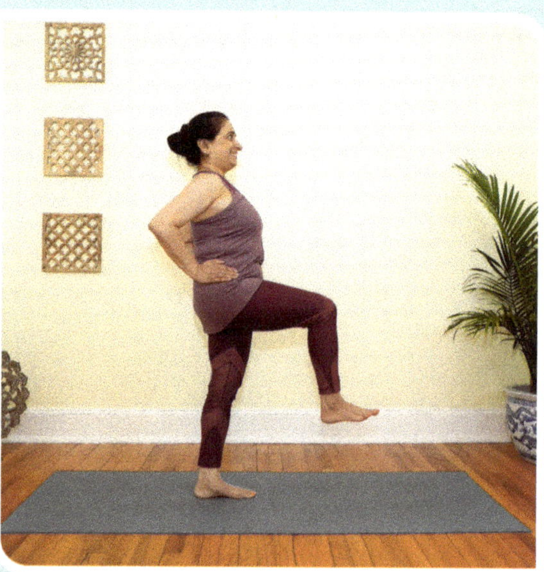
Variation with bent knee

Intense Raised-Leg Stretch Pose

ALSO CALLED: Uttana Padasana, Extended Fish Pose

WHAT IT DOES FOR YOUR THIGHS AND HIP FLEXORS: This pose requires strong thigh, hip flexor, and abdominal muscles. Your knees and ankles are completely extended and only your hips are flexed.

TUNE IT UP: It's important to take your time and start by doing this pose with tools. If your back, abdominal, and leg muscles are not strong enough, excessive weight will fall into your head, neck, and lower back. Do not rush to do the fully lifted variation until you feel very strong in the supported variation.

First, build the strength needed to protect the small vertebrae in your neck by putting a block under your shoulders and lifting only your arms (see photo). Press your palms firmly together and point your toes as much as you possibly can.

Engage your thigh muscles. Your legs should not be lazy and limp just because they're on the floor and there's support under your shoulders.

Use the supported variation to develop strength and focus. Don't waste the time you spend on your yoga mat lying around like a wet noodle. Get the most out of it that you can.

When you do feel ready to lift your legs, press your heels and inner thighs firmly together. To protect your low back from strain, draw your lower back slightly down toward the floor when you lift your legs, and keep that gentle downward action in your low back until your legs come back down to the floor.

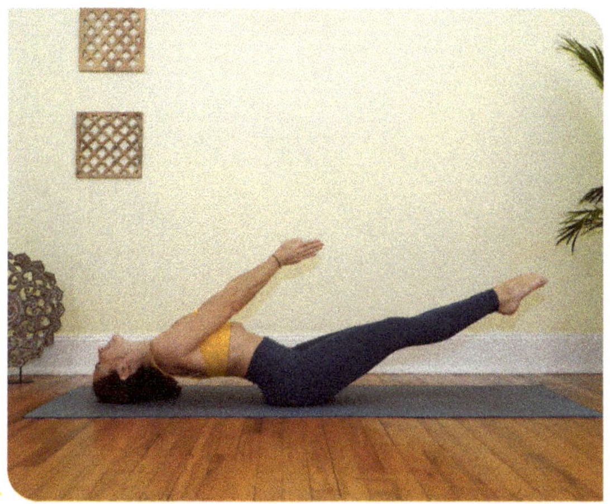

Intense Raised-Leg Stretch Pose

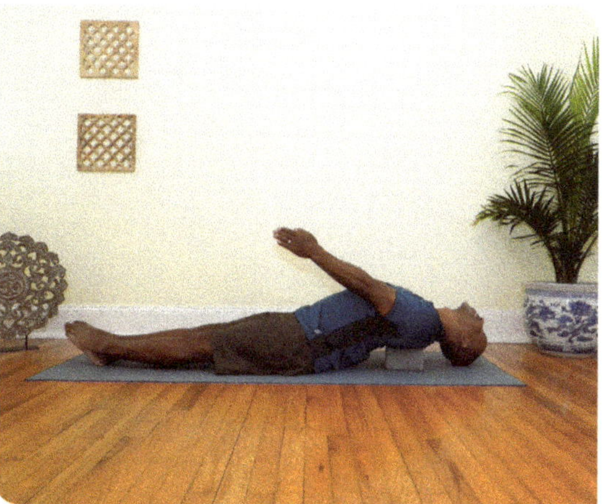

Variation with block and legs lowered

Wide-Legged Seated Balance Pose, B

ALSO CALLED: Upavistha Konasana, B

WHAT IT DOES FOR YOUR THIGHS AND HIP FLEXORS: This is a great pose for building strength in your hip flexors and quadriceps. Your ankles and hips are flexed while your knees are extended.

TUNE IT UP: Most people cannot hold the outer sides of their feet when they start trying this pose (not pictured). Don't worry; start by holding the backs of your legs anywhere that you can reach without slumping your shoulders (see photo).

Focus on lifting your chest and straightening your elbows and knees. It takes a lot of focus to balance on your butt.

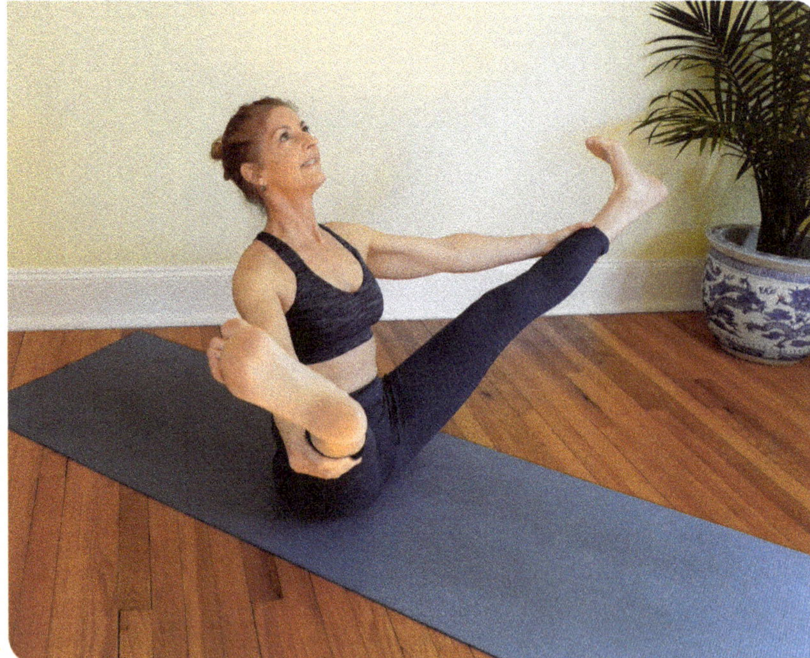

Wide-Legged Seated Balance Pose, B, variation holding shins

Head Stand Pose, B

ALSO CALLED: Sirsasana, variation B

WHAT IT DOES FOR YOUR THIGHS AND HIP FLEXORS: This is considered an advanced pose, because it requires so much physical strength and mental focus to do safely and effectively. The thighs and hip flexors work very hard to hold your legs at a right-angle in front of your body. Similar to Extended Hand to Big Toe Pose, D, you have to use your entire core to hold your legs out in front of your torso.

TUNE IT UP: Start slowly. Do not be overly eager to try this pose. Be humble and honest with yourself.

You *must* be very comfortable entering, holding, and exiting Head Stand Pose, A (Sirsasana, A) before you try version B. If you try this version before you're very strong and comfortable in Head Stand A, you can injure your neck and shoulders. (See Head Stand Pose in chapter 5, page 260.) Version B requires your hips to shift backward (behind your head) to counter-balance the weight of your legs lowering forward. Be careful; if you are not engaging your shoulders and upper back correctly, too much weight will fall into your neck vertebrae. Don't injure your neck. Be sure you are super-comfy in Head Stand A before moving into Head Stand B! When you do lower your legs forward, move extremely slowly. Don't try to go all the way down to 90-degrees at the start. Take it in small steps. You must remain keenly focused on every tiny shift in body weight as you enter, hold, and exit this pose.

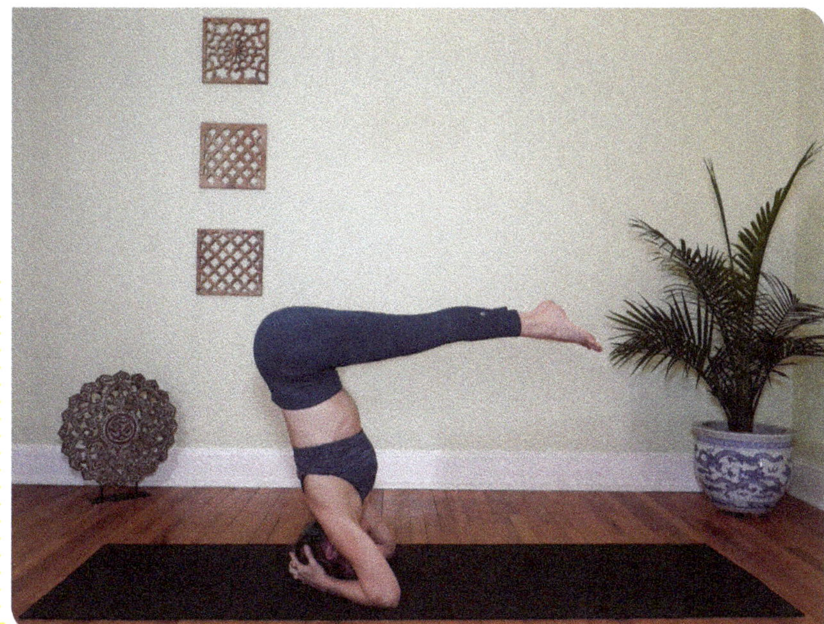

Head Stand Pose, B

Standing Forward Fold Pose

ALSO CALLED: Uttanasana

WHAT IT DOES FOR YOUR HAMSTRINGS: This pose is repeated often in yoga classes. It's a big stretch for your back and hamstrings because the hips are in full flexion, bringing the entire weight of your torso to pull downward on the back of the pelvis.

TUNE IT UP: If your hamstrings are tight, this pose can irritate your low back. So it's helpful to keep a couple of blocks at the front of your mat (one on each side) to put your hands on for back support. This keeps some of the weight of your arms, shoulders, and torso from pulling on your low back (see photo).

As your hamstrings get longer, keep your hands on the blocks but bend your elbows toward the back of your mat (not out to the sides). This will slightly increase the hamstring stretch without putting all that weight on your low back.

Eventually, you'll be able to do this pose without blocks. You can either hold the backs of your legs, put your hands on the fronts of your shins, or touch your fingertips to the floor. In all variations, draw your shoulders up, away from the floor, onto your back. Do not let your hips drift back too far behind your heels. Keep shifting weight toward the fronts of your feet.

Many people mistakenly think that touching the floor is the goal here. It is not! If you strain to reach the floor, your shoulders will round toward your neck, and your pelvis will duplicate this action by tucking under, increasing your risk of back strain and reducing the hamstring stretch you want. Keep lifting your shoulder blades up toward the ceiling (when you are upside-down, it's helpful to think of pulling your shoulders back toward the waistband of your pants). This action encourages your sitting bones to copy-cat by tipping upward, creating a more ideal stretch for your hamstrings.

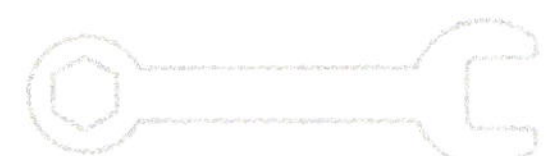

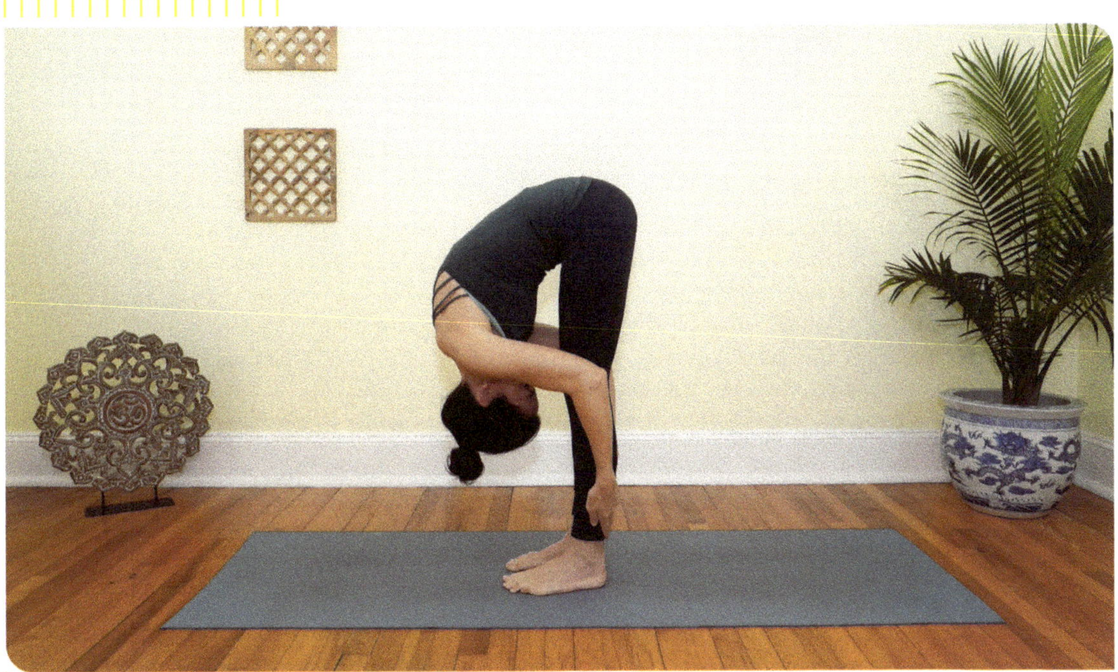

Standing Forward Fold Pose

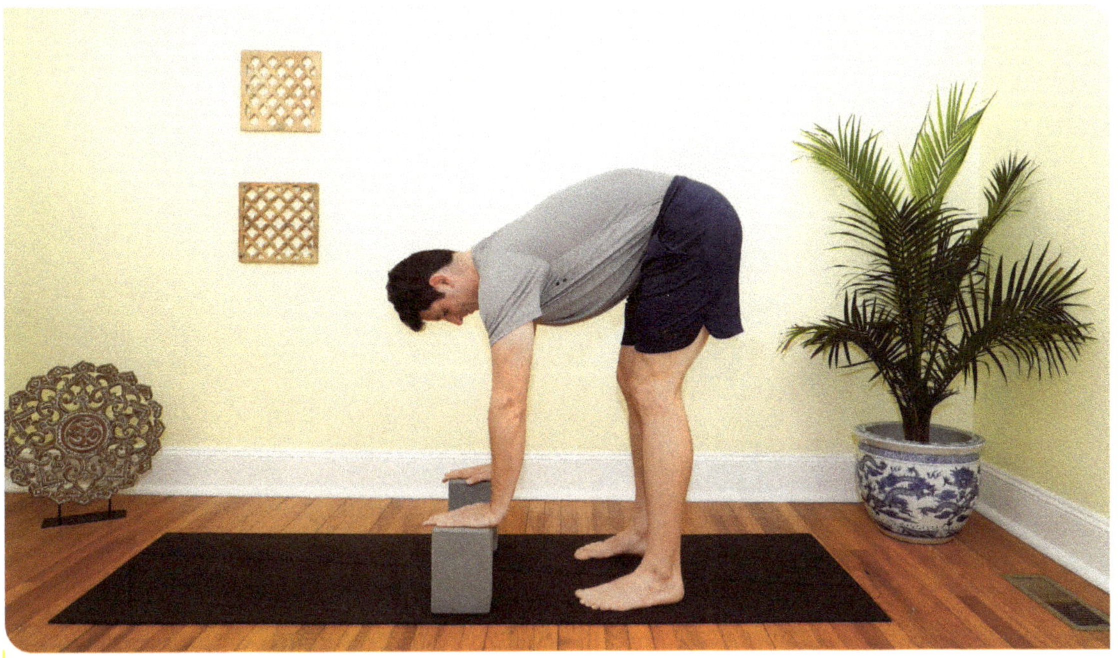

Variation with blocks

Hand Under Foot Pose

ALSO CALLED: Padahastasana

WHAT IT DOES FOR YOUR HAMSTRINGS: This is a more intense hamstring stretch than some other poses, because your hands are bound under your feet.

TUNE IT UP: If your hamstrings are tight, bend your knees to tuck your hands under.

Keep drawing your shoulders up away from the floor, toward the waistband of your pants. Do not force your knees to straighten, because that can strain your back.

Focus on pulling your low belly inward, and keeping your shoulders lifted back away from your neck. Breathe. This pose requires a great deal of patience. Be patient and wait for your hamstrings to lengthen. They will, give it time.

In standing forward folding poses with one foot forward (like Pyramid, see next pose, or Triangle), it's important to avoid shifting your hips back as you lean forward. Instead of bending your front knee, press your back foot down and backwards as if you're trying to stretch your mat longer. This action will shift your pelvis forward until it's centered between your feet. With your weight centered, you can safely work on straightening your front knee without the risk of hyperextending the ligaments behind it. Remember, central alignment means the weight should move down the centers of the bones and joints in your front leg, not into the back of your front knee.

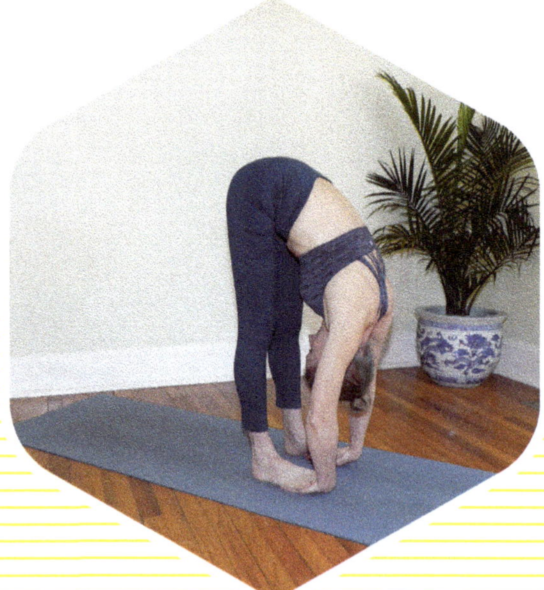

Hand Under Foot Pose

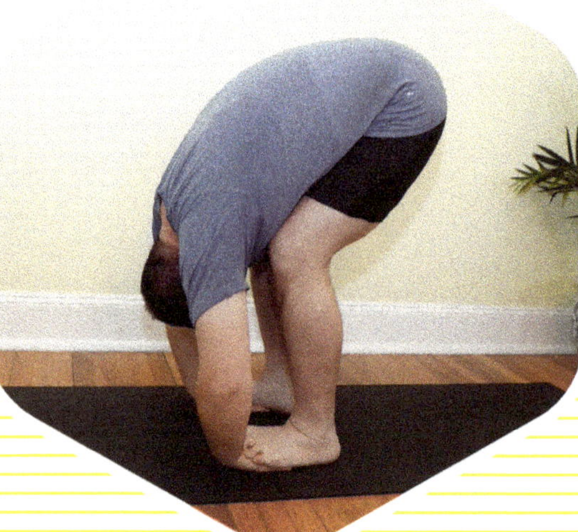

Variation with bent knees

Intense Side Stretch Pose

ALSO CALLED: Parsvottanasana, Pyramid Pose

WHAT IT DOES FOR YOUR HAMSTRINGS: This is an intense stretch for your hamstrings, outer thighs (outer quad, vastus lateralis), and hip stabilizers (ilio-tibial band and TFL) on the front leg.

TUNE IT UP: If your hamstrings are tight, put your hands on blocks to reduce strain on your low back (see photo). Correct (central) alignment is essential to stretch these muscles effectively without stressing your low back.

Although Pyramid Pose is often taught with the hands reaching toward the floor, the classical version calls for clasping your hands behind your back. There are important reasons for this. It creates a balance challenge that helps focus your mind on what you're doing; it reduces the temptation to let your shoulders round toward the floor; it increases shoulder-blade mobility; and it strengthens your upper-back muscles.

There are lots of ways you can choose to clasp your hands behind. You can make two fists and bump them knuckles-to-knuckles; interlace your fingers; hold opposite elbows (eventually wrapping your palms around the ends of your elbows); or touch your fingertips (eventually bringing the heels of your hands together in reverse prayer).

Whatever arm position you choose, when you bend forward, focus on correctly aligning your legs and torso. Do not focus on getting down close to your leg or the floor. If your arms are not bound behind your back, rounding your shoulders and reaching for the floor will reduce—not increase—the hamstring stretch, because your pelvis will copy-cat your rounded shoulders and tuck under.

Turn the toes of the back foot forward to about a 45-degree angle to protect your back knee and hip. This forward-facing position of your back foot, and the muscular action of drawing your upper thighs toward each other, will turn your pelvis to face the front of your mat.

To protect against hyper-extending the front knee, many instructors advise students to bend their front knee. This does reduce the risk of over-stretching the ligaments in the back of that knee, but it does not correct your basic alignment problem, your hips are in the wrong place—shifted too far back. Rock your hips carefully toward your front foot until the weight of your torso is centered between your feet, not dumping into the back leg.

Fold over your front shin by reaching your chest forward from your hips. It's a common mistake to fold your chest into the space between your feet. This is incorrect. Instead, line up the center of your chest with the center of your front shin, so there is a very slight rotation toward the front leg as you fold. As soon as you make this slight turn toward the front leg, you'll understand why the word "intense" is in the name of this pose. Do not fold into the space between your feet. Keep drawing your shoulders up away from the floor.

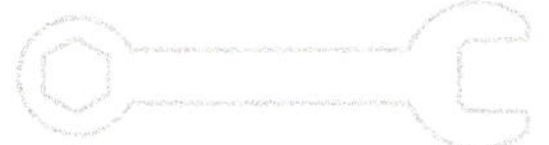

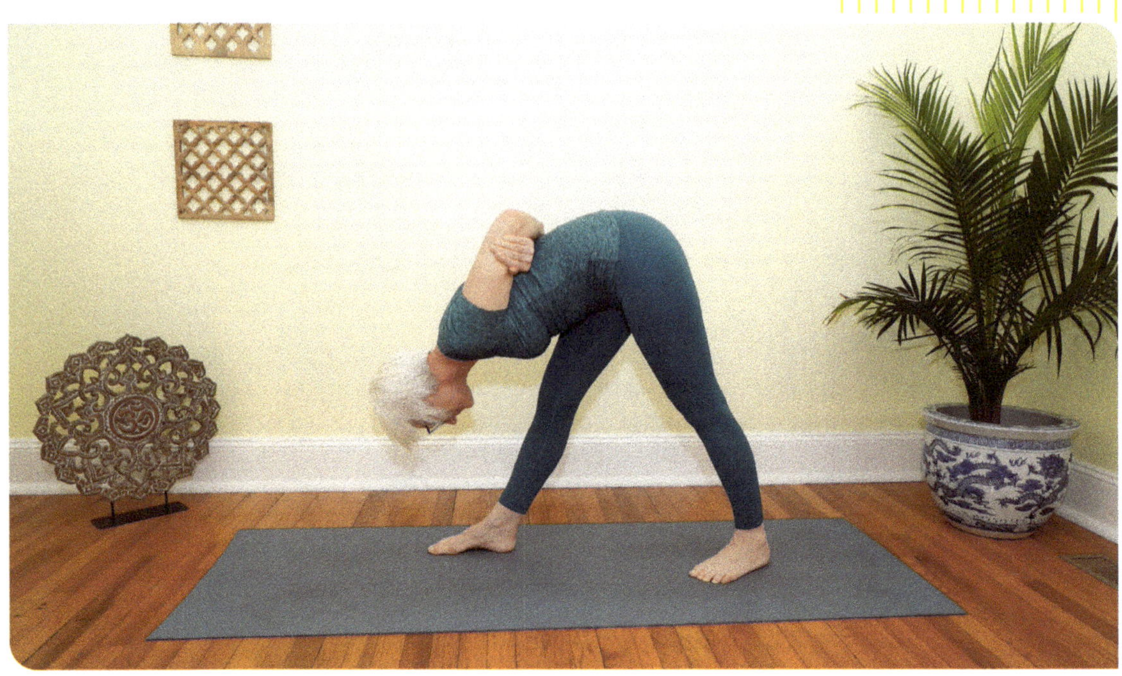

Pyramid Pose

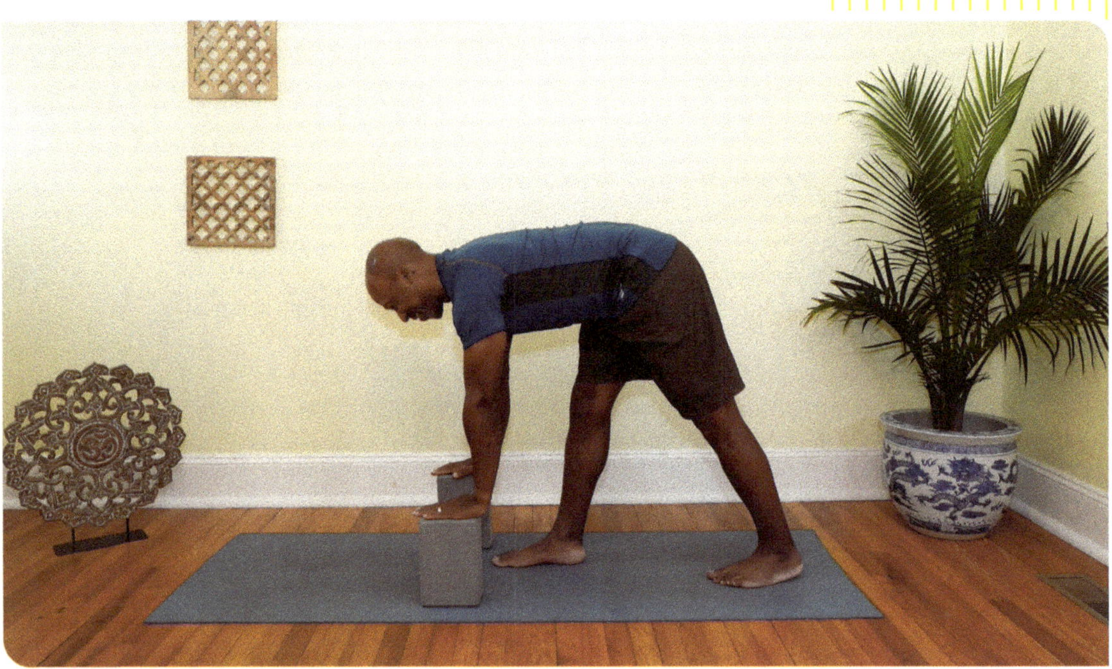

Variation with blocks

Spread-Legged Forward Fold, A and D

ALSO CALLED: Prasarita Padottanasana, A and D

WHAT THEY DO FOR YOUR HAMSTRINGS: These poses are excellent hamstring stretches that bring your hips into full flexion while extending your back. They also strengthen your hamstrings during the entry and exit movement as you lower and lift the weight of your torso primarily using your hamstrings.

TUNE IT UP: As with Pyramid Pose, if your hamstrings are tight, use blocks to raise your hands and reduce the weight pulling on your low back. Keep reaching your chest forward, away from your hips.

Many people mistakenly think that the goal of these poses is to put your head on the floor. It is not. If your head touches the floor, you should move your feet closer together, until there is at least a small space between the top of your head and your mat when you're fully folded. With space below your head, you have room to stretch your spine and chest forward and down. (The exception to not resting your head on the floor, of course, would be if you are using the pose to enter a headstand.)

In version D, turn your wrists to face each other, and draw your elbows out to either side (don't let them fall in toward your legs). Draw your shoulders toward your hips, away from your neck.

As in all forward folds (standing and seated), draw your shoulders towards your waist and away from your neck. Do not round your back and shoulders.

In all standing forward folds, there's a tendency to shift our hips backward as we lean forward—it's a natural, counter-balancing instinct. But this creates incorrect alignment, because your weight does not stay centered between both legs. Letting your hips swing back in this pose risks hyper-extending your knee joints. Carefully, shift some weight toward the fronts of your feet until the weight of your torso is centered between your feet, not dumping into the back of your knee joints.

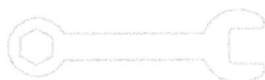

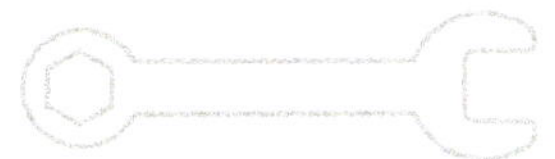

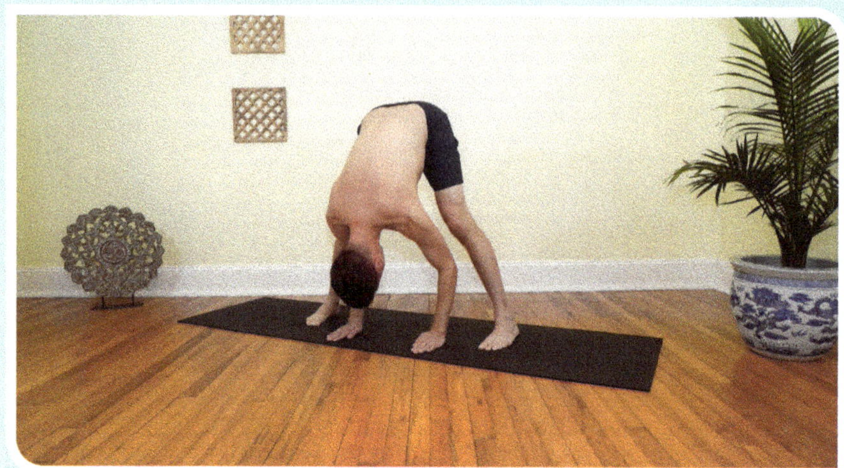

Spread-Legged Forward Fold, A

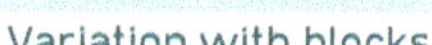

Variation with blocks

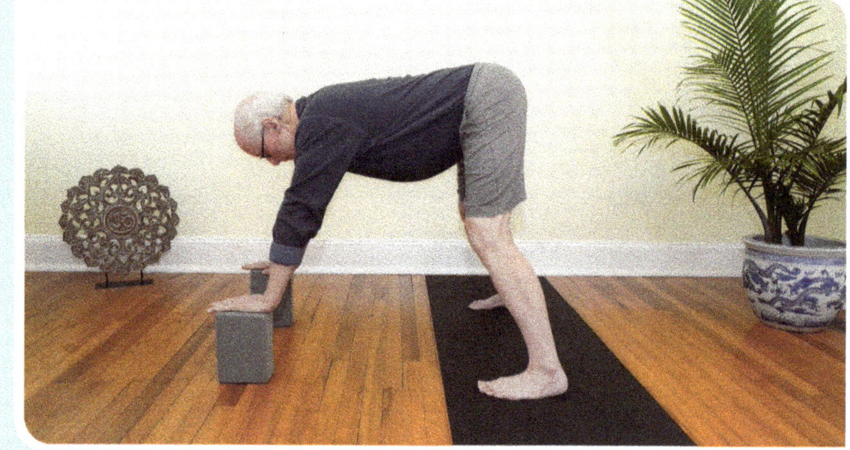

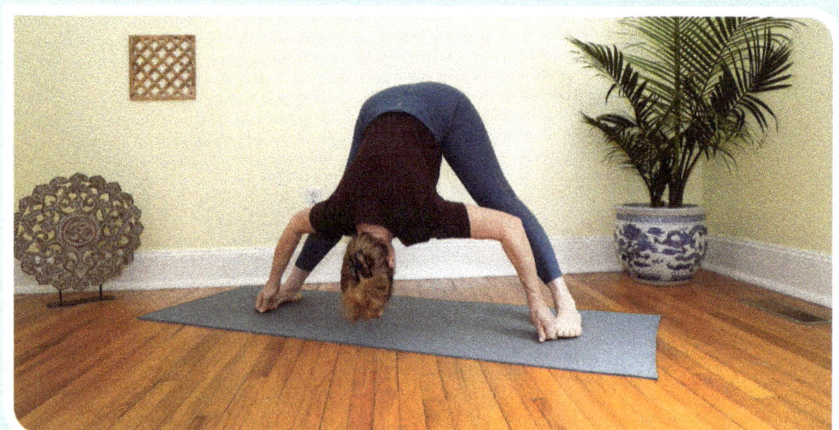

Spread-Legged Forward Fold, D

Seated Forward Fold

ALSO CALLED: Paschimottansana

WHAT IT DOES FOR YOUR HAMSTRINGS: This pose flexes the hips and ankles with the knees extended. Like all forward folds, it is a big stretch for your back muscles and hamstrings.

TUNE IT UP: This pose is more difficult than it looks, because it requires two opposing actions. First, you must firm up your thigh muscles and press the backs of your legs down into the floor. Folding forward over limp, lazy legs will hurt your back. Second, you must draw your shoulders away from the floor even as you fold forward over your legs. This will send your sitting bones back (stretching your hamstrings), and activate your belly muscles to support your back.

Turning your upper, inner thighs slightly inward and pressing the sides of your big toe mounds gently together will also help activate your low belly muscles.

Be patient. Changing your muscles takes time. Build good alignment habits, and then focus on long steady deep breathing and keeping your eyes still. Do not let your eyes jump all around the room. Be still. Focus your mind and observe.

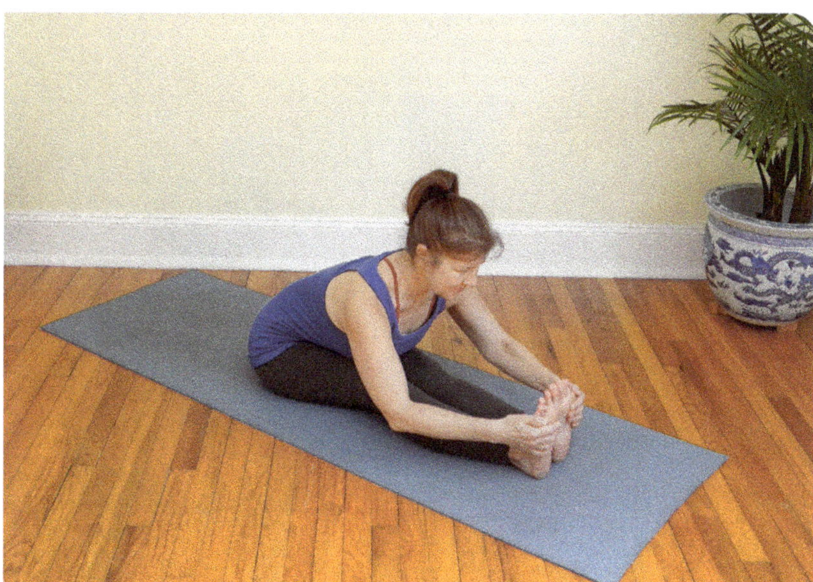

Seated Forward Fold

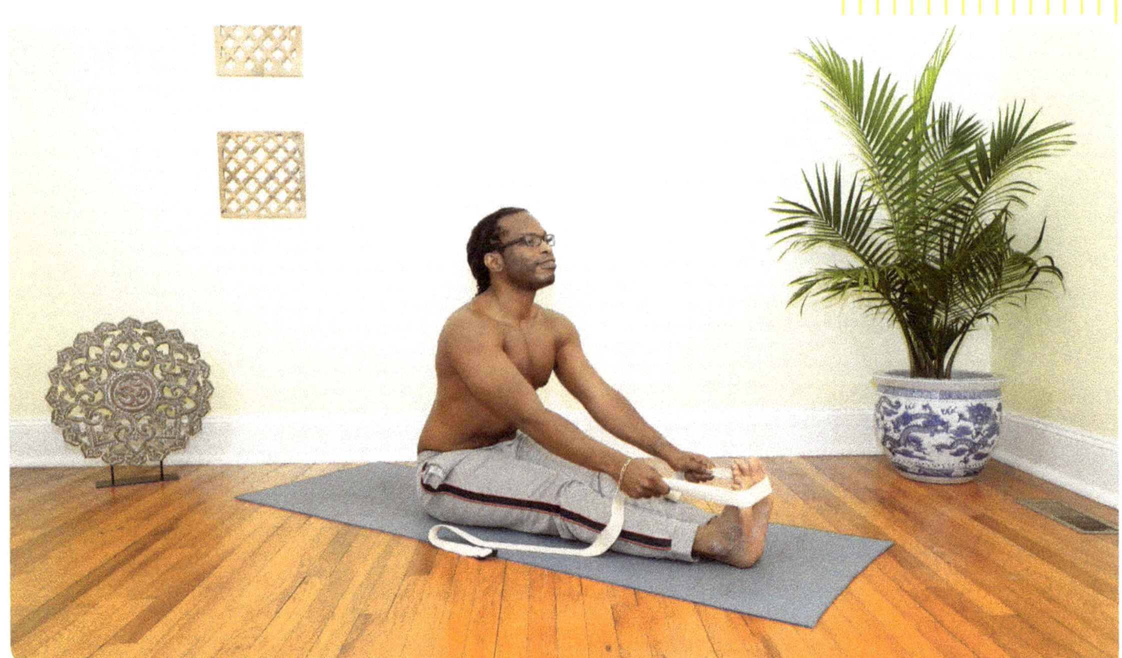

Variation with strap

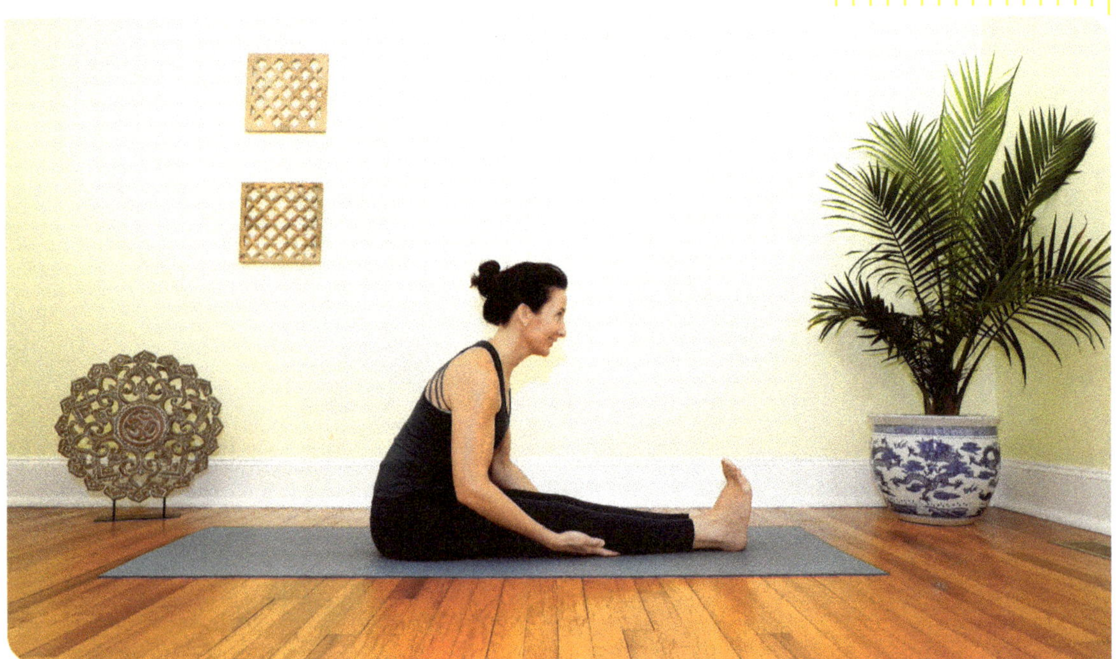

Variation with fingertips tucked

Head of Knee Pose, A

ALSO CALLED: Janu Sirsasana, A

WHAT IT DOES FOR YOUR HAMSTRINGS: This pose stretches the hamstrings and, like other seated forward folds, it also stretches the back muscles. With practice, over time, you will eventually be able to reach the foot on your extended leg. At that point, you can begin to use the hand-to-foot bind to increase the stretch all the way down your back from shoulders to the lumbar area. So as your hamstrings become long enough, the focus of this pose shifts from stretching your hamstrings to stretching your back muscles.

TUNE IT UP: This pose is often translated as Head *to* Knee Pose. But I greatly prefer the translation Head *of* Knee Pose, because it reminds you to focus on maintaining muscular activity in the bent leg. That will help protect your low back from strain.

Draw the bent knee forward (as if trying to point it toward the front of your mat) and press the bent knee and the pinky-toe side of that foot down as you fold. Keeping your leg muscles engaged and active recruits your low belly muscles to help protect your back.

The Head *to* Knee Pose translation is also a problem because it reinforces the mistaken idea that the goal is to put your head on your knee. It is not. Attempting to put your head on your knee makes your back and shoulders round—and the pelvis tucks under to copy, producing an ineffective hamstring stretch. Instead, reach your chest forward and lift your shoulders up away from the floor. Focus on building the core strength needed to do this pose safely and effectively.

Think chest forward, not head downward. The first thing that (eventually) touches your leg will be your low belly, not your face. Remember, when your shoulders round, your pelvis tucks under, releasing the hamstring stretch.

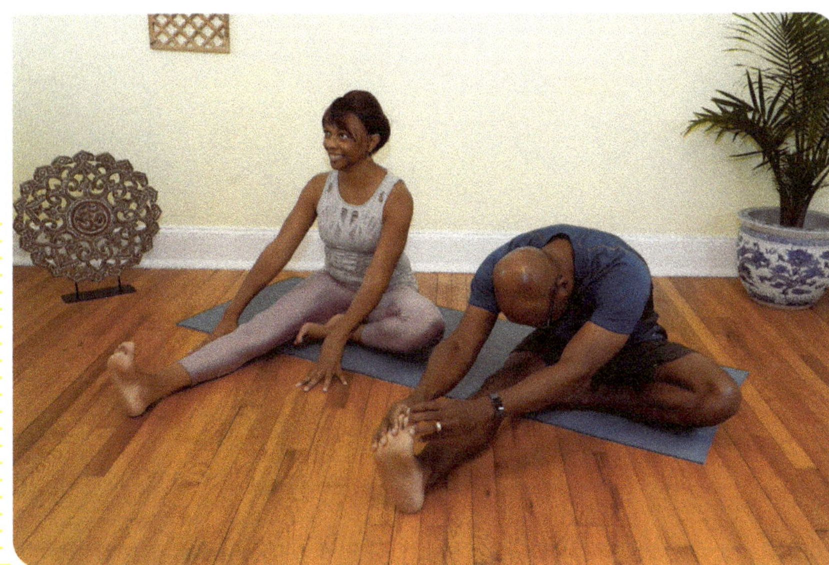

Head of Knee Pose. Correct alignment is on the left; putting your head on your knee is not the goal. Don't be a downer!

Half Monkey Pose

ALSO CALLED: Ardha Hanumanasana, Half Split Pose

WHAT IT DOES FOR YOUR HAMSTRINGS: Keeping the extended foot strongly flexed increases the hamstring stretching benefits. This is another hamstring stretching pose that tempts you to round your back.

TUNE IT UP: I highly recommend putting your hands on blocks to remove that downward temptation. Extend your chest forward toward your front ankle by reaching your ribs away from your hips.

Even as your hamstrings get longer, keep using the blocks for a while, and bend your elbows back toward the back of your mat (not out to the sides). This will keep you focused on reaching forward. Avoid bending your elbows outward; your upper arms will tend to rotate inward and cause your shoulders to round down. Focus on keeping your back straight and lengthening your waist.

It's also important to draw your inner, upper thighs toward each other to square your pelvis forward. Many people who have been doing this pose for a long time get a big surprise when they firmly draw their thighs inward, because the hamstring stretch is much more intense when you really have your hips squared forward. Your body is very clever at making little "work-around" adjustments to avoid stretching where it's tight or strengthening where it's weak. Small shifts—like pulling the inner thighs together—make a big difference.

Strongly flex the extended foot, pulling your toes toward your face. Don't let your straight leg be limp and lazy. Take big, slow breaths.

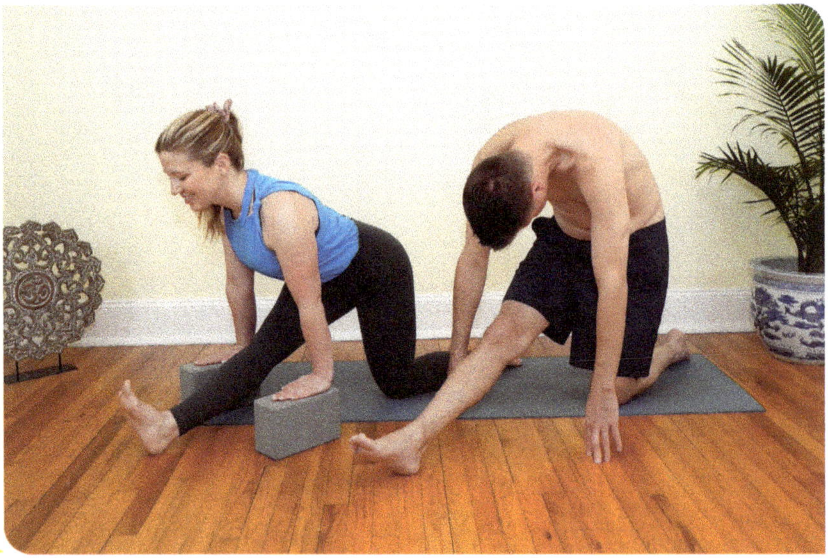

Half Monkey Pose. Correct alignment is on the left. Don't be a downer!

Reclined Hand to Big Toe Pose, A

ALSO CALLED: Supta Padangustasana, A

WHAT IT DOES FOR YOUR HAMSTRINGS: These are slightly easier versions than the standing pose (Utthita Hasta Padangustasana, A; see next pose). The reclined version takes the balancing component out, and the floor provides firm support for your back as you stretch your hamstrings.

TUNE IT UP: If you have tight hamstrings or back problems, it's a good idea to start with this reclined version, to build the strength and flexibility you'll need to try the standing pose sometime in the future.

In Reclined Hand to Big Toe, press down very firmly with the lower leg, shoulder, and hand. Focus on your alignment and deep breathing. In both the reclined and standing versions, focus on keeping both knees and elbows straight.

If your hamstrings are too tight to straighten your knee, use a strap and hold it so that both your elbow and knee are straight. No bent elbows. No bent knees. Your free hand should firmly press down into the thigh of the lower leg. Do not let that elbow rest on the floor. To better engage the oblique muscles in your waist, your lower arm should be kept straight and firm.

The knee of the non-raised leg will want to bend, and turn outward, which is usually due to tight hip flexors and weak waist and low belly muscles. So focus on pressing your lower leg straight, and keeping that kneecap pointed directly up at the ceiling.

When you're able to do the A version with your head lowered on the floor and with correct alignment and steady breathing, the next step is to lift your head, chest, and shoulders up off the floor. Draw the lifted leg closer by bending your elbow (keeping the raised leg, lowered leg, and elbow on the lowered arm straight). Moving into the lifted version intensifies both the hamstring stretch and core strengthening benefits of this pose. Many people hold their breath when they lift up. It's a natural tendency, because all of the auxiliary muscles of breathing are working very hard to hold this pose. Strengthen them by focusing on breathing deeply, steadily, and continuously. There's no sense in adding the challenge of lifting up if you are struggling to hold correct alignment in the lowered version. Do the first pose, and then add the lifting action as you gain strength and flexibility.

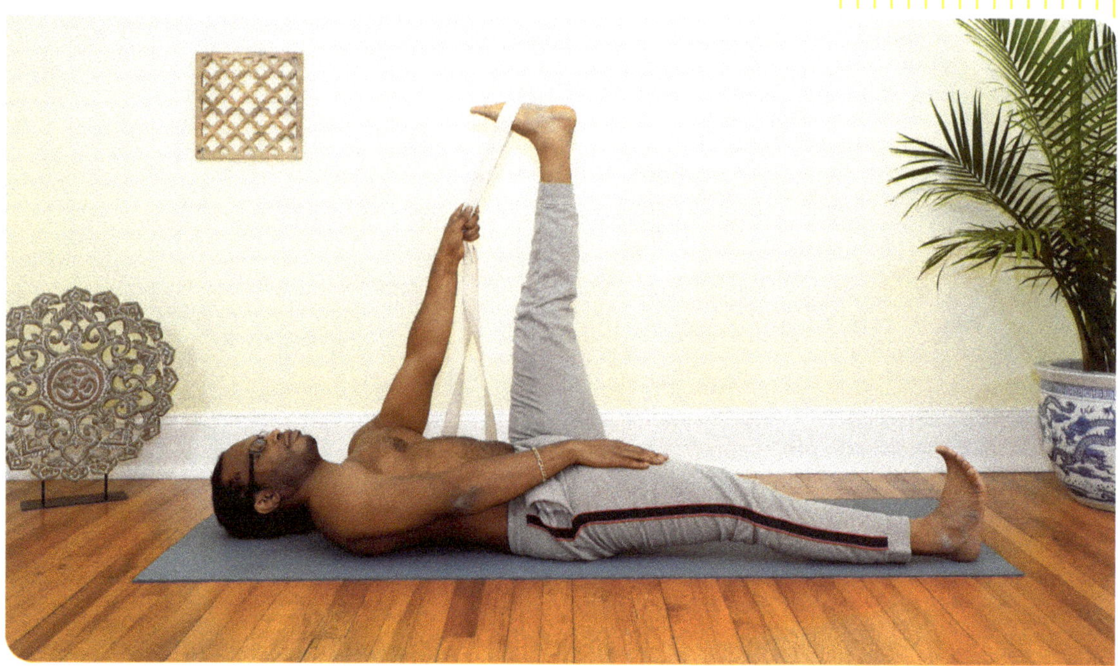

Reclined Hand to Big Toe Pose, A, variation with strap and head down

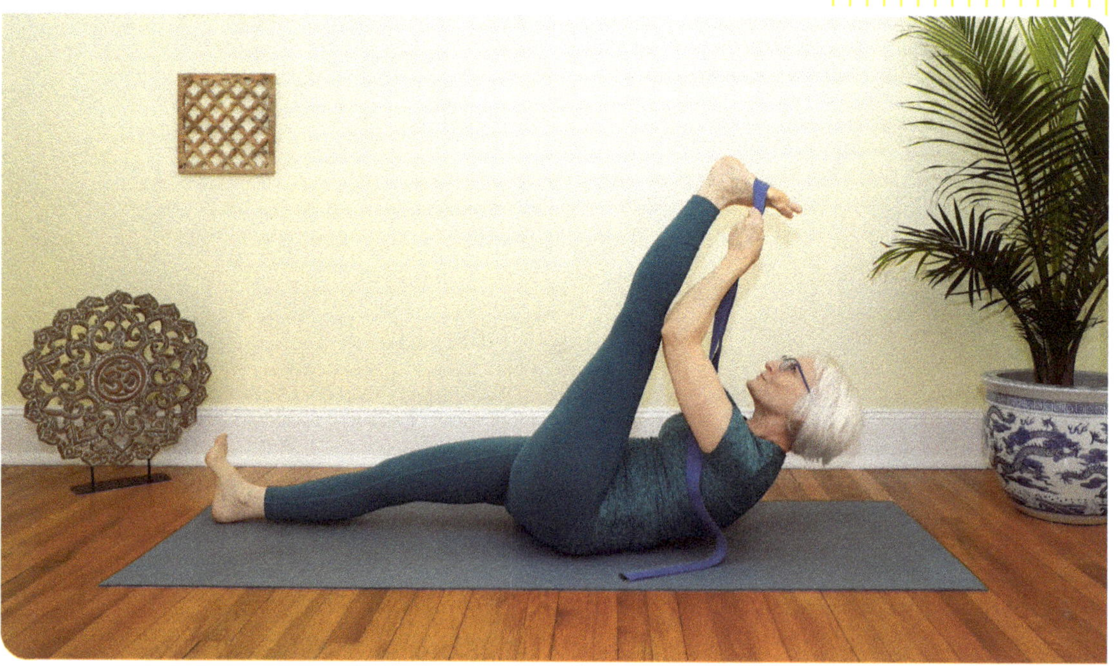

Reclined Hand to Big Toe Pose, A, variation with strap

Extended Hand to Big Toe Pose, A

ALSO CALLED: Utthita Hasta Padangustasana, A

WHAT IT DOES FOR YOUR HAMSTRINGS: Stretches your hamstrings and calf muscles on the lifted leg. Like all standing balance poses that are done on one foot, it also strengthens the hamstrings, quads, and hip stabilizers on the standing leg.

TUNE IT UP: If your hamstrings are very tight, you can practice this pose by holding your bent knee. This helps develop flexibility in your hip joint and strength in your standing leg, abdominal muscles, and shoulders while you wait for your hamstrings to get longer. You can also use a strap on the ball of the lifted foot if you can't reach it. Using a strap will stretch your hamstrings more than holding the bent knee, but extending the leg does make balancing more difficult.

In all versions, draw your inner thighs toward each other to activate your groin and low belly muscles, and steady your balance.

Always draw your shoulders back and lift your chest. Look forward, not down at the floor. Remember, your head weighs eight to twelve pounds. It's heavy! When you look down, your entire body has to compensate to support your heavy head. Keep your ears over your shoulders. Imagine you're looking out at the horizon. I think of this as *looking the world straight in the eye*. Keep your eyes steady on one point.

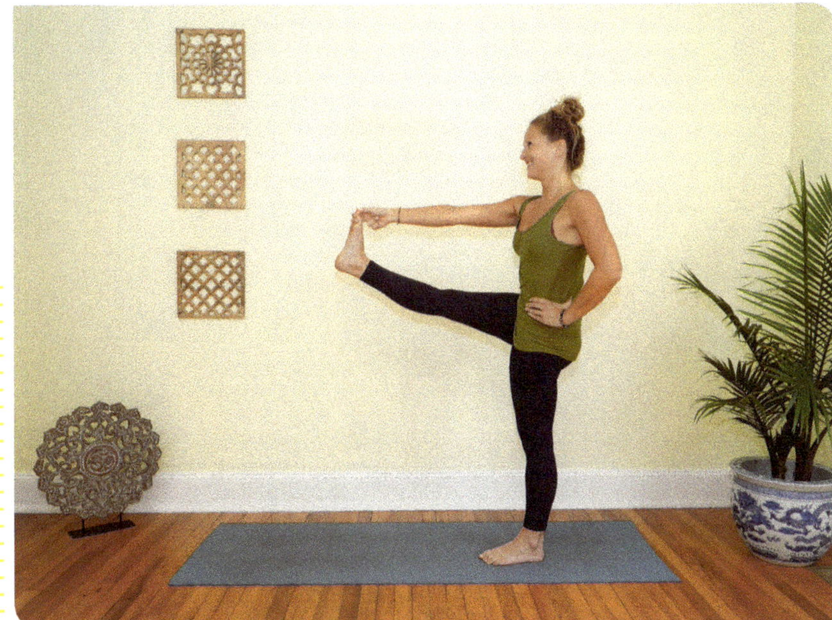

Extended Hand to Big Toe Pose, A

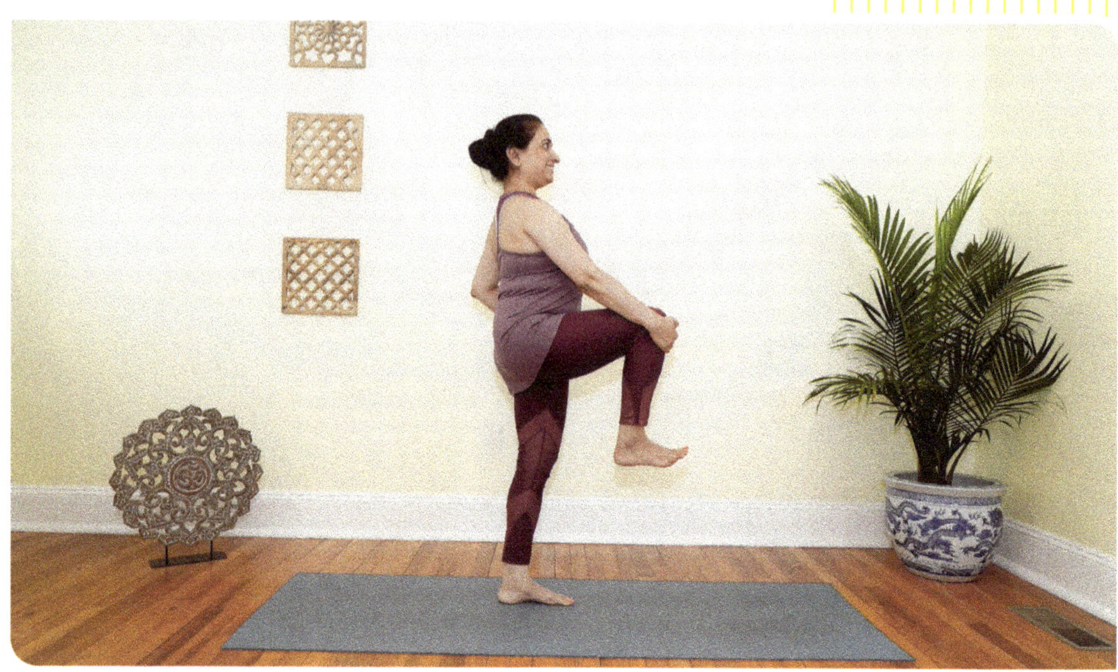

Variation holding knee

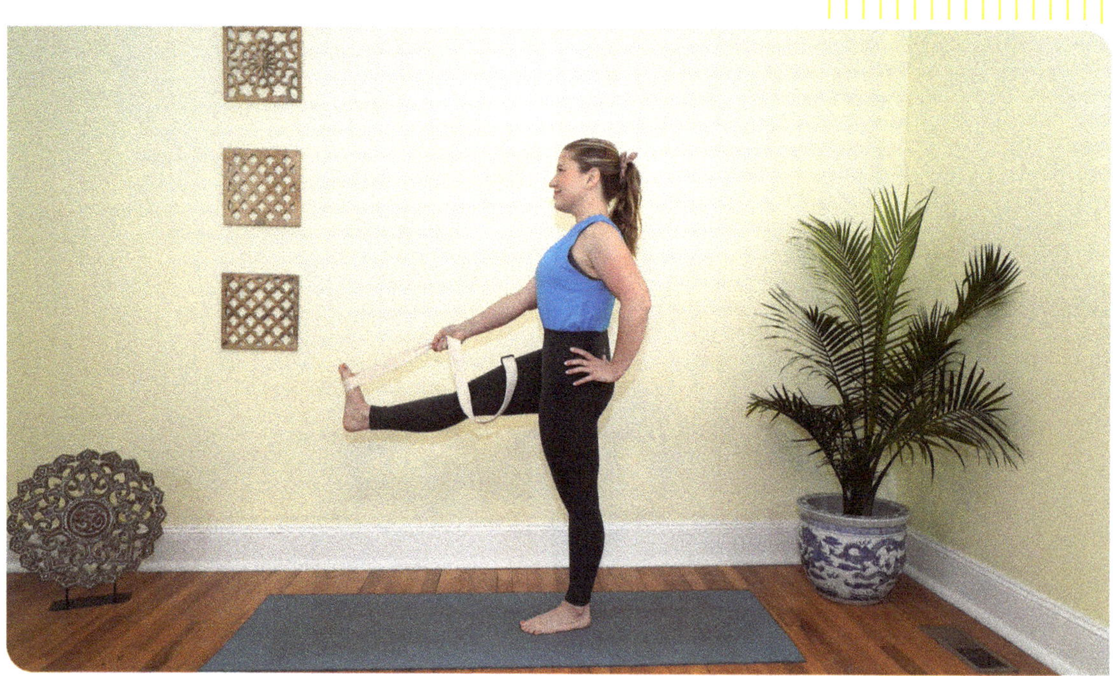

Variation with strap

Upward Facing Intense Stretch Pose

ALSO CALLED: Urdhva Mukha Pachimottansana

WHAT IT DOES FOR YOUR HAMSTRINGS: Stretches your hamstrings and calves, and because it's a balancing pose also builds focus.

TUNE IT UP: If your hamstrings are tight, use a strap. You can also keep one knee bent with your foot on the floor (see photos). This enables you to stretch one set of hamstrings at a time while you're building strength in your thighs, hip flexors, back, and abdominal muscles.

In all versions, your elbows and the lifted knee(s) should be straight. Reach high enough up the strap to get your elbows straight.

Focus on lifting your chest and drawing your shoulder blades down toward your waist. Draw your inner thighs toward each other.

Breathe. Observe what's happening in your body and in your mind. Keep your eyes still. Don't look all over the room as you practice.

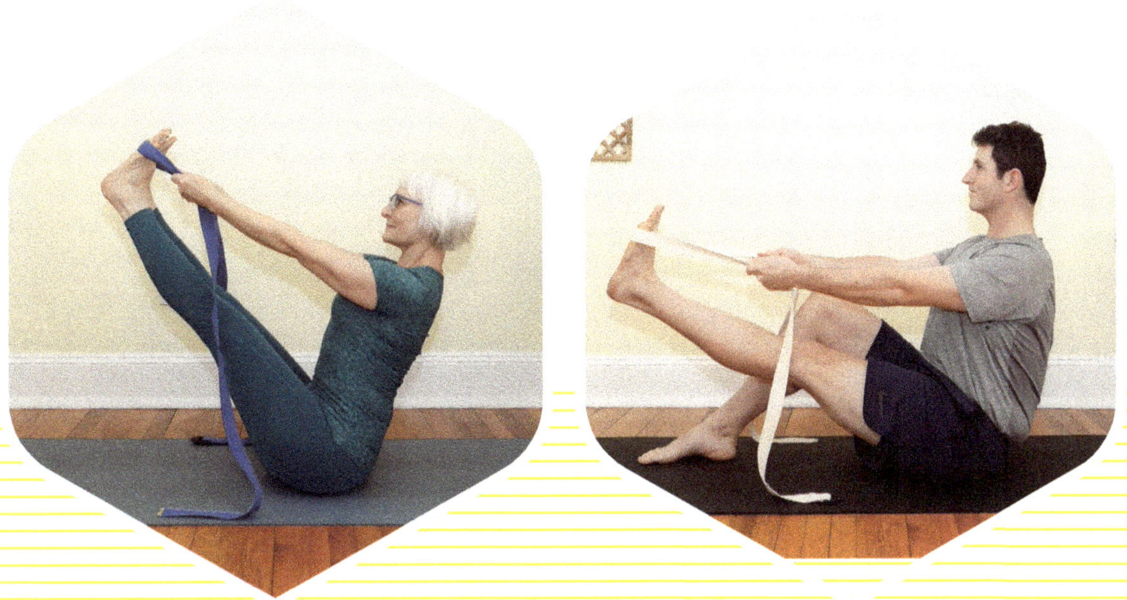

Upward Facing Intense Stretch Pose, variation with strap

Variation with strap and bent knee

Half Standing Forward Fold Pose

ALSO CALLED: Ardha Uttanasana

WHAT IT DOES FOR YOUR HAMSTRINGS: This pose is repeated often in yoga classes, because it is part of the traditional sun-salute sequence that's commonly used as a warm-up. It builds strength in your hamstrings because they contract to lift and lower the weight of your head, shoulders, and torso.

TUNE IT UP: If your low back and hamstrings are weak or tight, or if your low back is easily irritated, bend your knees and press your palms firmly into your thighs. This uses your arm strength to reduce the amount of weight your back muscles have to lift.

The most important actions of Half Standing Forward Fold are to draw your shoulders up onto your back and extend your chest forward. But because this pose usually comes in the middle of a fast, flowing sequence, it's easy to forget those two crucial actions. Try to be mindful of doing them.

You should also recruit your other leg muscles—primarily the stabilizers on the outer hips—to help protect your back. To engage these other leg muscles, press your feet outward, as if sliding them away from each other. This outward action of the feet will turn on large muscles in your upper legs and hips, and take some load off your low back.

A lot of people mistakenly think that the goal of this pose is to touch the floor. It's not. Eventually your hands may reach the floor, but that's not the focus. Keep drawing your shoulders up onto your back, and extending your chest forward. Do not round your back trying to touch the floor. There's nothing magic down there.

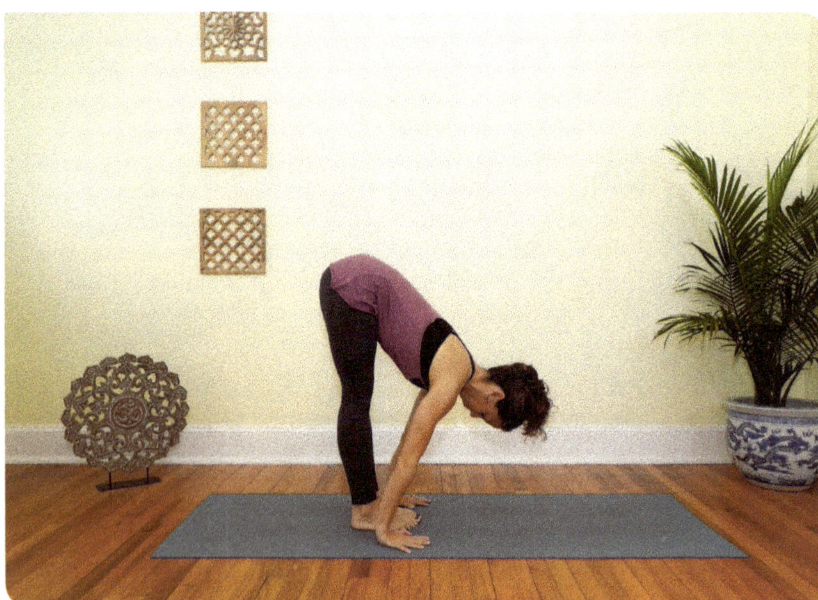

Half Standing Forward Fold Pose

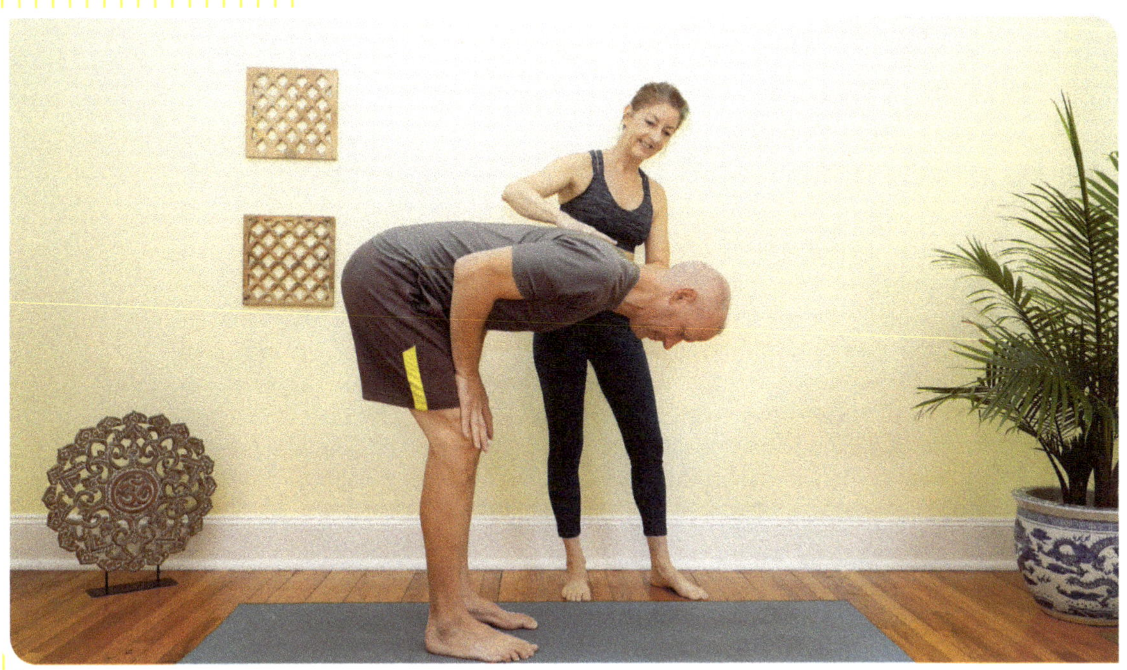

Variation with knees and elbows bent

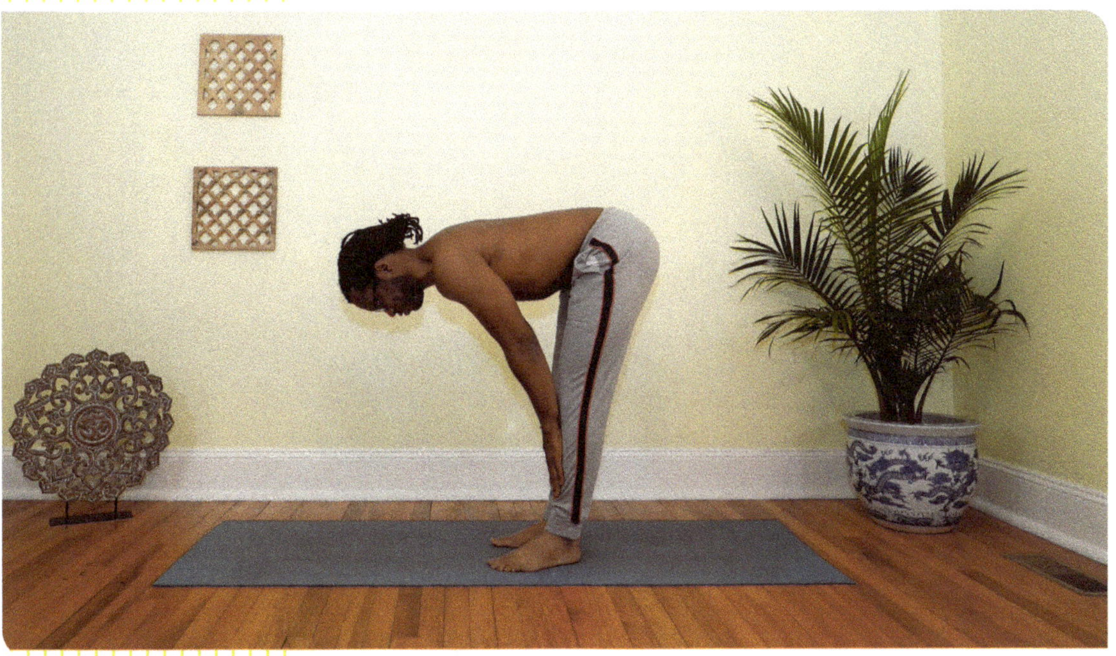

Touching the floor is not the goal!

Upward Plank Pose

ALSO CALLED: Purvottanasana, Reverse Plank Pose

WHAT IT DOES FOR YOUR HAMSTRINGS: This pose is a good way to build strength in the hamstrings and glutes, but it calls for a lot of flexibility across the chest, shoulders, and upper arms.

TUNE IT UP: If your hamstrings are weak or your chest and shoulders are tight, bend one or both knees to recruit your thigh muscles (your quadriceps) to help lift your hips. Eventually, you'll be able to keep both knees straight and your toes pointed forward.

One day, when your hips get high enough, your toes will touch the floor. But that's not the goal. Press your heels down and pull them back toward you as if you're trying to drag them toward your hands (they won't actually move).

Pull your shoulder blades toward the center of your back to help lift your chest from the back. This is a big stretch on the front of your upper arms (your biceps). Breathe.

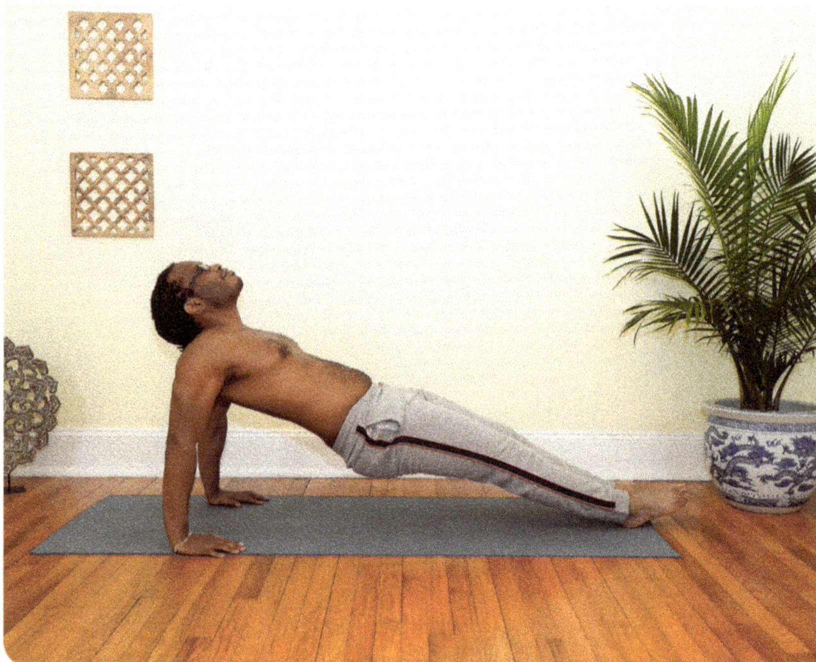

Upward Plank Pose

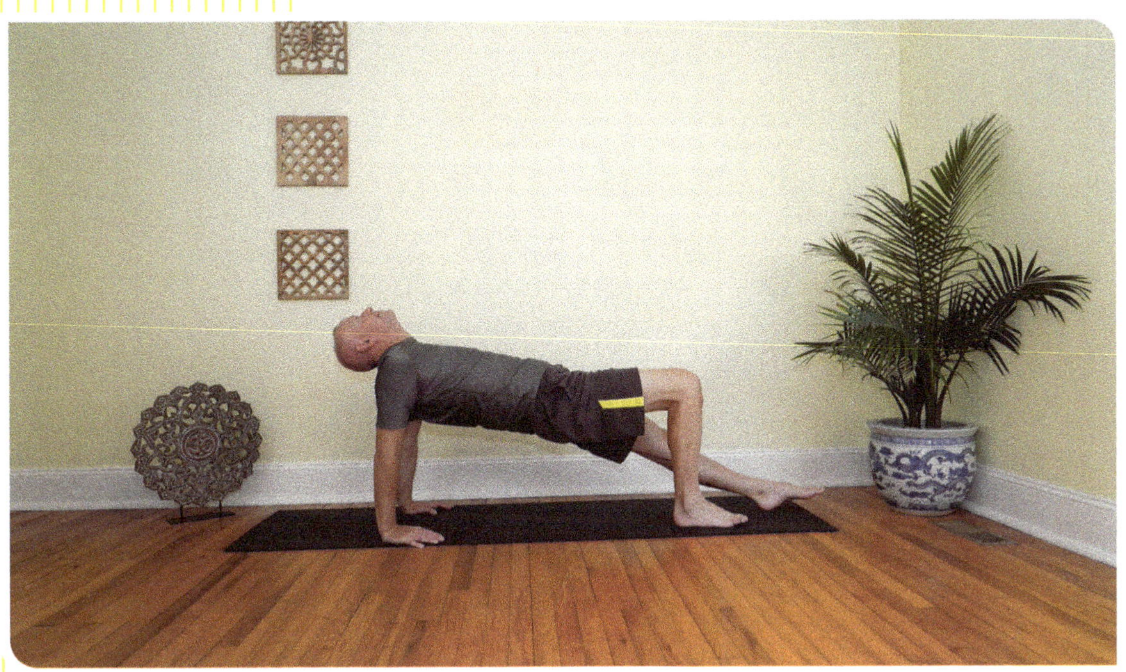

Variation with bent knee

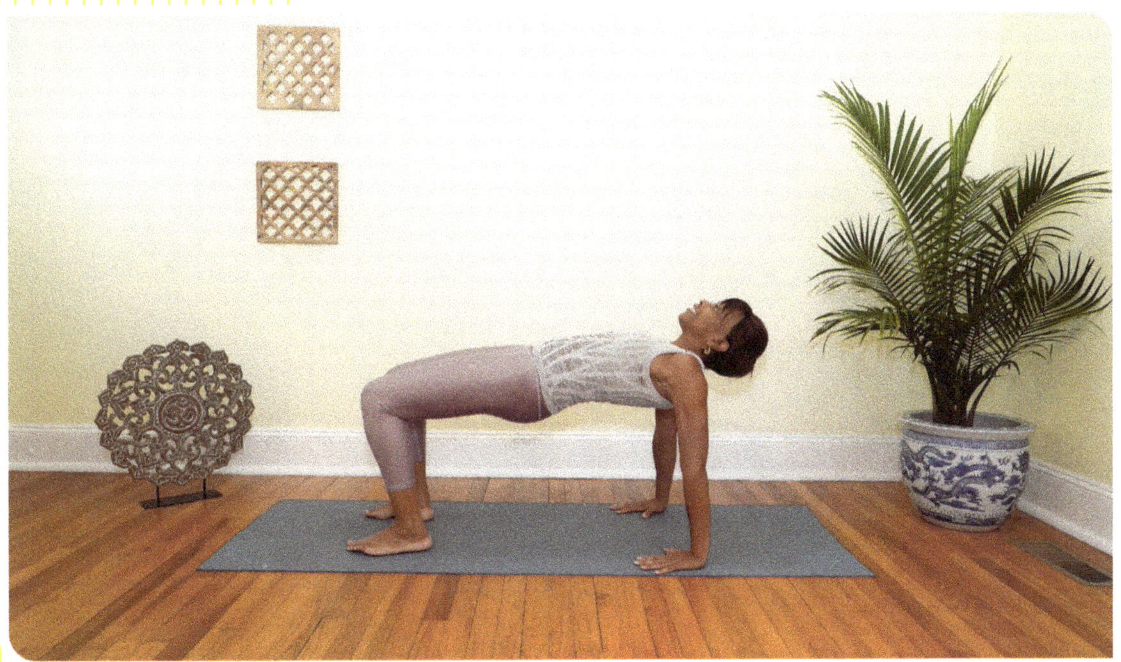

Variation with both knees bent

One-Legged Bridge Pose

ALSO CALLED: Eka Pada Setu Bandhasana

Locust Pose, variation

ALSO CALLED: Salabhasana, variation

WHAT THEY DO FOR YOUR HAMSTRINGS: These poses strengthen your hamstrings and glutes. If your shoulders are weak or your chest is tight, both of these poses will help strengthen and stretch them as well.

TUNE IT UP: In One-Legged Bridge Pose, press the foot on the floor down and forward. You can hold a strap running across the mat, under your body, one side in each hand (hold it with your palms turned up toward the ceiling). Or grab the edges of your mat, pulling outward to increase the strengthening and stretching benefits.

In Locust Pose, variation, bend your knees and flex your feet firmly, keeping the soles parallel to the floor. If your hamstrings and shoulders are weak, or your chest is very tight, you can keep your forehead, hands, and thighs on the floor. For a more intense challenge, lift your forehead, hands, and thighs a few inches off the floor (see photo).

Keep your elbows straight in both poses, and draw your shoulder blades toward the center of your back. It's very difficult to breathe in these poses, so focus on steadying your breath and keeping your eyes on one point. Keeping your eyes still will help steady your mind as well.

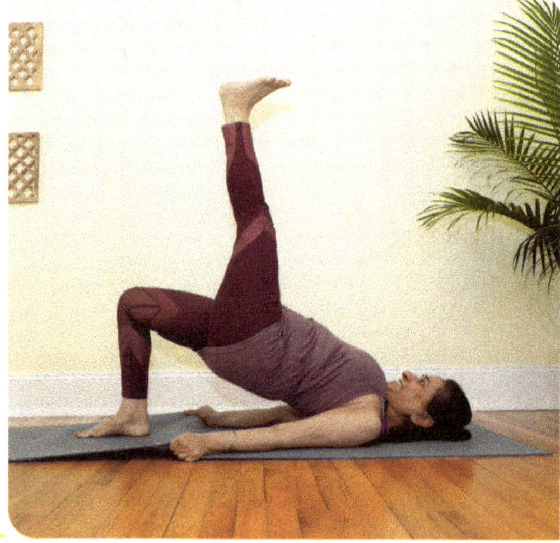

One-Legged Bridge Pose, holding mat

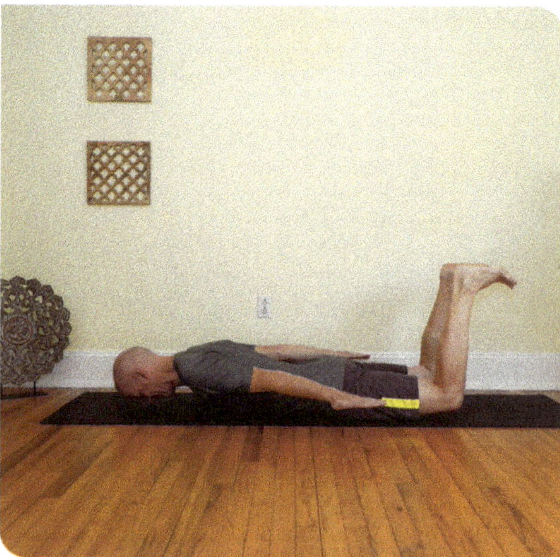

Locust Pose, variation

Half-Bound Lotus Standing Forward Fold Pose

ALSO CALLED: Ardha Baddha Padmottanasana

WHAT IT DOES FOR YOUR HAMSTRINGS: Like all standing forward folds, this pose strengthens your hamstrings, especially as you enter and exit the pose. Your hamstrings must be quite strong for this pose, because you can use only one set of hamstrings to lower and come back upright. Your other leg is out of the equation. The hamstrings on your standing leg have to contract to control the descending weight of your torso, head, and shoulders, and then lift all that weight back up again. This pose is also a big outer hip stretch on the bent leg side.

TUNE IT UP: It helps to bend your standing knee a little to recruit your thigh and glute muscles to help carry these loads.

When you first start trying this pose, put a block under your lower hand to reduce how far you have to lower and lift your torso weight. At first, put a small bend in your standing knee; don't fold all the way down, and set your gaze slightly forward to help with balance. By looking forward, your neck and upper back will also lift the weight of your head (that's 8-12 pounds), which takes some of the stretching force off of your hamstrings.

As you progress, you'll change how you do this pose bit by bit. Eventually you'll lower your head enough to look at the back of your mat, or even up toward the ceiling behind you. Make this change in head position, and gazing point, slowly.

It will take several months for your body to develop an ability to balance while upside down. It will also take a while to develop the flexibility to reach the lifted foot behind your back. Don't struggle to grab your foot. Work on building the strength and length to enter, balance, and exit. Be patient, and give your body time to learn how to do it. Over time, this pose will make your legs and your mental focus very strong.

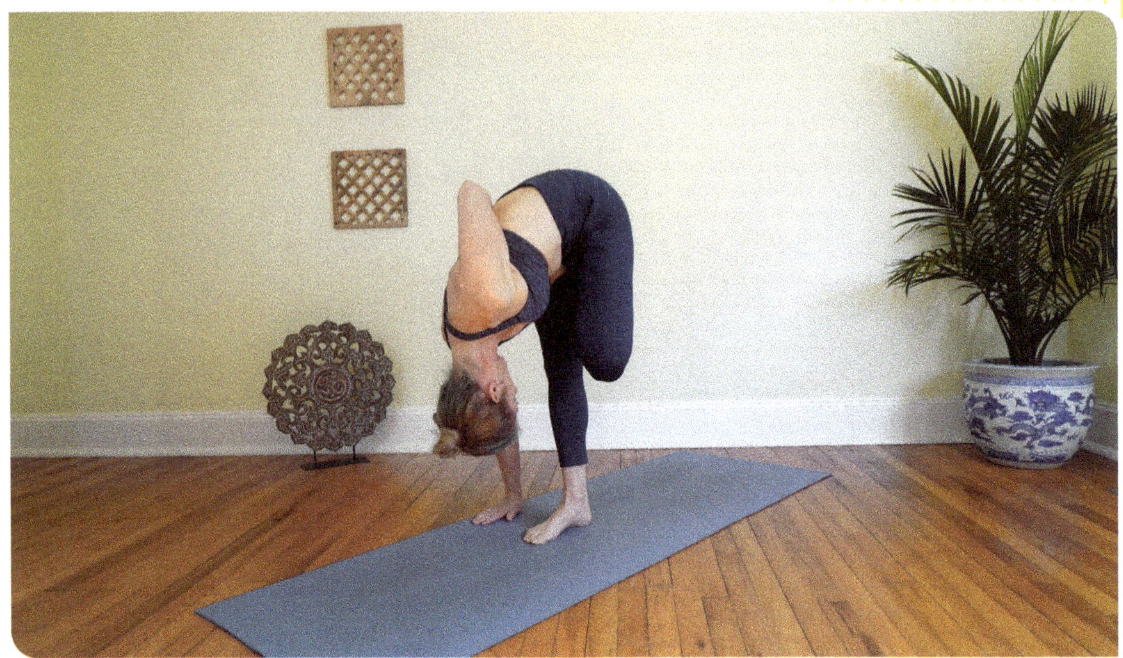

Half-Bound Lotus Standing Forward Fold Pose

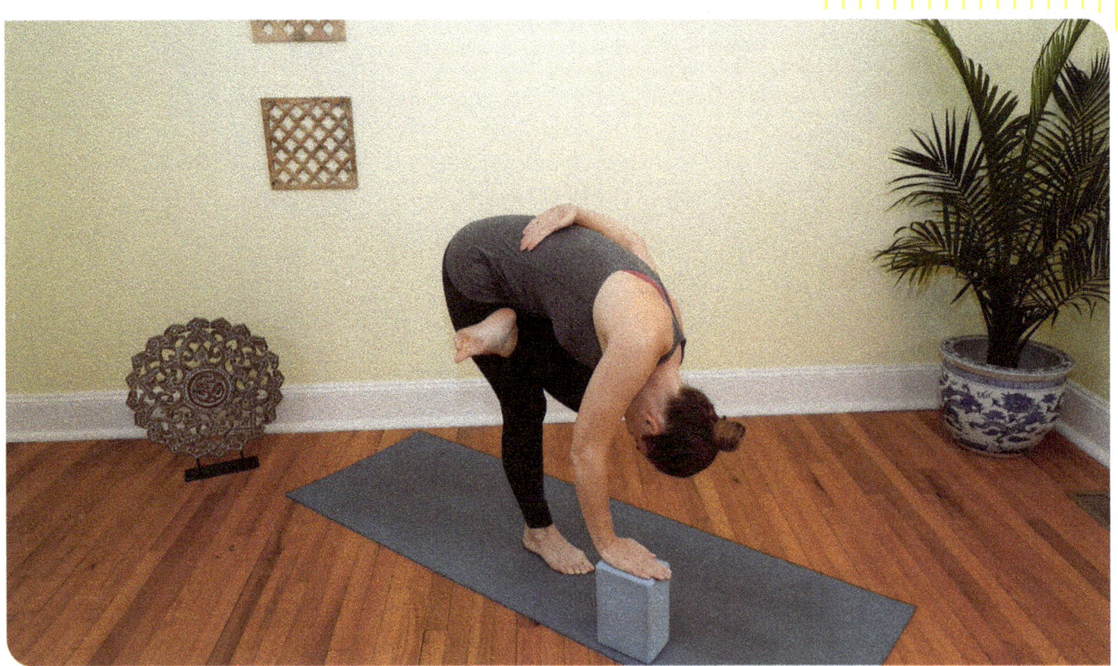

Variation with bent knee and block

Revolved Lunge Pose

ALSO CALLED: Parivrtta Anjaneyasana

WHAT IT DOES FOR YOUR OUTER HIPS: Strengthens the quads and hamstrings, and stretches the glutes, TFL, and IT-band on your front leg, by turning the centerline of your torso toward your front thigh.

TUNE IT UP: You can do Revolved Lunge Pose either with your back knee on the floor, or lifted. When your back knee is on the floor, balancing becomes easier, but turning your torso to hook your elbow over your front knee becomes more difficult (because your pelvis is less able to help turn your torso). When your back knee is lifted off the floor, balancing gets trickier, but the revolving action becomes easier (because your pelvis and back hip are free to turn and help rotate your torso).

If your back knee is lifted, work to keep it straight. Do not let your back knee bend (unless it's on the floor, of course).

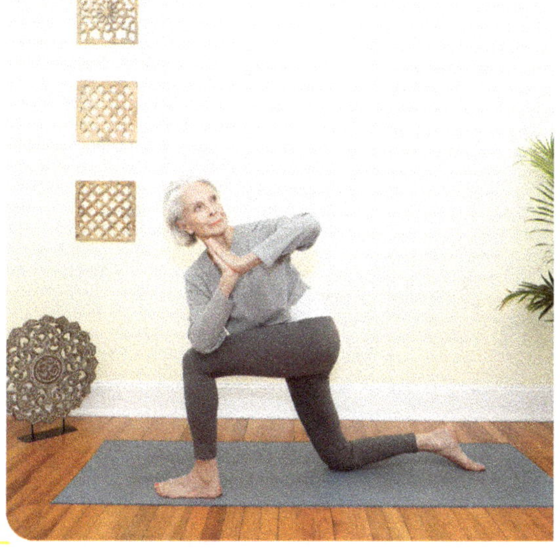

Revolved Low Lunge Pose

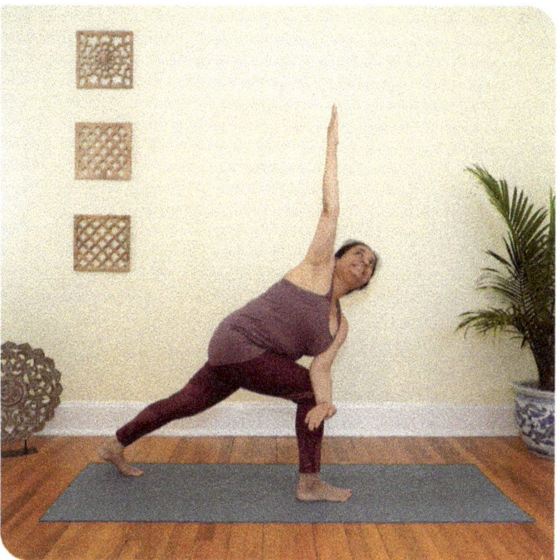

Revolved High Lunge Pose, variation

Revolved Triangle Pose

ALSO CALLED: Parivrtta Trikonasana

WHAT IT DOES FOR YOUR OUTER HIPS: Stretches the glutes and IT-band on your front leg by turning the centerline of your torso toward your front thigh.

TUNE IT UP: The most important actions for this pose are turning your back thigh inward (to turn your pelvis and low back), and extending your chest forward. There's a tendency to let your chest curl down toward the floor, and for your back hip to turn outward. You must rotate your torso using your back inner thigh and low belly. Draw your inner thighs firmly toward each other.

Do not use your arms and hands to crank your way into this turn. That won't work. Use your legs and pelvis to turn your torso instead.

When you first start trying this pose, raise your bottom hand by putting a block under it. Do not strain to touch the floor. That's not the goal, and it's counter-productive, because focusing on trying to reach the floor will make your chest curl downward. Remember, when your shoulders round down, your pelvis tucks under. Your chest should be extending forward, away from your hips. Your spine should be moving toward a straight position, not hunching or rounded.

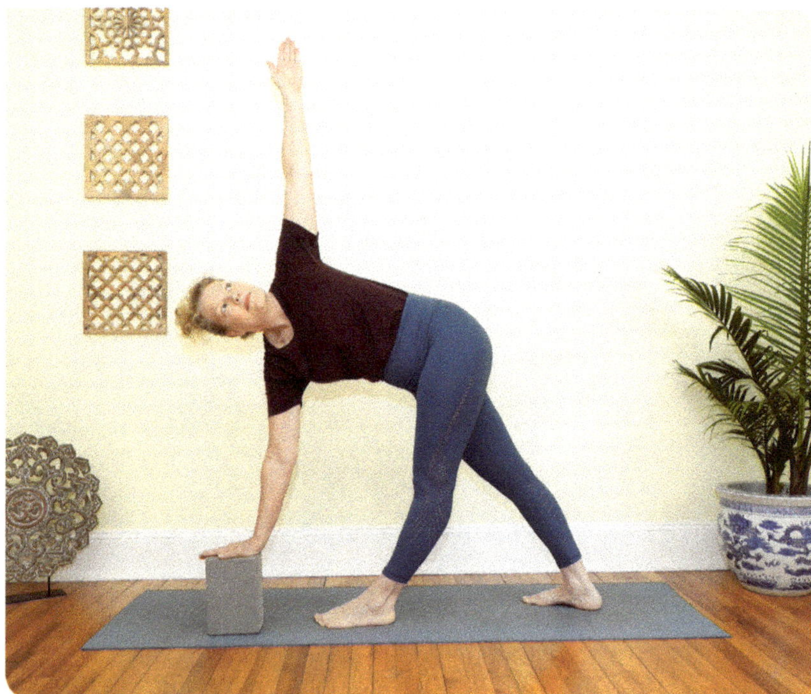

Revolved Triangle Pose, variation with block

Revolved Chair Pose

ALSO CALLED: Parivrtta Utkatasana

WHAT IT DOES FOR YOUR OUTER HIPS: Stretches the glutes, TFL, and IT-band on your front leg by turning the centerline of your torso toward one thigh.

TUNE IT UP: The traditional instruction in Revolved Chair Pose is to keep your knees lined up side by side, but be aware that you can't rotate as far with your knees level and your pelvis turned to face forward toward the front of your mat. You can intensify the stretch in your outer hip by drawing the knee that you are turning toward (the one your elbow is on) back, and letting the other knee slide forward. This pulls one hip toward the back of your mat and creates a more intense gluteal stretch. Neither way is right or wrong, as long as you maintain overall central alignment with the weight or force moving through the centers of the bones and joints. So choose how you do it based on what you want to accomplish. If you want to stretch your outer hip, let your knees be uneven. Don't worry. You won't get a ticket from the yoga police if you draw one knee back, and your glutes and low back will thank you.

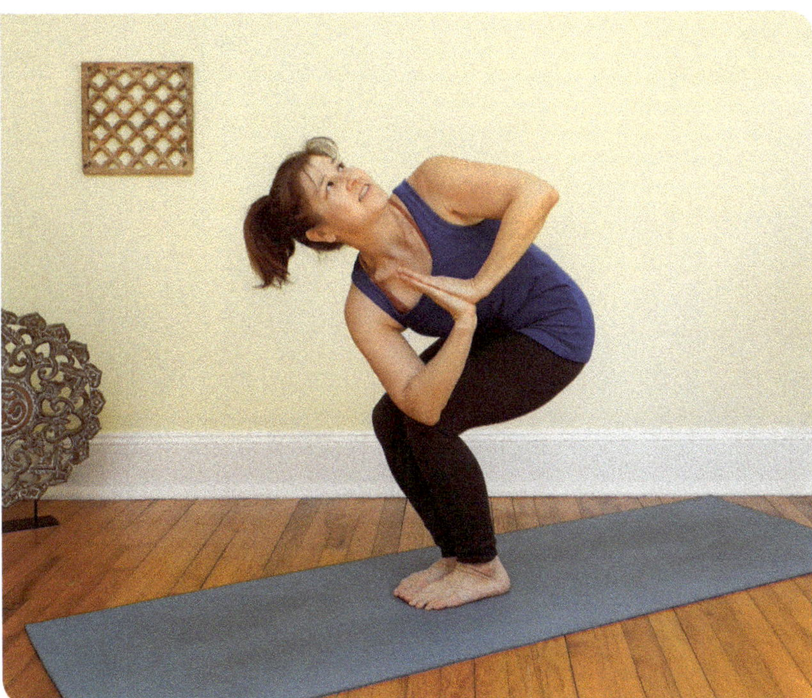

Revolved Chair Pose

Revolved Hand to Big Toe Pose

ALSO CALLED: Parivrtta Hasta Padangusthasana

WHAT IT DOES FOR YOUR OUTER HIPS: Stretches your glutes and IT-band by turning your torso toward the lifted leg.

TUNE IT UP: If you have tight hips, start by lying on your back, and use a strap to hold the lifted foot. In this supine variation, you'll have to work hard to keep the hip of the lifted leg down on the mat. Many people mistakenly think that the goal is to touch the lifted foot to the floor on the other side of their body. Nope. Don't roll sideways and let the hip come off the floor to follow the movement of the lifted leg. This is pointless, because it erases the benefits of this pose. When your hip rolls up off the floor, both the glute stretch and the strengthening work of holding that side of your body down are released.

The seated version requires even more abdominal strength, because you must lift your chest and ribs away from your hips while you turn. Even if you can do the seated or standing variations of this pose, there are advantages to doing the supine (lying down) variation. It allows you to focus on stretching your glutes and outer hip stabilizers while protecting your low back, as you build strength in your abdominal muscles.

In all versions, work to keep both knees and elbows straight. If you use a strap to reach your foot, hold onto the strap close enough to your foot to get your elbow straight. If you have tight hamstrings but choose to hold your foot (not using a strap), your knee will be bent; still keep trying to straighten both knees.

Do not let the lifted leg be lazy—keep pressing it forward. This action takes a lot of effort, and will also tend to pull your shoulder up off the floor or forward. Work to pull that shoulder back over your hip or down to the floor.

In all variations, the action is to push with your foot, and pull back with your shoulder (not with your biceps). Keep your elbows straight. Explore the sensations of effort and stretch. Breathe fully.

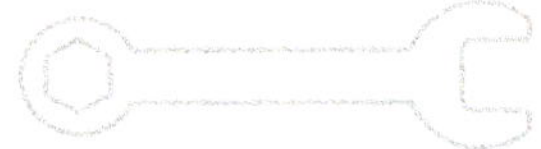

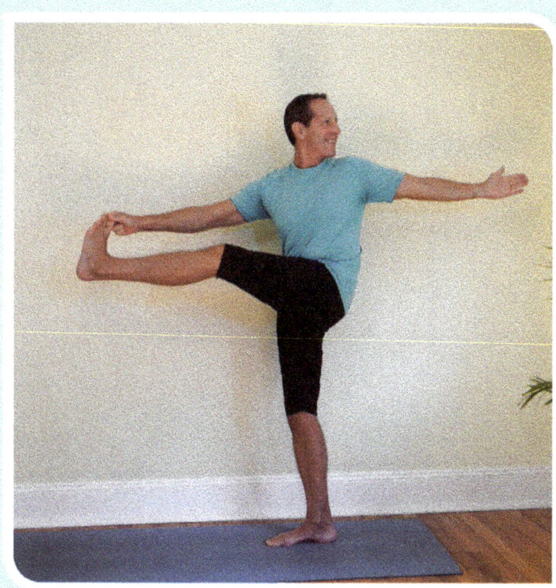
Revolved Hand to Big Toe Pose

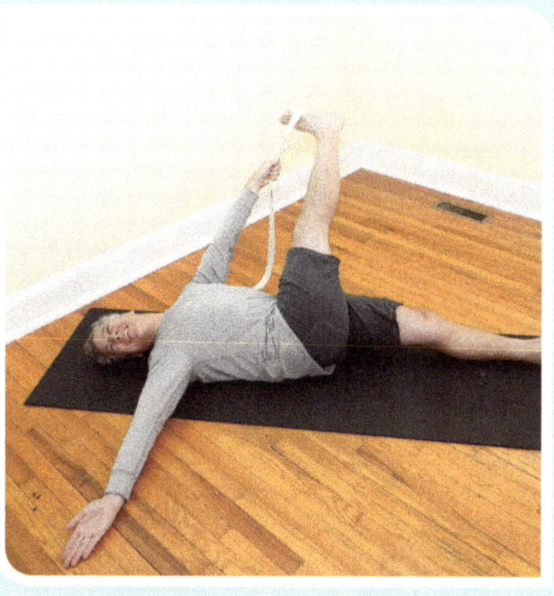
Supine variation with strap

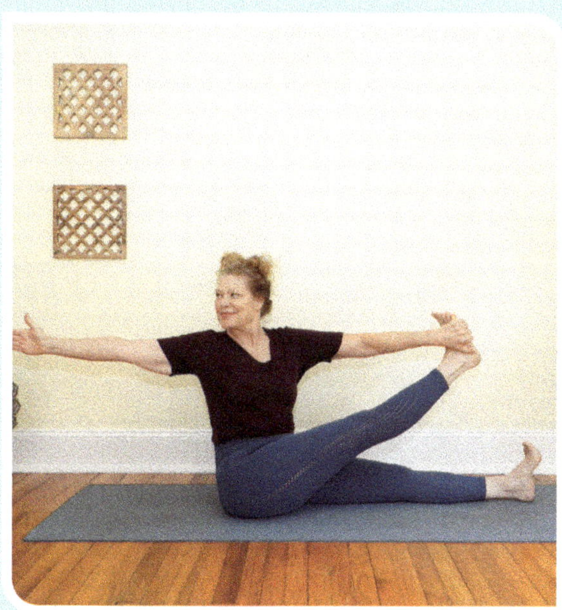
Seated variation

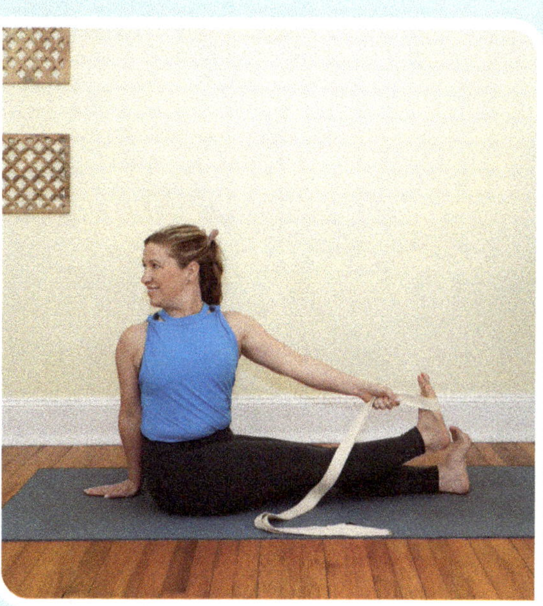
Seated variation with strap

Seated and Supine Spinal Twist Poses

ALSO CALLED: Ardha Matsyendrasana, Half Lord of the Fishes Pose and Supta Matsyendrasana, Supine Lord of the Fishes Pose

WHAT THEY DO FOR YOUR OUTER HIPS: Stretch your glutes, TFL, and IT-band by drawing your thigh across the centerline of your torso with different degrees of intensity.

TUNE IT UP: This twist can be done seated or lying down (supine). You can also do this pose with the bottom leg straight. The legs are very important for supporting your low back in both versions. In both versions, draw your inner thighs firmly toward each other and press the outer edge of your bottom foot (pinky-toe-side) down into the floor. Pulling your inner thighs together will help activate your abdominal muscles and stabilize your lower back. In the supine version, you can relieve any sensation of excess compression or pinching in your lower back by tucking your sitting bones very slightly toward your feet. Focus on lifting your chest away from your hips in both versions to increase the stretch.

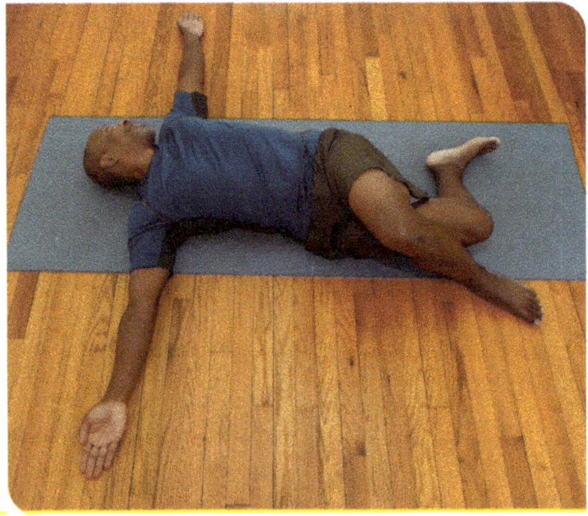

Supine Spinal Twist Pose

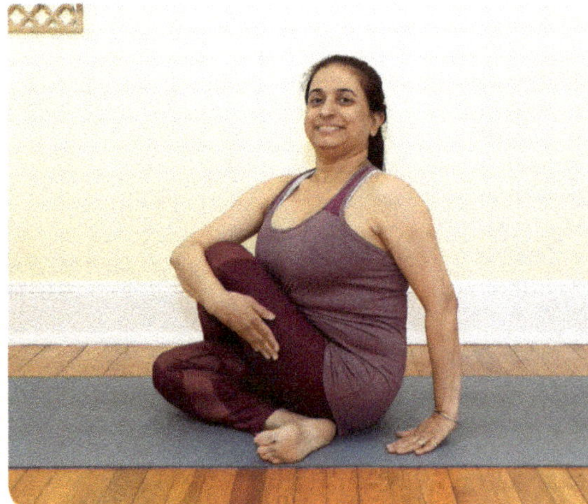

Seated Spinal Twist Pose

The Sage's Pose, C

ALSO CALLED: Marichyasana, C

WHAT IT DOES FOR YOUR OUTER HIPS: Stretches your glutes, TFL, and IT-band by drawing your thigh across the centerline of your torso. It also strengthens your groins through drawing your inner thighs toward each other.

TUNE IT UP: This pose requires a lot of abdominal strength and outer-hip flexibility, because your front arm is bound around the bent knee with your hands (eventually) clasped behind your back. This bound variation draws your thigh as far as possible across the centerline of your torso, creating a very intense stretch in your glutes on the bent knee side. If you cannot clasp your hands behind your back, or if your abs and back are weak or tight, you can keep the back hand on the floor. Have a straight elbow and sit up as tall as you can (see photo).

In all of these glute-stretching poses and variations, focus on lifting your chest away from your hips and drawing your spine upright. Do not get overly focused on turning around. That rotation will come in time, as your glutes open and your abdominal muscles become stronger.

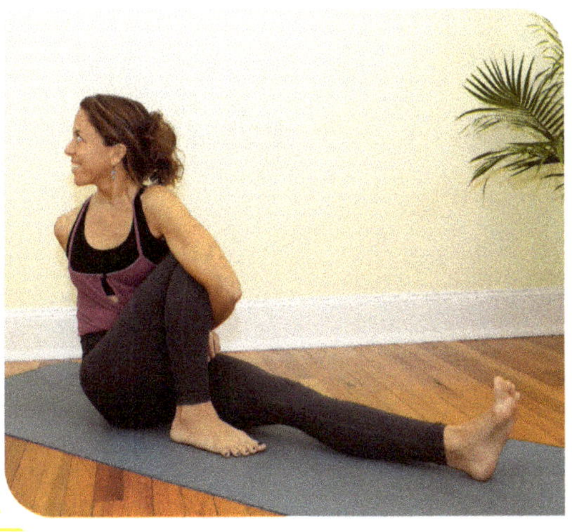

The Sage's Pose, C

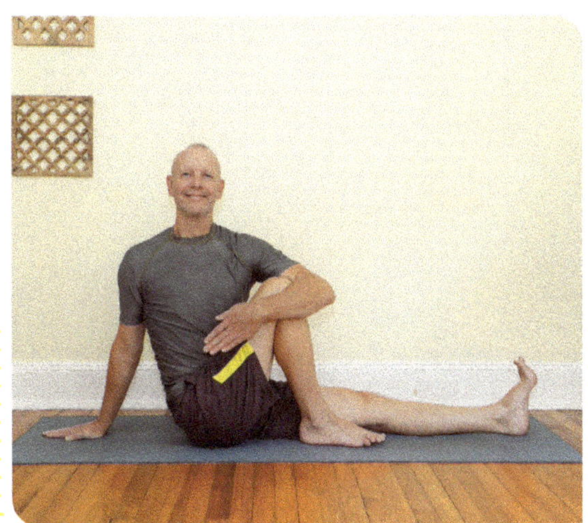

The Sage's Pose, C, variation with hand on floor and forearm in front

MECHANIC'S NOTE: Seated and Standing Twists

Many people make the mistake of positioning their legs and immediately turning around as far as they can into seated twists like The Sage's Pose as well as standing twists like Revolved Lunge. I highly recommend moving into these types of deep twists very slowly, and in a step-by-step manner. First, while facing forward, sit or stand up tall and firmly pull your inner thighs toward each other. Second, roll your back shoulder open, and turn your chest while still facing forward with your head. Last, turn your head and neck. Resist the urge to crank yourself around using your hands and arms, or to move quickly into the turn; those actions can injure your back. Using your arms too much also prevents you from building the core and leg strength it takes to do these poses safely and effectively.

Focus on sitting or standing up as straight as possible, and let the revolving action happen naturally starting from the hips and moving up. Be patient. Breathe deeply and steady your eyes on one point. Do not force your way into these poses. Respect your wonderful body and treat it with care.

The Sage's Pose, A and B

ALSO CALLED: Marichyasana, A and B

WHAT THEY DO FOR YOUR OUTER HIPS: Stretch your glutes by rotating the thigh bones inside your hip sockets in the pelvis. In version A, you stretch the glutes on the bent leg side. In version B, you stretch the glutes on both legs, because the leg that was straight in version A is now rotated outward with the foot tucked into your hip crease. Both versions also stretch the groins (your adductors).

TUNE IT UP: Eventually, you'll be able to clasp your hands behind your back in both versions. But it takes a really long time to develop the shoulder blade mobility needed for that. In the meantime, hold a strap behind your back, and pull your hands backward, straightening your elbows if possible.

When you first start trying this pose, stay upright—don't worry about folding forward. Later, as you develop more gluteal and shoulder flexibility, and more abdominal strength, start to fold forward just a few inches and stop. Take it little by little over many months. Approach these poses with care and patience. Breathe. Do not force your way into these complex poses, you'll be sorry. Just take it slow and steady.

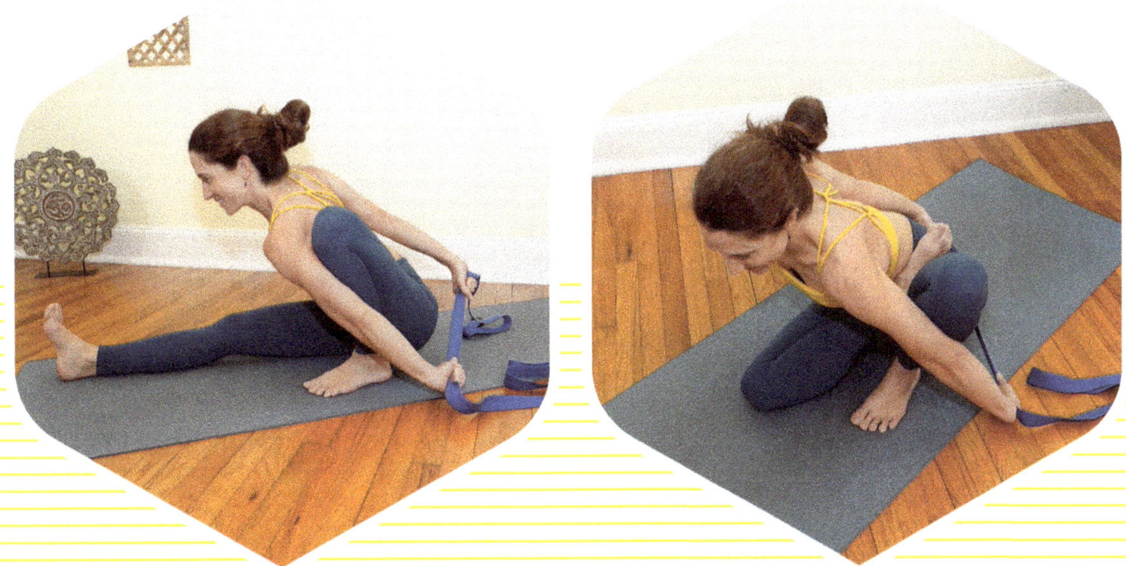

The Sage's Pose, A, variation with strap

The Sage's Pose, B, variation with strap

Cow Face Pose

ALSO CALLED: Gomukhasana

WHAT IT DOES FOR YOUR OUTER HIPS: Uses outward (external) rotation of the thigh bones to stretch your glutes and TFL.

TUNE IT UP: If you have very tight glutes, limited knee flexion, or low back weakness or pain, do this pose lying on the floor, holding onto your feet, ankles, shins, or knees.

You can also sit up on one or more blocks to reduce the amount of weight pressing down on your hip, knee, and ankle joints.

If you're flexible enough to sit flat on the floor with no hip, knee, or ankle discomfort, you can begin to fold forward. How far you fold is determined by the flexibility of your glutes and strength of your back and abdominal muscles. Squeeze your upper inner thighs toward each other and, if seated, press the outer edges of your feet into the floor to help support your back. Do not round your shoulders. As you lean forward, keep lifting your chest and drawing your shoulders up, away from the floor. Notice the sensations of stretching and strengthening. Go slow. Remain calm. Breathe.

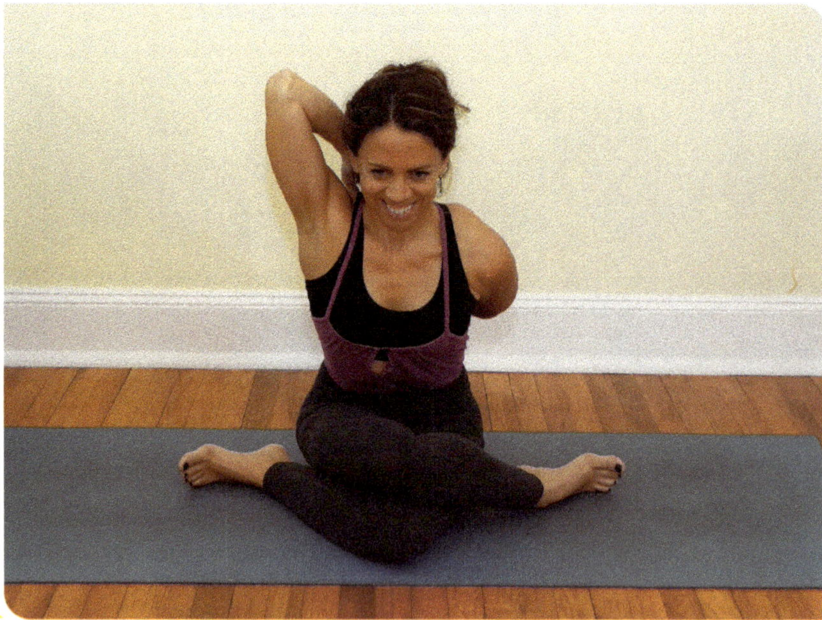

Cow Face Pose

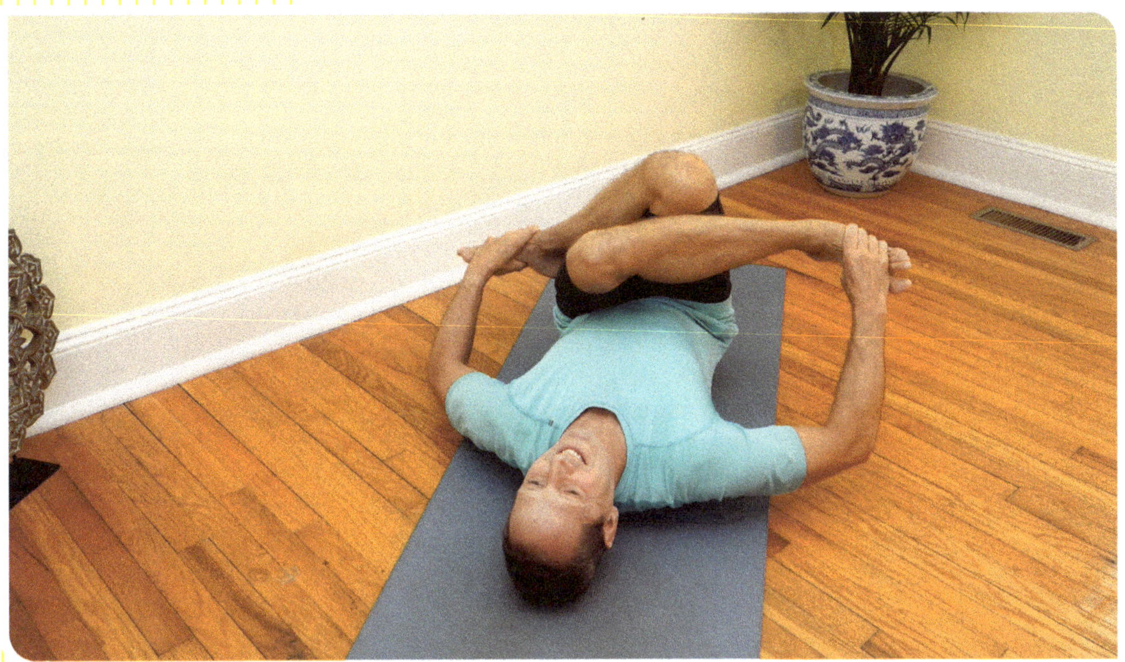

Supine variation

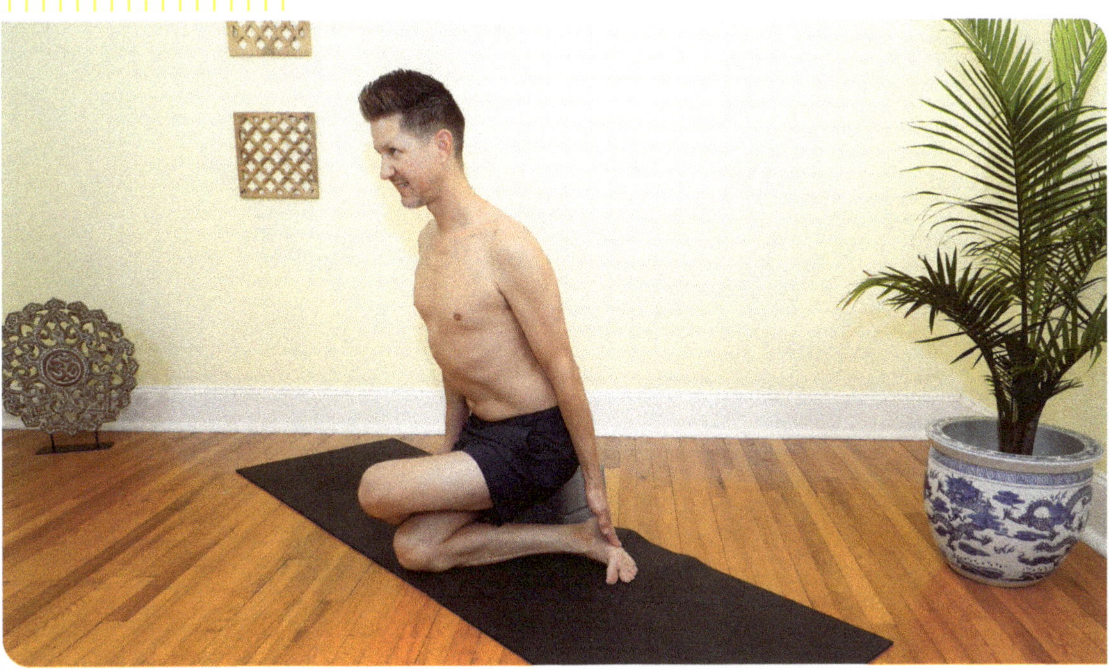

Variation with blocks and arms lowered

One-Legged King Pigeon Pose

ALSO CALLED: Eka Pada Rajakapotasana, or simply, Kapotasana

WHAT IT DOES FOR YOUR OUTER HIPS: Stretches your glutes on the front leg (bent knee side) by rotating that thigh bone outward (externally). Stretches the groins on both legs and your hip flexors on the back leg.

TUNE IT UP: If your glutes are very tight, support your hip and the bent knee on a rolled blanket or a bolster. Both the hip and knee should be elevated higher than the front foot to prevent rotational forces from sneaking into the knee joint. Pulling your front foot in close to your inner thigh will also reduce the rotational forces in your hip and knee. Moving the front foot forward (until your foot knee and hip are at a 90-degree angle) increases the rotational forces in this pose. So move the front foot forward with caution and be very aware of any rotation that may start falling into your knee joint. Keep all rotation at the hip joint.

Remember, only the hip joint can rotate. Your knee is a hinge joint. Respect your body. Practice carefully and patiently. Lift your chest and ribs away from your hips and breathe.

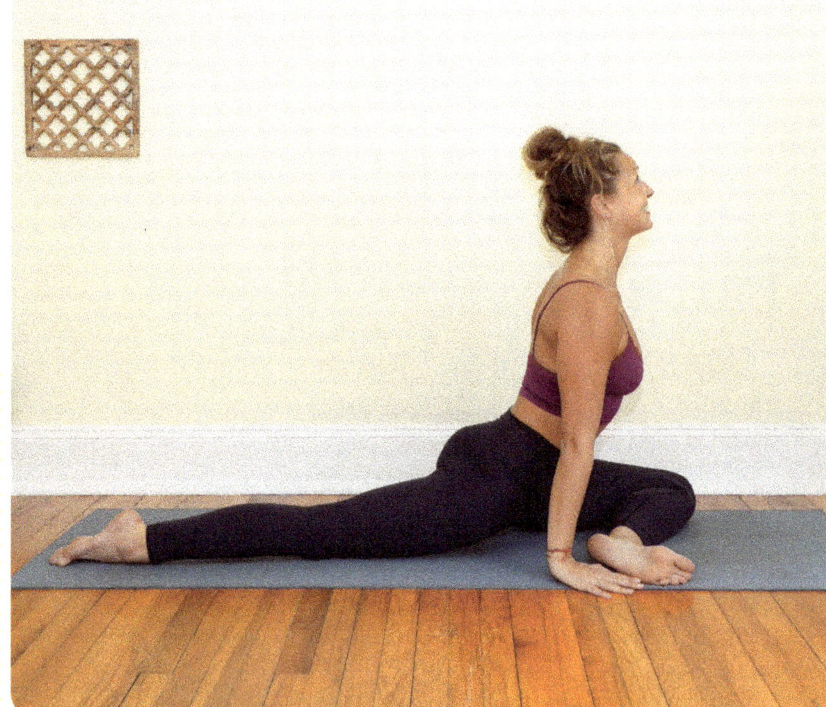

One-Legged King Pigeon Pose

High Lunge Pose

ALSO CALLED: Anjaneyasana

WHAT IT DOES FOR YOUR OUTER HIPS: Primarily strengthens the glutes, quads, TFL, and IT band on your front (bent) leg. That said, the effort of keeping your back knee straight also strengthens the thigh muscles and hamstrings on that leg.

TUNE IT UP: Draw your inner, upper thighs toward each other to square your pelvis toward the front of your mat and engage your groins (adductors). This pose strengthens them, too. As always, lift your chest and ribs up away from your hips. It's a common tendency to look down at the floor in this pose. Break that bad habit and learn to look the world straight in the eye.

Because all standing yoga poses require weight bearing by your legs, they all strengthen your glutes, TFL, and IT bands. The most effective ones call for bending one or both knees, or standing on one leg, because these actions focus the weight-bearing directly in your glutes and quads.

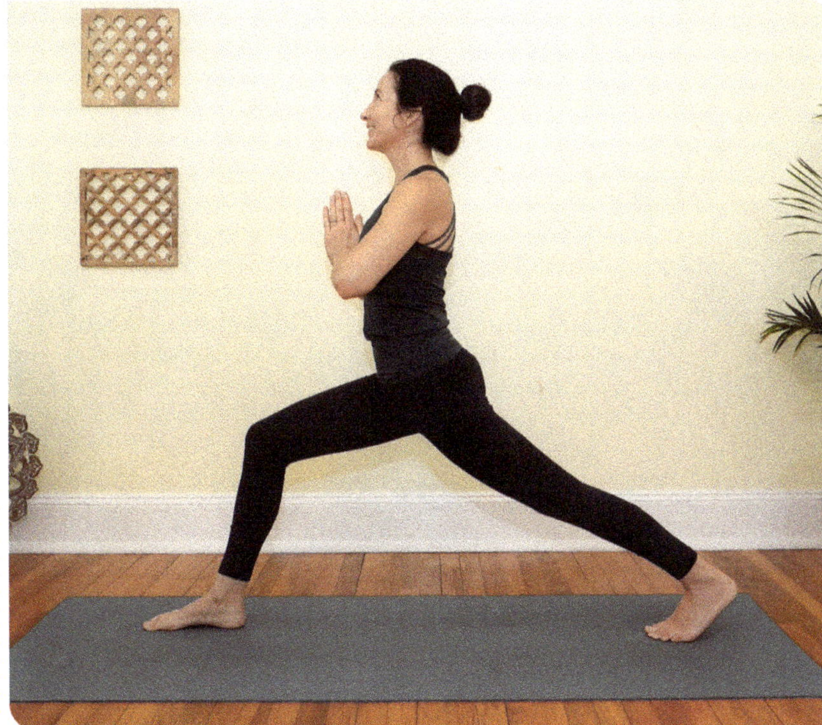

High Lunge Pose

Chair Pose

ALSO CALLED: Utkatasana, Fierce Pose

WHAT IT DOES FOR YOUR OUTER HIPS: Strengthens the glutes, quads, adductors, TFL, and IT bands on both legs.

TUNE IT UP: Squeeze your knees toward each other to recruit and strengthen your adductors (your groin muscles). At the same time, pull your ankles slightly apart. This action strengthens your outer shin muscles (your peroneals), and the anterior tibialis on the front shin.

In both this pose and High Lunge Pose (previous), focus on lifting your chest and drawing your shoulder blades into the center of your upper back. Do not let your shoulders come up toward your neck.

Your gaze should be aimed forward, or slightly upward. Resist the temptation to look at the floor, this puts your ears in front of your shoulders and misaligns your head and neck. Breathe. Feel what's happening in your body. Where is it strengthening, and where is it stretching?

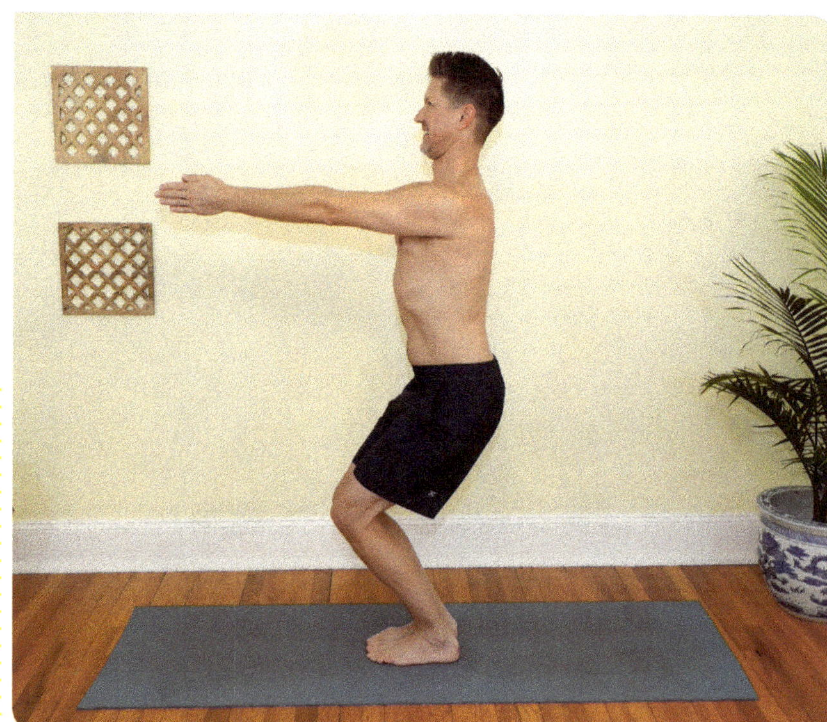

Chair Pose, arms forward

One-Legged Downward Facing Dog Pose

ALSO CALLED: Eka Pada Adho Mukha Svanasana, Three-Legged Dog Pose

Warrior Three Pose

ALSO CALLED: Virabhadrasana Three

WHAT THEY DO FOR YOUR OUTER HIPS: Build strength in the glutes, quads, and hamstrings on both your lifted and standing legs, and strengthen the IT band and TFL on your standing leg.

TUNE IT UP: In both of these poses, reach your chest forward away from your hips, and resist the tendency for the lifted leg to turn outward. Keep the toes of the raised leg turned straight down toward the floor.

In Warrior Three, focus your eyes on a spot slightly ahead of you on the floor. Do not drop your head. Keep the back of your neck and spine as straight as possible.

In One-Legged Downward-Facing Dog Pose, the heel of your standing foot will want to lift up. Draw the heel down and gently wrap the outer ankle toward the floor. Stabilize your shoulders by wrapping your outer armpits down around your outer ribs—don't sag your shoulders and chest down toward the floor. Reach your chest slightly forward toward your thumbs while bringing your chin slightly in toward your chest, and breathe.

In Warrior Three Pose, your hands can stay in front of your chest (in a prayer or palms together position, called anjali mudra), or you can extend your arms back alongside your hips, or forward out in front of you. If you extend your arms forward, your elbows should be straight (see chapter 4, page 176). If you can't straighten your elbows, move your hands further apart until your elbows straighten. Extending your arms not only makes balancing in this pose more challenging, it builds tremendous strength in your back and abdominal muscles. Start with your hands far apart and, over time, you'll build enough strength to bring your palms together with your arms extended in front of you. Be patient.

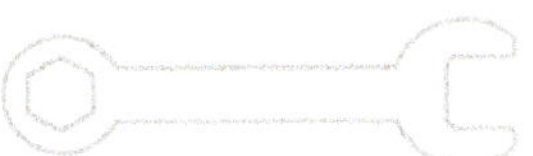

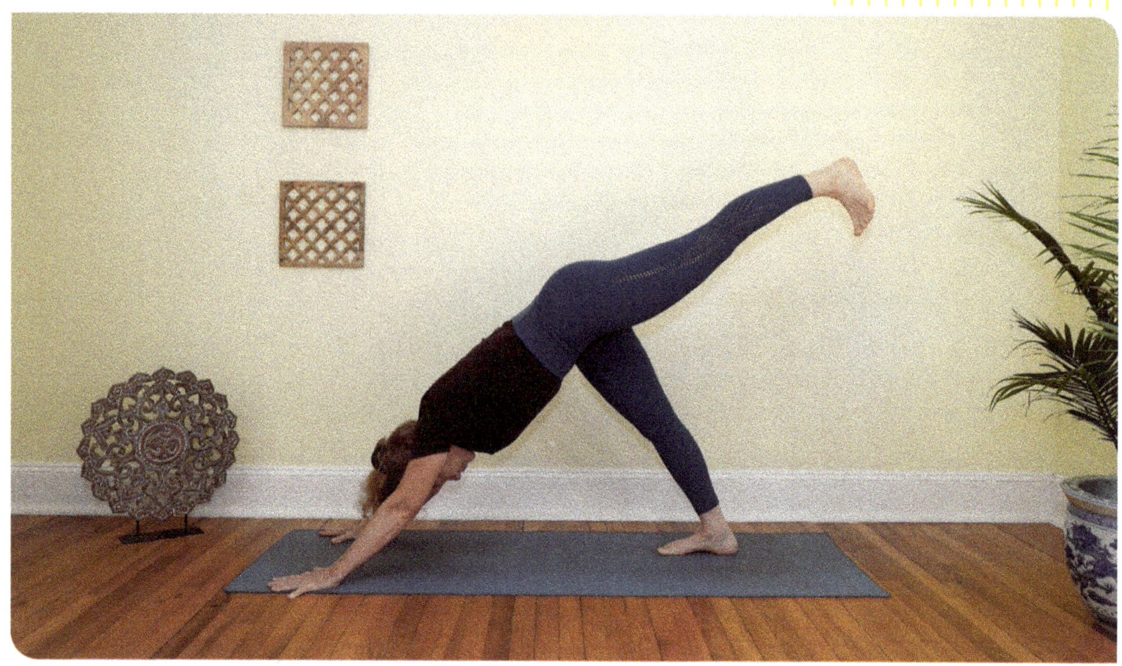

One-Legged Downward-Facing Dog Pose

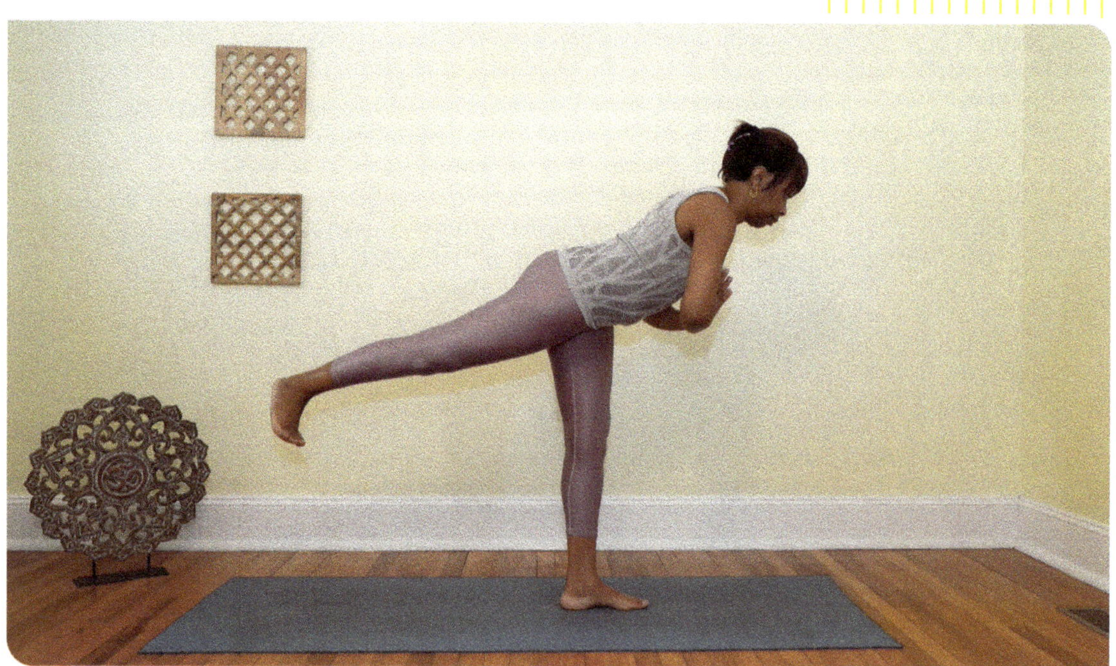

Warrior Three Pose, hands at chest

Extended Side Angle Pose

ALSO CALLED: Utthita Parsvokonasana

Warrior Two Pose

ALSO CALLED: Virabhadrasana Two

WHAT THEY DO FOR YOUR OUTER HIPS: Build a lot of strength in the glutes, quads, TFL, IT-band, and adductors especially in your front (bent) leg.

TUNE IT UP: Extended Side Angle Pose has the widest stance (distance between your feet) of all of the standing poses in yoga. With your feet placed so far apart, your leg muscles must work very hard. There is a tendency to stand with more weight in your front foot than your back foot. You'll need to pay attention to distributing your weight evenly, and finding correct (central) alignment in this pose.

Many people tend to lean their chest forward, and stick their butt out behind them, in this pose. Try to stay centrally aligned. Pull your front hip in toward the center of your mat to put it directly behind your front heel.

Start Extended Side Angle with your front elbow on your front thigh, and focus on lifting your chest toward the top of your mat. Spend several weeks or months doing this pose with your lower elbow on your knee, and your top arm raised to the ceiling or the front of your mat. This will build your strength and flexibility before you try lowering your bottom hand to a block, to your front ankle, or, eventually, to the floor.

Many people mistakenly think that the goal of this pose is to touch the floor with your bottom hand. That's not the point. Do not turn your chest downward or let your hips swing back just to reach the floor; there's nothing magic down there. Straining to reach the floor is a fool's errand. If you don't have the strength and flexibility to easily place your hand on the floor, straining to do it will simply ruin your alignment and

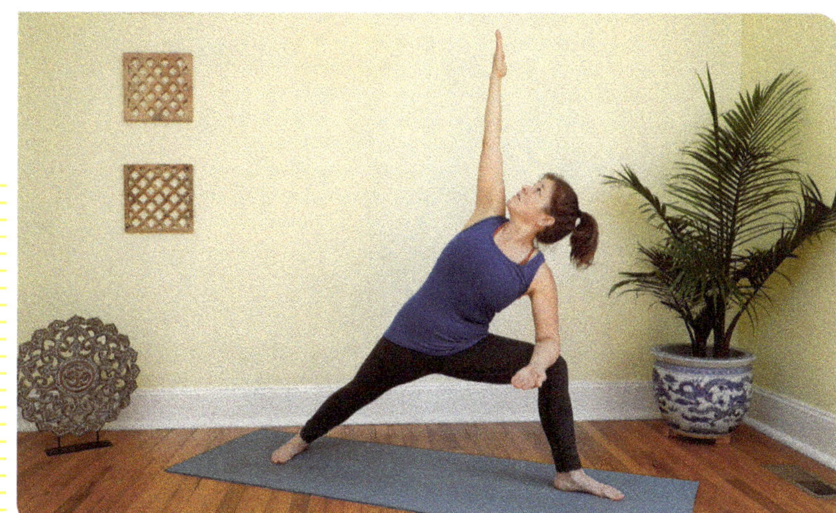

Extended Side Angle Pose, variation with elbow on thigh

increase your risk for injury. Remember, incorrect alignment also erases many of the strengthening and stretching benefits of the pose.

As your glutes, thighs, and abdominals become stronger, and your side waist (obliques) and groin muscles (adductors) become more flexible, you'll be able to bend your front knee deeper, and slide your back foot further back to spread your stance wider. This lowers your hips and brings the floor within reach. Widening your stance with correct alignment is how your bottom hand eventually reaches the mat. Don't hurry. Don't worry! Spend time letting your body adjust to what you are asking of it. Forcing these challenging poses only leads to frustration and injury.

Warrior Two presents many of the same challenges as Extended Right Angle Pose, but your feet are not quite so wide apart, and your torso remains upright. Make sure your back hip is not cranked up higher than your front hip—you may need to unbend your front knee a little to keep your hips level. Also, don't let your torso extend forward over your front thigh. Stay upright and centered between your feet. There's a common tendency to let the back shoulder roll slightly forward. Draw it back and feel your chest open toward the long edge of your mat. Keep gently tilting your sitting bones down toward the floor between your heels. Lift your chest and breathe.

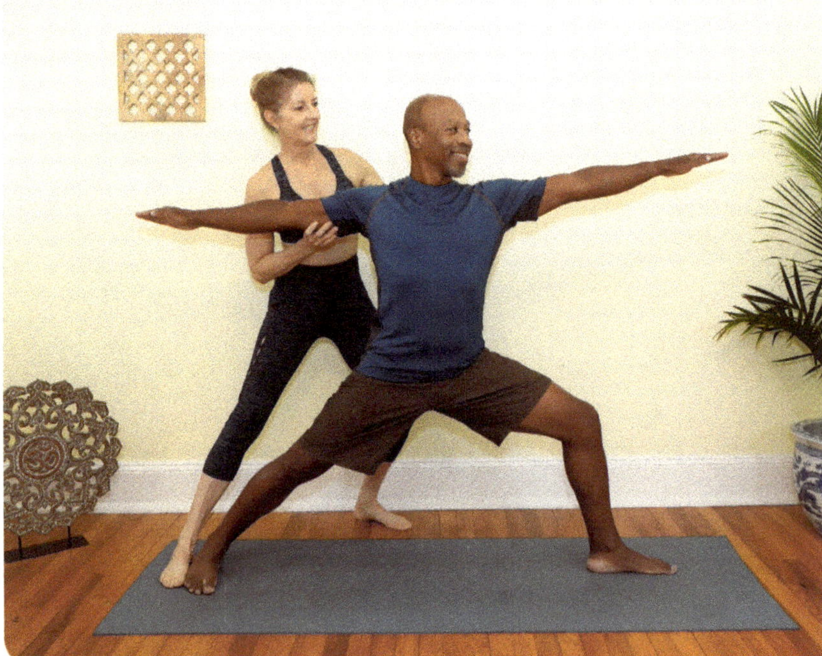

Warrior Two Pose

One-Legged Bridge Pose

ALSO CALLED: Eka Pada Setu Bandhasana

WHAT IT DOES: All variations of Bridge Pose build strength in your glutes, quads, TFL, hamstrings, and IT bands.

TUNE IT UP: Press your foot firmly down and forward on the floor like you are trying to stretch your mat longer. This action in the legs will roll your chest back over your shoulders. Pull your shoulder blades together.

If you have weak thigh or upper back muscles, use blocks to support some of the weight (see photo). Focus on pressing the back edge of your armpits into the floor to lift your chest and pull your upper, inner thighs slightly toward each other.

Do not let the bent leg be lazy. Use your legs and your shoulders to lift your chest from the back. Many people mistakenly think thrusting the hips upward as high as possible is the point of this pose. It's not. This pose is a preparatory position for shoulder stand, and focuses on building flexibility in the chest and strength in the upper back. If you push your hips up too hard, you'll strain your low back. Focus on using your leg strength to roll your chest backwards toward the alignment of your shoulders. Steady your gaze up at the ceiling, or cast your eyes slightly back toward the wall behind you. Don't take a nap just because most of your body weight is supported on blocks! Build strength and flexibility by engaging your muscles where you can. You already made the effort to get on your mat, you might as well get the most benefit possible.

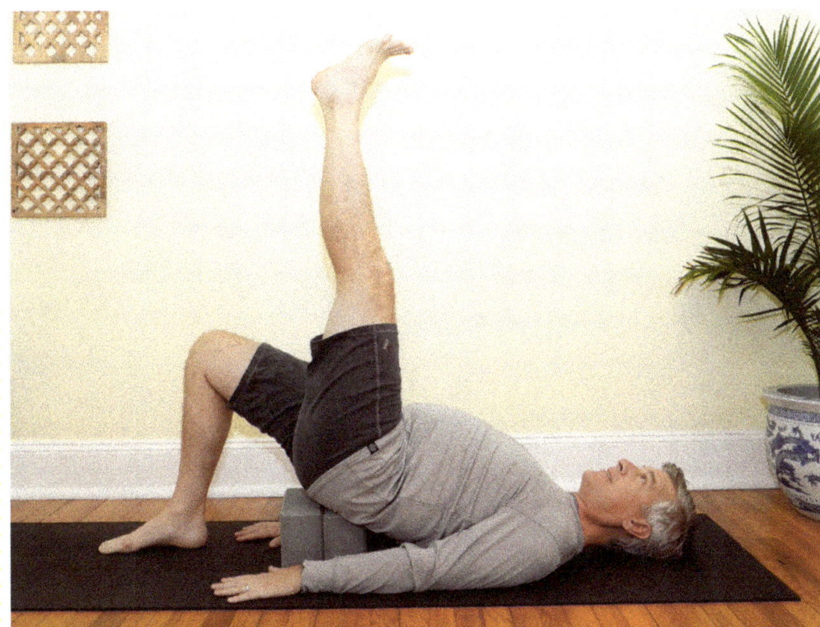

One-Legged Bridge Pose, variation with blocks

Half Moon Pose

ALSO CALLED: Ardha Chandrasana

Eagle Pose

ALSO CALLED: Garudasana

WHAT THEY DO FOR YOUR OUTER HIPS: Strengthen your glutes, quads, adductors, TFL, and IT bands—especially on the standing leg. Like all of the one-legged standing balance poses, these poses also build mental focus because you must balance on one foot.

TUNE IT UP: In both poses, flex the lifted foot to help keep the muscles of that leg engaged and active. It is essential to use the muscles in both legs to balance—even the one that is off the floor. Do not let the lifted leg be limp.

You'll be tempted to look down at the floor for balance. Don't do that. Instead, train yourself to look forward or slightly upward in these poses. Get used to moving your gaze off the floor, first by only moving your eyes slightly forward instead downward. After a month or two of moving only your eyes, begin to move your face a little bit in that direction. Moving your eyes first tells your brain that you'll eventually be moving your head (which weighs a lot), and gives your body time to prepare to shift this heavy weight. So start slowly and shift your head position gradually. This is slow but important work, because if you keep looking down at the floor, your chest and upper back will want to curl downward, too.

Lift your chest away from your hips. Take steady, deep inhales and smooth, complete exhales.

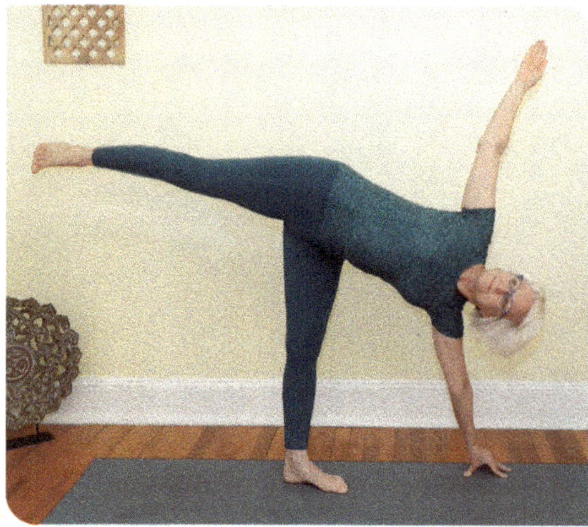

Half Moon Pose

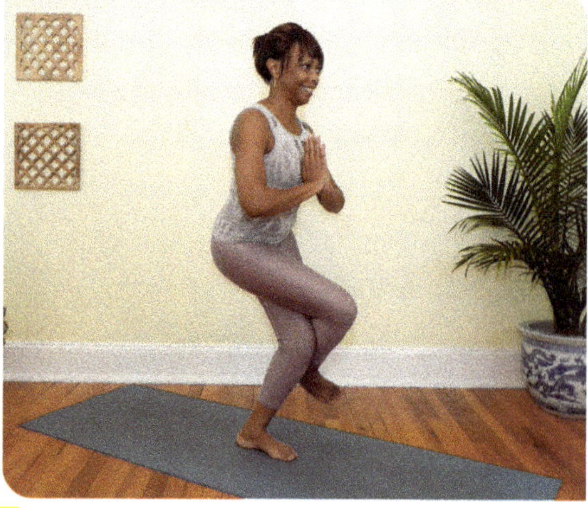

Eagle Pose, variation with hands in front of chest

Comfortable Seated Pose

ALSO CALLED: Sukhasana

Lotus Pose

ALSO CALLED: Padmasana

WHAT THEY DO FOR YOUR INNER HIPS: Both poses stretch your groin muscles.

TUNE IT UP: There's a lot more going on in these poses than it appears. First, do not force your legs into Lotus Pose if your adductors and glutes are tight. Forcing your way into it can produce uneven (unaligned) forces in your knee and ankle joints that can injure them. Remember, hips rotate; knees and ankles do not.

If your groin muscles are tight, when you try to sit cross-legged on the floor your low back will tend to round backward, your pelvis will tuck under, and your knees will be pointing up (instead of out to the side). If that's you—don't worry. Sit up on a bolster, block, or folded blanket. Raising your hips will reduce pressure in your low back and tension in your hip flexors, and will give your thigh bones (femurs) some room to begin gradually dropping down. Focus on lifting your ribs up and gently pressing your thighs down.

Also use the very subtle action of pulling your thighs slightly together, which gently draws your knees toward the front of your mat. This action may not produce any visible change in your leg position, but it turns on a group of very deep, low belly (your transverse abdominus) and pelvic floor muscles that help support your spine and the weight of your torso. This subtle, inward action of the thighs is how you can begin to find the deep small muscles of the low belly (you might have heard these called the "root lock," or mula bandha). When you engage more muscle groups to support your body weight, your torso will feel lighter and your seated position more comfortable. It will feel like your lungs and chest are riding freely above your hips and legs. Breathe.

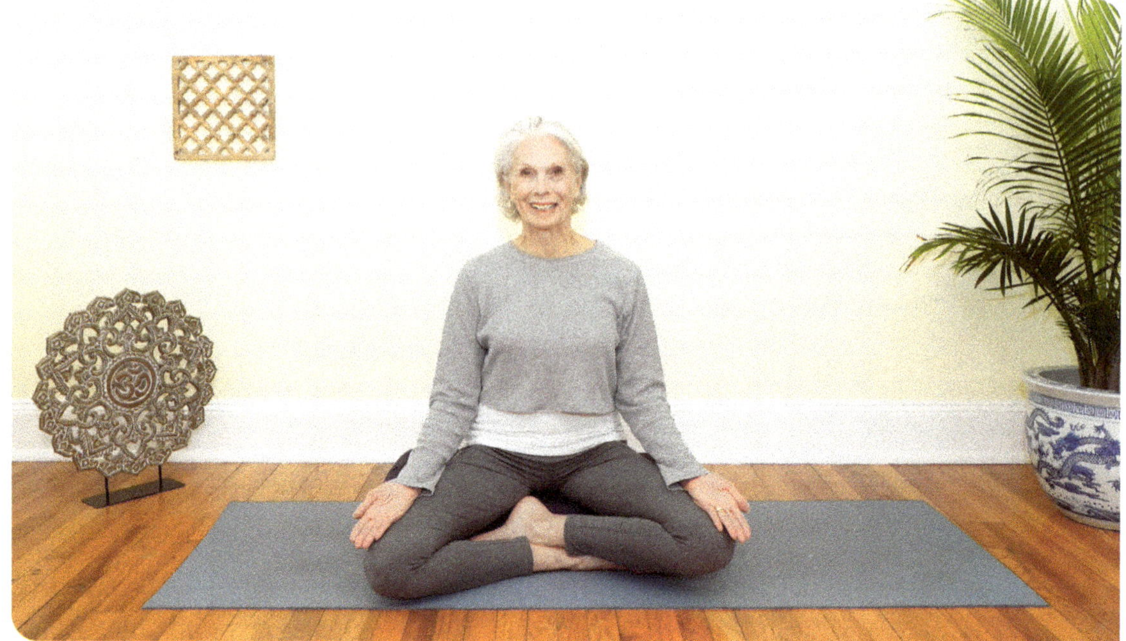

Comfortable Seated Pose with bolster

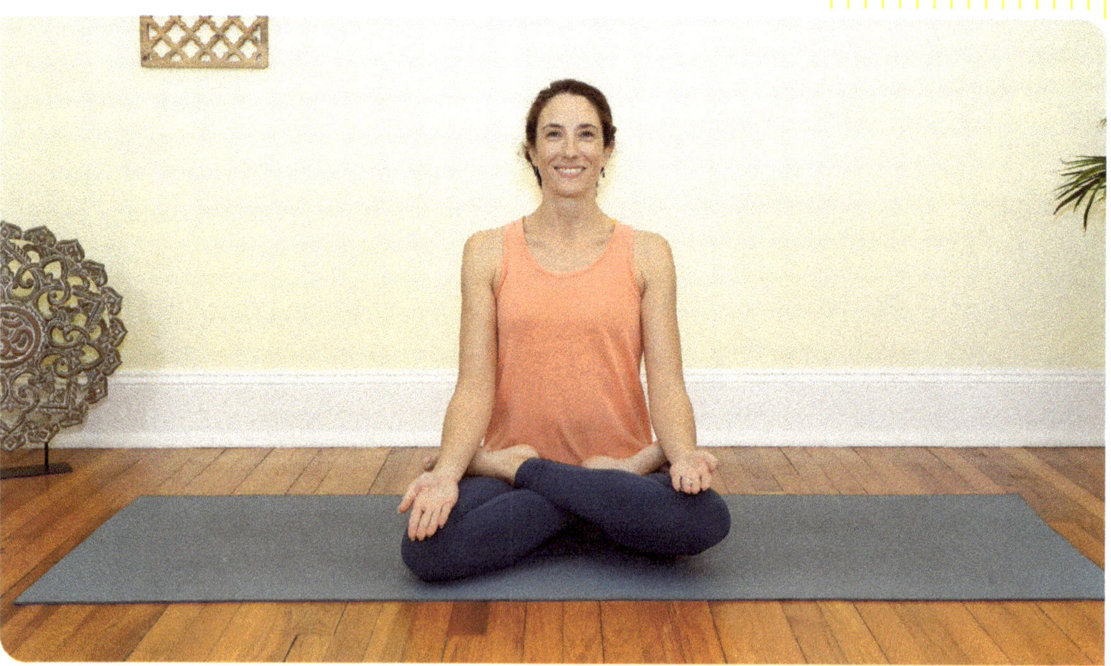

Lotus Pose

Bound Angle Pose, A

ALSO CALLED: Baddha Konasana, A; Butterfly Pose; Cobbler's Pose

WHAT IT DOES FOR YOUR INNER HIPS: This is an intense stretch for your groins (your adductors) and glutes.

TUNE IT UP: Keep your back as straight as possible and gently pull on your feet or ankles as if drawing them back toward you (they will not visibly move).

If your hips and groin muscles are tight, sit up on a block, bolster, or rolled blanket. You can also try elevating your heels on a rolled blanket (but not your toes, keep them on the floor). This increases the outward rotation at your hip joint while protecting your knee joints. Raising your hips up off of the floor will also help protect your low back from strain as you lean forward.

Don't let your shoulders and chest round downward. Keep reaching your ribs forward, away from your hips. Also, do not pull too hard on your feet in this pose. Focus on reaching your chest forward and pressing your thigh bones down. Pressing the pinky-toe edges of your feet firmly together and letting your big toes roll away from each other will help lower your thighs.

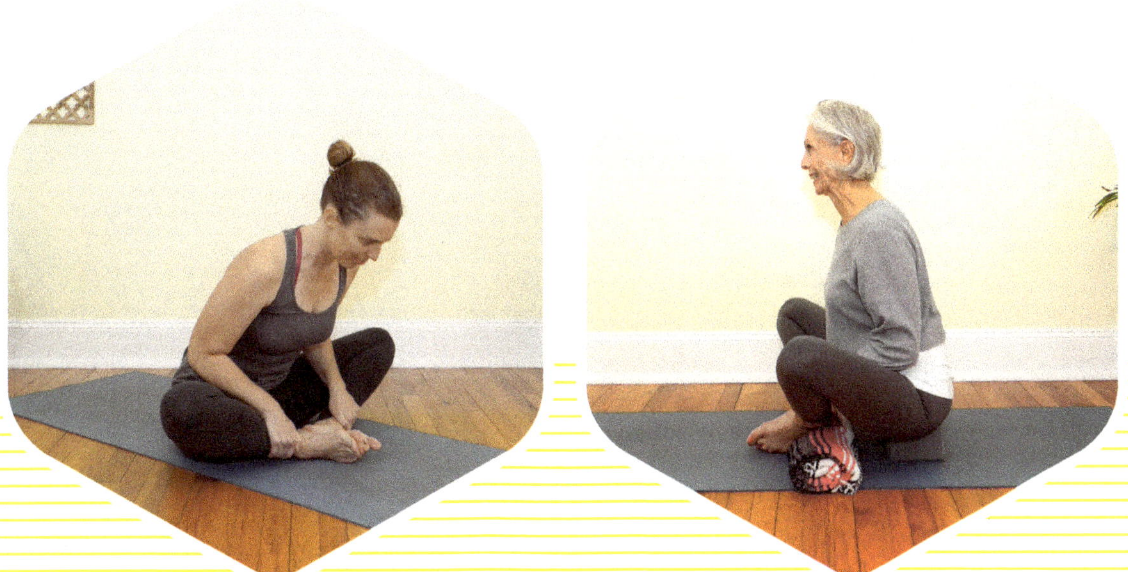

Bound Angle Pose, A

Variation with block and blanket

Wide Angle Seated Forward Fold Pose

ALSO CALLED: Upavistha Konasana

WHAT IT DOES FOR YOUR INNER HIPS: This is a great stretch for your groin muscles, but it's wise to approach this pose gradually. Tight groins are common, and take a long time to become more flexible.

TUNE IT UP: As with most seated forward folding poses, the temptation is to reach your hands forward, drop your head, and round your back. Don't do any of that. Focus on keeping your legs absolutely straight by pressing your heels outward. Keep your thigh muscles very firm while you do this pose, to help protect your low back joints.

If your groin muscles are tight (and for most people, they are), put your palms flat on the floor or on some blocks with straight elbows, and press down to lift your chest.

Breathe. Eventually, as your groins (your adductors) become longer, you'll begin reaching your chest slightly further forward. Keep your arms and legs straight, and your back as flat as possible. Keep stretching forward. Remember, there are no downward folding poses in yoga. Don't be a downer!

As you begin to make progress, you can reduce the risk of straining your low back by supporting your head on blocks as well (see photo). Be patient.

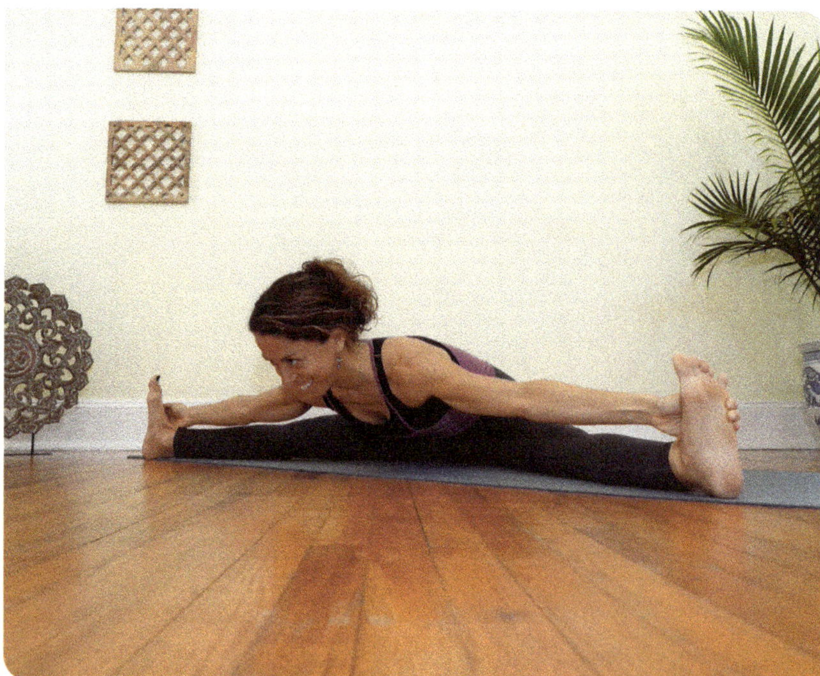

Wide-Angle Seated Forward Fold Pose

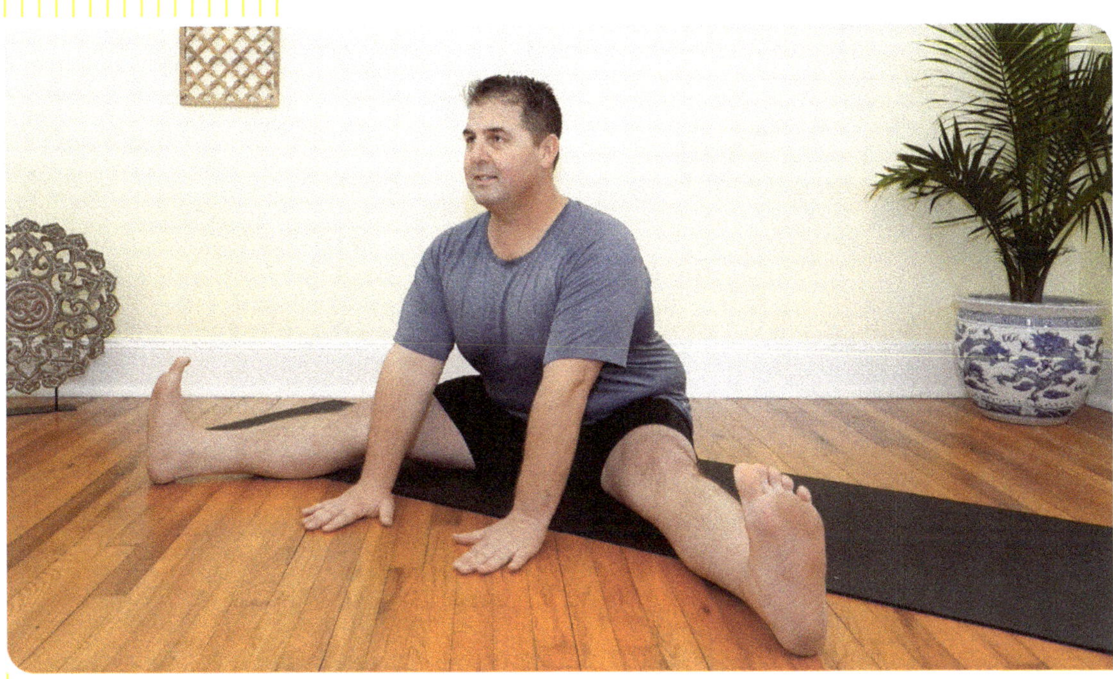

Variation pressing palms to floor

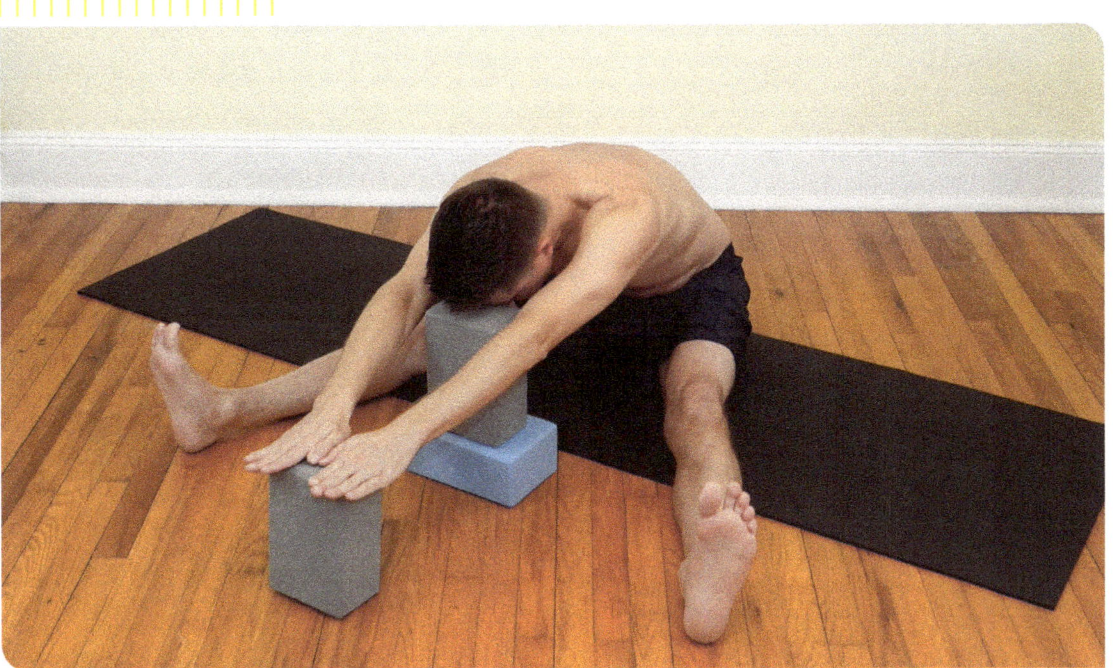

Variation with blocks

MECHANIC'S NOTE: Chest up Chin in

If your back is easily irritated, you can do Wide-Angle Seated Forward Fold Pose lying on your back (supine), and get the same groin-stretching and abdominal-strengthening benefits. Lie down on your back, pull your knees in toward your belly, and then extend your legs out to either side. Use your hands to support the backs of your legs, or let your hands rest on your inner thighs. Focus on pressing outward through your heels and getting your knees as straight as possible. This supine variation is very effective for stretching the groins while protecting the low back.

There's a tendency to stick your chin up to the ceiling and let your chest sag down into the floor in this and other supine poses. If you're doing that, draw your chin slightly toward your throat to lengthen the back of your neck and imagine lifting your chest up to engage your core muscles. Of course, tensing the back of your neck and sticking out your chin doesn't help stretch your groins. The action is chest up/chin in for every pose, whether you are standing, seated, or lying down. So, you notice and then adjust. We do that in every yoga pose: notice what we're doing and determine if it's helping or hindering us. If it's a hindrance, work on changing it.

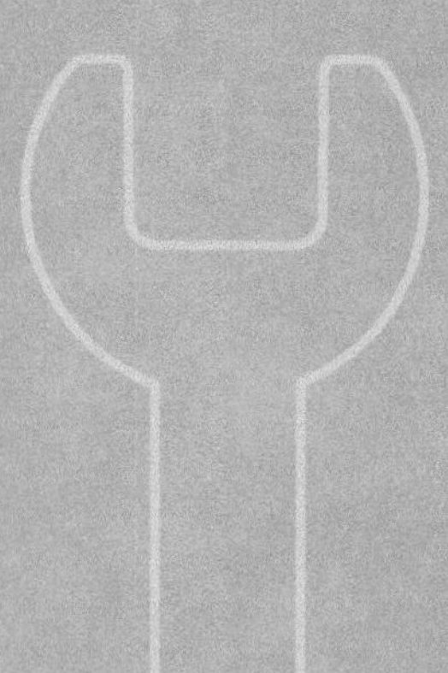

Extended Hand to Foot Pose, B

ALSO CALLED: Utthita Hasta Padangusthasana, B

WHAT IT DOES: Stretches your groins while building strength in the standing leg (especially in your glutes, TFL, and IT band). Like all balances, this pose also builds mental focus.

TUNE IT UP: If you have tight groin muscles, bend your lifted knee and hold there. Or use a strap looped around the ball of your foot and straighten your knee, holding the strap far enough out that your elbow can be straight. (See photos.) Don't bend your elbow. Focus on pressing firmly outward through the lifted leg.

Do not let the lifted foot go limp. The action in this pose is to press outward with the foot, and pull back against that force with your shoulder blade. Work from your upper back, not from your biceps, to draw the leg back. This push-pull action will help you balance.

Steady your gaze and breathe. Do not look down at the floor. Keep your gaze forward or slightly upward. This will help lift your chest and ribs up away from your hips. Eventually, you will shift your gaze to the side away from the lifted leg.

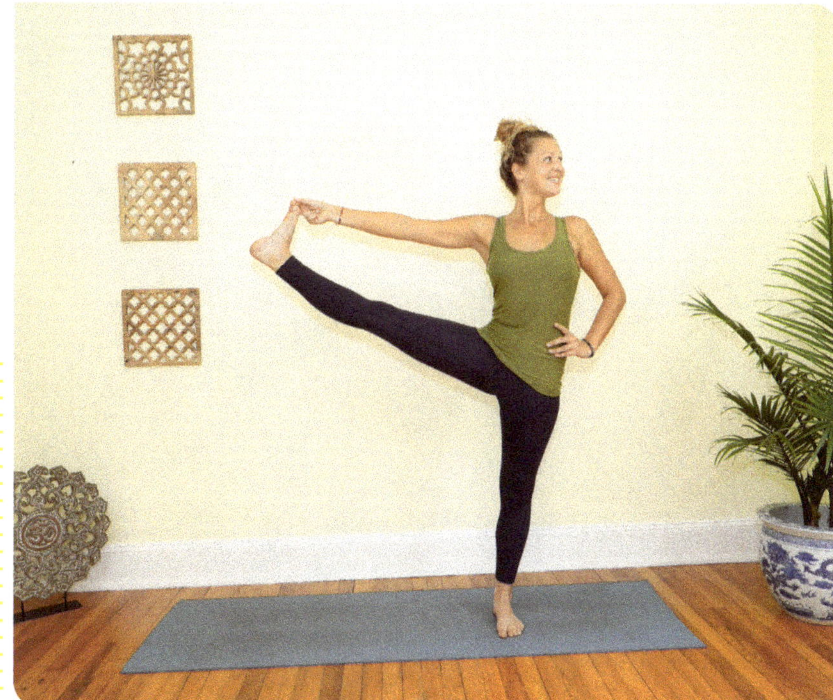

Extended Hand to Foot Pose, B

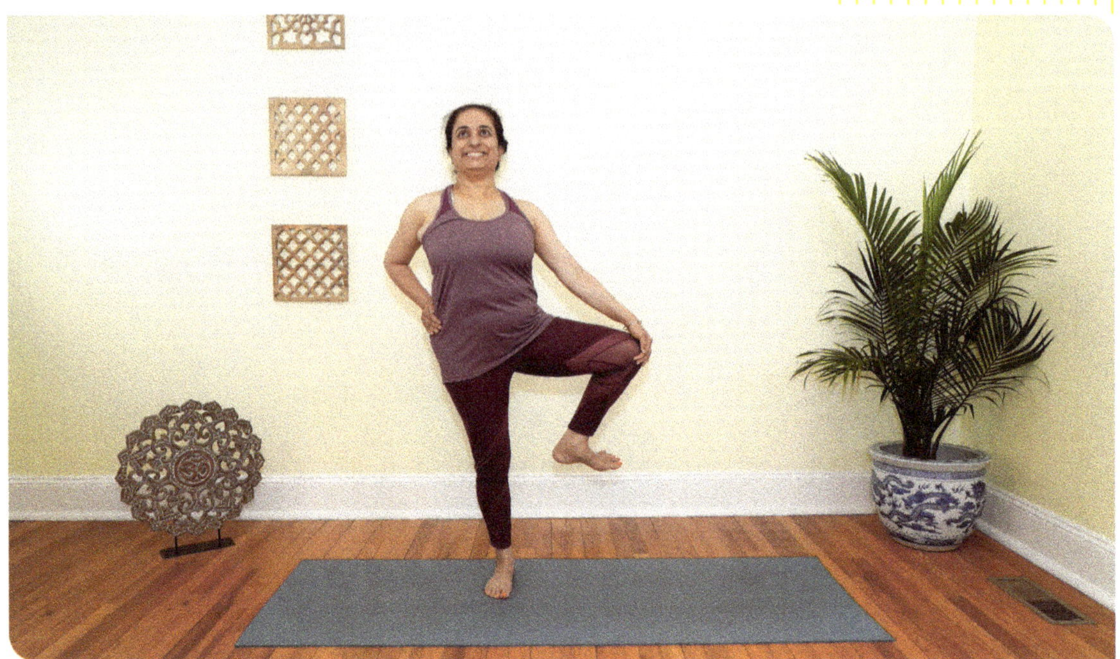

Variation with knee bent and only eyes (drishti) moving to the side

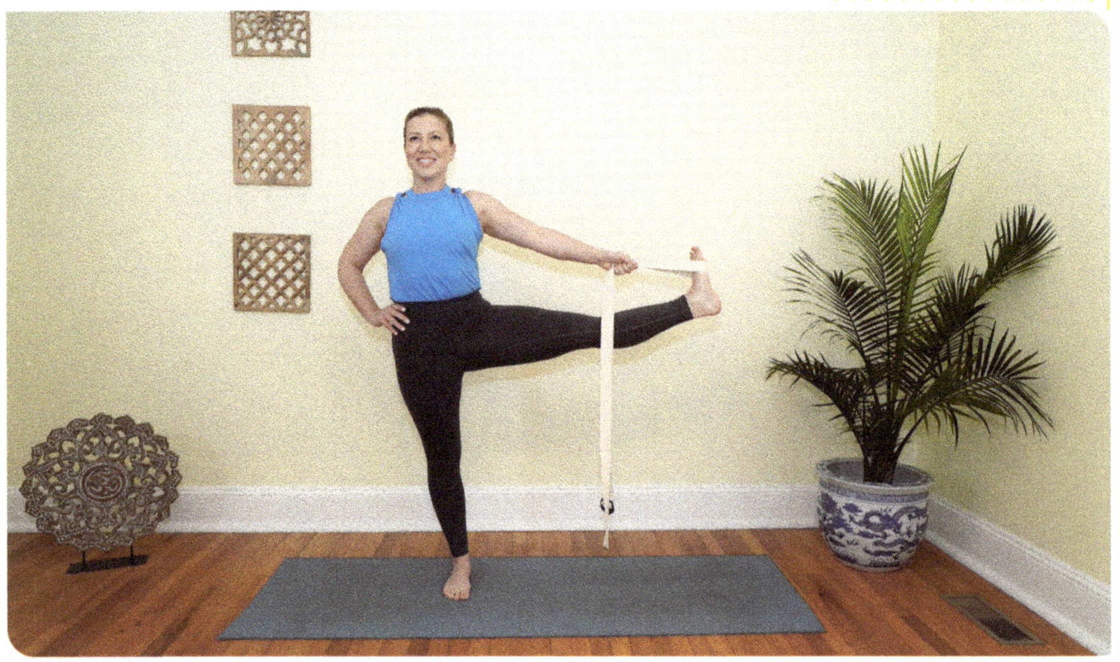

Variation with strap and gaze (drishti) forward

Reclined Hand to Foot Pose, B

ALSO CALLED: Supta Padangusthasana, B

WHAT IT DOES FOR YOUR INNER HIPS: Stretches the groins, hip flexors, and hamstrings. Builds a great deal of strength in the abdominal muscles, which must work to press the opposite side of your body down, and not let it roll up off the floor to follow your leg.

TUNE IT UP: As with Extended Hand to Foot Pose, you can use a strap to reach the foot if your hamstrings and groins are tight, but hold the strap with a straight arm. Do not bend your elbows or your knees.

Keep both arms and both legs straight. The hand that is not holding your foot (or strap) should be straight, and pressed firmly down on the other thigh.

Press forward through both heels and try to hold the leg on the floor straight. It will want to bend, especially if you have tight hip flexors, and will also tend to roll out to the side if you have weak abdominal and groin muscles. Don't let it.

Do not rest either elbow on the floor. It builds abdominal strength to hold your arms straight, and off the floor.

There's a tendency to hold your breath in this pose. That doesn't help either. Breathe.

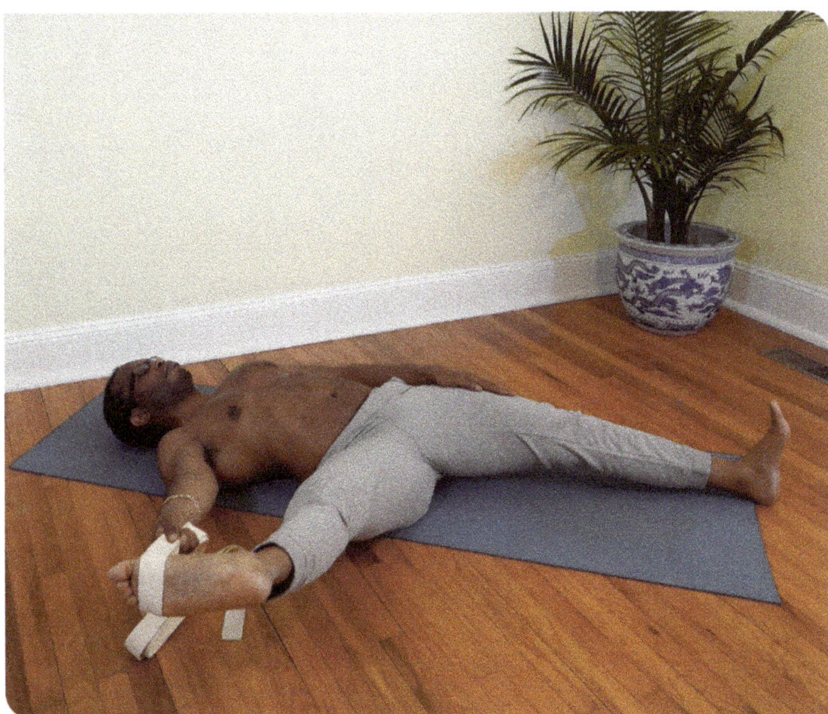

Reclined Hand to Foot Pose, B, with strap and gaze (drishti) forward

Wide-Legged Forward Fold Pose, B

ALSO CALLED: Prasarita Padottanasana, B

WHAT IT DOES FOR YOUR INNER HIPS: Like the other standing poses that place your feet wide apart, this is a good groin stretch. It also strengthens your upper back and mental focus because your hands stay on your hips.

TUNE IT UP: Extend your spine, keeping it as straight and flat as possible. Focus on reaching your chest forward and hinging from the hips. Do not let your back and shoulders round. As always in standing poses, you can bend your knees, a little or a lot, to reduce the force pulling on your low back and hamstrings. If you bend your knees deeply, stop at the halfway folded point and focus on stretching your sitting bones up and back as you reach your chest forward.

Your toes should be pointing directly forward, or turned slightly inward. Do not turn your toes outward; that introduces too much pressure into the inner side of your knee joints.

Keep your thigh muscles firmly engaged throughout this pose (while entering, holding, and exiting it).

To reduce strain in your low back, press your hands firmly down onto your hip creases when entering and exiting this pose. Your hip creases are slightly below your hips. If you sit in a chair, they are the bend-line where your legs meet your torso.

Use your arm strength. In any standing forward fold, you can reduce pressure on your low back muscles by using the strength of your arms to help lift and lower the weight of your torso, by pressing your hands into your hips and making your arms do some of the work. It also helps to press outward on your feet with bent knees.

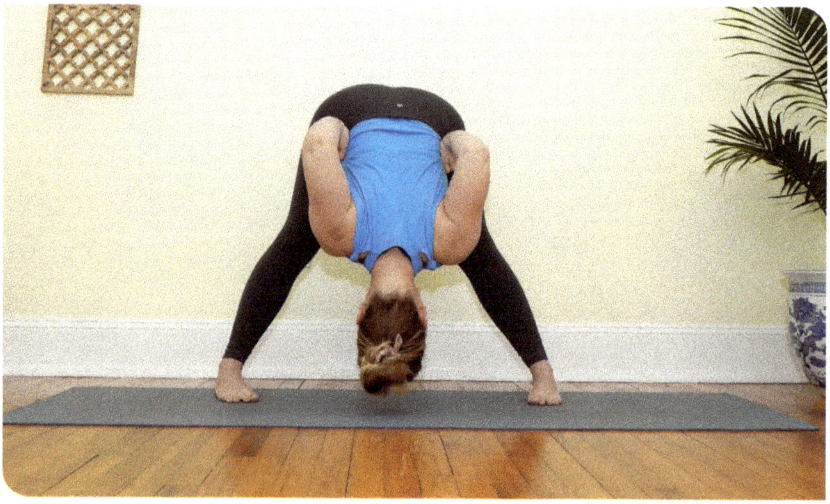

Wide-Legged Forward Fold Pose, B

Extended Side Angle Pose

ALSO CALLED: Utthita Parsvakonasana

Warrior Two Pose

ALSO CALLED: Virabhadrasana Two

WHAT THEY DO FOR YOUR INNER HIPS: Poses that place your feet wide apart are excellent stretches for your groin muscles (adductors).

TUNE IT UP: In both poses, resist the urge to lean forward and stick your butt out behind you. Instead, focus on keeping torso directly above your legs. Lift your chest away from your hips, and draw your shoulder blades down and together on your upper back.

As your groin muscles get longer over time, you'll be able to widen your feet and bend your front knee deeper. In Warrior Two Pose, be careful to keep your back hip down level with the front one because raising your back hip releases the groin stretch. In Side Angle Pose, your feet will eventually be so far apart that your bottom hand can easily reach a block or the floor. But remember, touching the floor is not your goal. You want to stretch your groins and strengthen your legs, back, and abdominals. Do not strain to touch the floor.

Steady your gaze. Breathe and focus on experiencing the sensations of the pose. Maybe they are pleasant. Maybe they are unpleasant. In either case, it will soon be over and in the past. Do each pose and then move on.

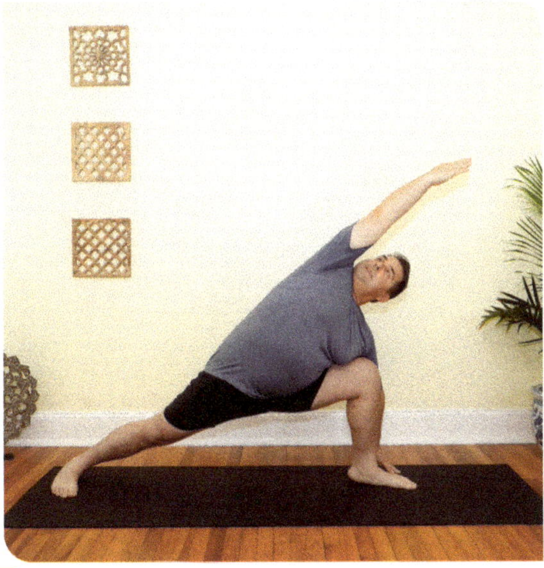

Extended Side Angle Pose

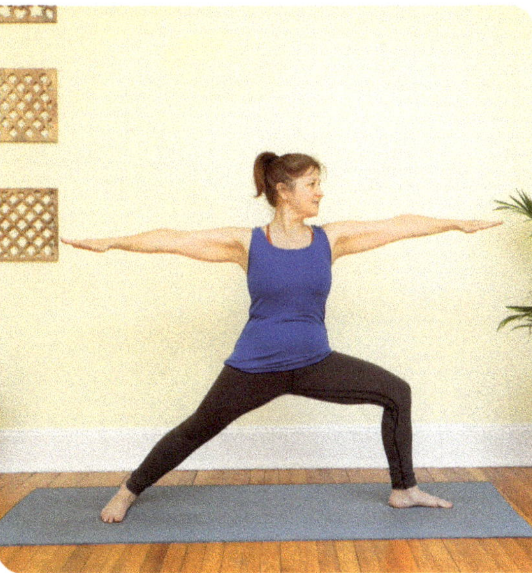

Warrior Two Pose

Warrior One Pose

ALSO CALLED: Virabhadrasana One

WHAT IT DOES FOR YOUR INNER HIPS: In this pose, the inner thighs (your adductors) draw toward each other to square your pelvis forward. This takes some doing, because your legs are going in opposite directions; one foot is forward and one is back.

TUNE IT UP: Keep your back leg straight and pull your upper thighs toward each other. This action also engages your low belly muscles (transverse abdominus) and can help you begin to find what's called your root lock (also known as mula bandha). Learning to use (and thereby strengthen) this group of deep abdominal muscles at the pelvic floor is key for doing more challenging yoga poses safely and effectively. I find that the easiest way to start finding your root lock in many poses is through the action of pulling your thigh bones (your femurs) toward each other.

Raising your arms and, eventually, touching your palms requires a lot of strength in the upper back and shoulders. Keep your elbows straight, no matter how wide your arms must be to do that.

Lift your low belly, ribs, and chest up, away from your hips. Breathe.

Poses that draw the inner thighs toward each other strengthen the groins. Standing poses that square your hips (your pelvis) toward the front of your mat require pulling the upper, inner thighs toward each other. Rotated or revolved standing poses also strengthen your groins (your adductors), because you must scissor your inner thighs toward each other to help turn your pelvis and low back (which sits on the bone at the back of your pelvis, called the sacrum).

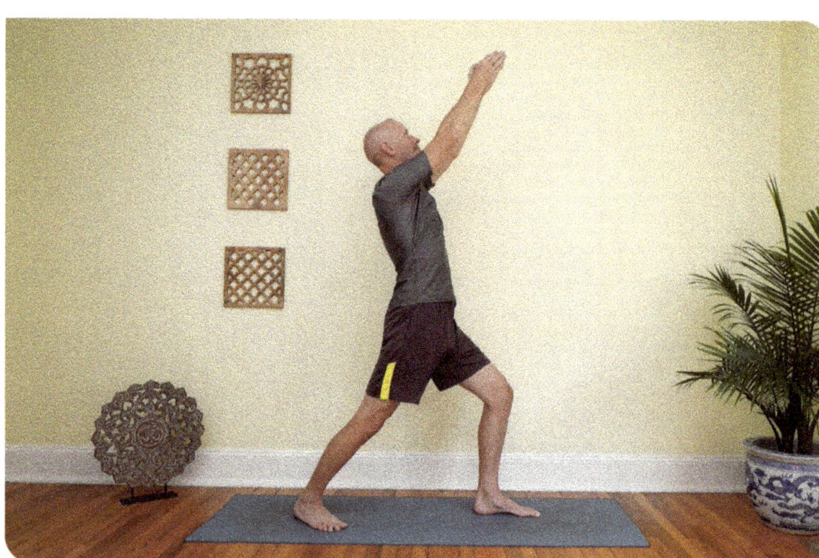

Warrior One Pose

Revolved Crescent Lunge, variation

ALSO CALLED: Parivrtta Anjaneyasana, variation

WHAT IT DOES FOR YOUR INNER HIPS: The scissoring action of drawing your upper inner thighs toward each other creates a lot of adductor (groin) strength.

TUNE IT UP: You must turn the entire structure of your lower back and pelvis as one unit to avoid injury. In fact, it's anatomically impossible to turn your lower back without turning your pelvis (your hips) too, because the vertebrae in your low back have almost no ability to rotate one-over-the-other, and they sit on your pelvis (at the sacrum). If you don't turn your hips, your low back cannot participate in the turn. Drawing your upper, inner thighs toward each other is essential to turn your pelvis and lower back. Turning the thigh of the back (extended) leg inward also helps rotate your pelvis toward your front thigh. This muscular action is essential to turn your entire torso.

Some people will be able to hook their opposite elbow over the front knee. If that's not you, use a strap from hand to hand, with one hand behind your back and the other over your front thigh (see photo). If you're holding a strap, don't let your arms be limp. Instead, pull your knuckles down toward the floor to straighten your elbows. The action of pulling down in the strap behind you and also where it crosses over your front thigh will help you rotate toward the front thigh.

In this pose, focus more on building strength in your leg and abdominal muscles and less on turning your torso. The twisting action will come. First build the strength needed to support that rotation with your leg and belly muscles. Be patient.

Many people mistakenly think that the goal in twisting poses is to crank your spine around as far as possible. This is dangerous and incorrect. Do not crank your back using your arm strength. That can injure your back. Instead, learn to use a scissoring action in your legs to turn your pelvis and low back, and use your core strength to turn your mid- and upper-back. Then place your arms wherever they reach. You should feel effort, but not strain.

If your balance feels unsteady, you can lower your back knee, and put a folded blanket under it if having your knee on the floor is uncomfortable. However, while lowering your back knee makes balancing easier, it makes turning your pelvis and low back more difficult. When you've developed stronger leg and abdominal muscles and a sharp mental focus, try to raise your back knee, and gradually work towards pressing back through that heel until your back leg is straight. Do not let your back knee stay bent in this pose through years and years of practice; work slowly and steadily to straighten it over time.

Be patient. Eventually, you'll be able to rotate your torso far enough to hook your elbow (or even your shoulder) outside your front knee. Resist the urge to use your elbow to crank yourself around the turn. Bring your palms together and gently press the heels of your hands downward to help lift your chest up. Turn using the strength of your leg and core abdominal muscles, not the leverage of your arms. Your low back will thank you.

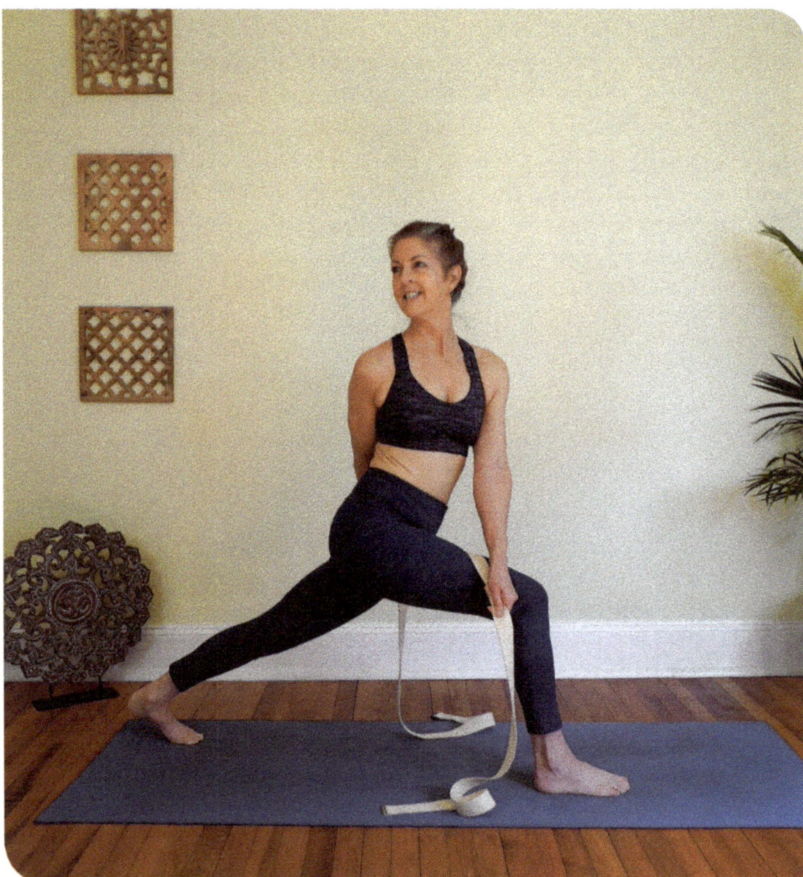

Revolved Crescent Lunge, variation with strap

Revolved Side Angle Pose

ALSO CALLED: Parivrtta Parsvokonasana

WHAT IT DOES FOR YOUR INNER HIPS: This pose is very similar to Revolved Crescent Lunge (previous), and uses the same muscular actions, but in a more physically and mentally challenging pattern. Do not be overly enthusiastic about doing this pose until you're very comfortable in Revolved Crescent Lunge Pose.

TUNE IT UP: One of the primary reasons this pose is so challenging is that it has the widest stance of any standing pose in yoga. Because your feet are so far apart, this pose requires a very strong inward action in both thighs. Your hip stabilizer, abdominal, shoulder, and back muscles must be very strong and flexible to protect your low back from harmful strain. As in Revolved Crescent Lunge, do not focus on hooking your elbow or shoulder over your front knee, and don't crank your spine into this twist using your arms. Be patient. Do not force your body to do movements that it is not prepared for.

Practice this pose step by step, and gradually build the needed strength and flexibility. Don't start by reaching for the floor. Instead, start learning this pose with your hands pressed together as if at prayer (anjali mudra), to hook your elbow over your knee.

Press your your top palm down into the bottom palm and draw the heels of both hands slightly toward the floor to help lift your chest. Eventually you will be able to lower your hips enough that your shoulder will cross your thigh, and you can release the palms and extend the lower hand to the floor. The upper hand can come to your back hip and, eventually, it will reach out overhead. This process takes time. Focus on using your leg and abdominal strength to turn your torso. This is a very intense pose. Go slowly.

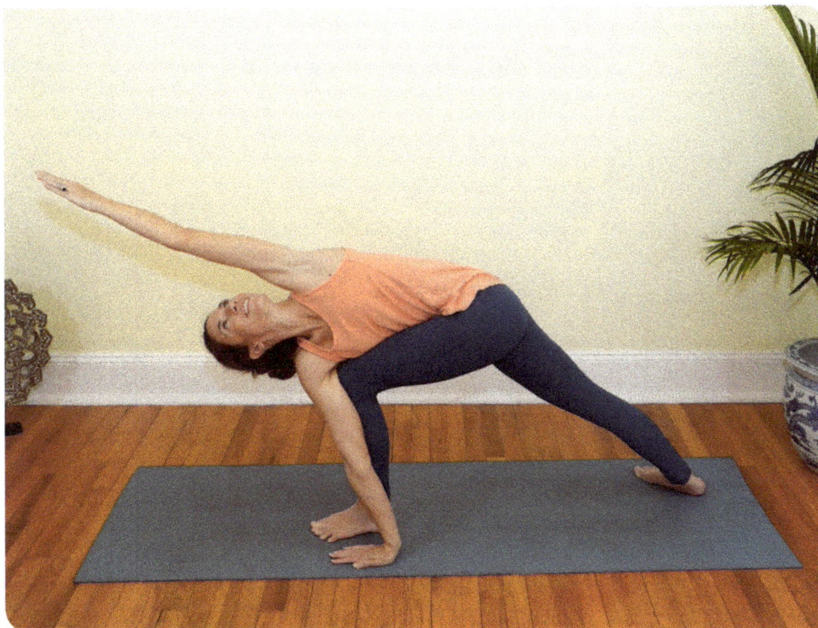

Revolved Side Angle Pose

Revolved Triangle Pose

ALSO CALLED: Parivtita Trikonasana

WHAT IT DOES FOR YOUR INNER HIPS: Like the other standing revolved poses, this one requires you to scissor your inner thighs and use your upper leg strength to turn your pelvis and torso.

TUNE IT UP: This pose, like others that strengthen the inner hip muscles, requires a strong inward action of your upper, inner thighs in order to rotate your pelvis. If your pelvis is not participating in the turn, you're risking too much compression at the lowest spinal joints that can actually rotate. (That's where your last thoracic vertebrae meets your first lumbar vertebrae, called the T-12 / L-1 junction. We'll talk more about the spine in chapter 4). Cranking your torso into a twist concentrates too much force into the discs and ligaments of the mid- and lower back.

Instead, rotate your torso gradually into the turn, using the strength of your leg and abdominal muscles. Draw your upper, inner thighs toward each other and stretch your chest forward. Do not let your chest turn down toward the floor.

It's a great idea to put a block under your bottom hand and keep your back hand on your hip (see photo), so you can focus on making the turn happen with your leg, hip, and belly muscles. Draw the lowest muscles in your belly firmly upward. Even if your hand can reach the floor, I highly recommend trying this pose with your hand on a block sometimes, so you can focus on reaching your chest forward and scissoring your thighs. You have to try something new to get something new.

Once you're able to comfortably rotate with your chest extending forward, think about raising your top hand, and maybe lowering your bottom hand a little closer to the floor (maybe to a lower block, or to your ankle).

Remember, there is nothing magic down on the floor to grab hold of. Do not strain to reach the floor. Be alert. Observe your muscles working. Breathe. Notice the awesome strength of your body, heart, and mind. Honor and respect your wonderful body.

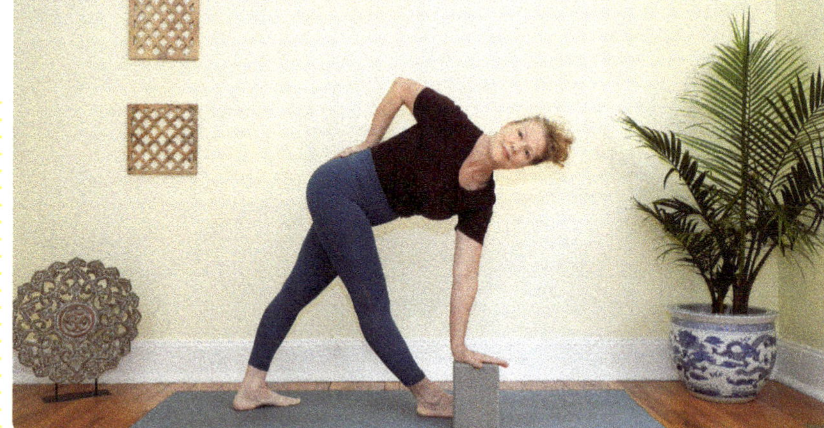

Revolved Triangle Pose, variation with block

Crow Pose

ALSO CALLED: Bakasana, Crane Pose

WHAT IT DOES FOR YOUR INNER HIPS: This is a great way to strengthen your groin muscles (adductors) because you have to squeeze your inner knees against your upper arms.

TUNE IT UP: You can build the groin and abdominal strength needed to do this pose by first trying it on your back. Doing this supine variation will also help build your awareness of the correct muscular actions in this pose. Whatever version you do, focus on strongly pressing your thighs against your arms. If you have a wrist injury, just do Crow Pose on your back until it heals. You might be surprised how hard this pose is to do even when you're lying down!

To try the upright version, start with your feet on a block (see photo) to get a feel for just how strong the inward leg action must be to keep your knees from sliding down your arms. Place your palms flat on the floor (shoulder distance or a little wider) and bend your elbows. Shift forward very, very slowly, to bring your face closer to the floor and your knees higher up your arms.

As you progress and your hips and shoulders start moving toward the front of your mat, your toes will eventually feel like they're about to lift off the block (or the floor). Now try raising one heel at a time toward your butt. One day, both toes may lift off and your crow will take flight.

As your groin, shoulder, and abdominal muscles get stronger, you'll be able to draw your heels closer and closer to your butt and straighten your elbows. These actions take years. Don't worry. Don't hurry. Just enjoy your flight.

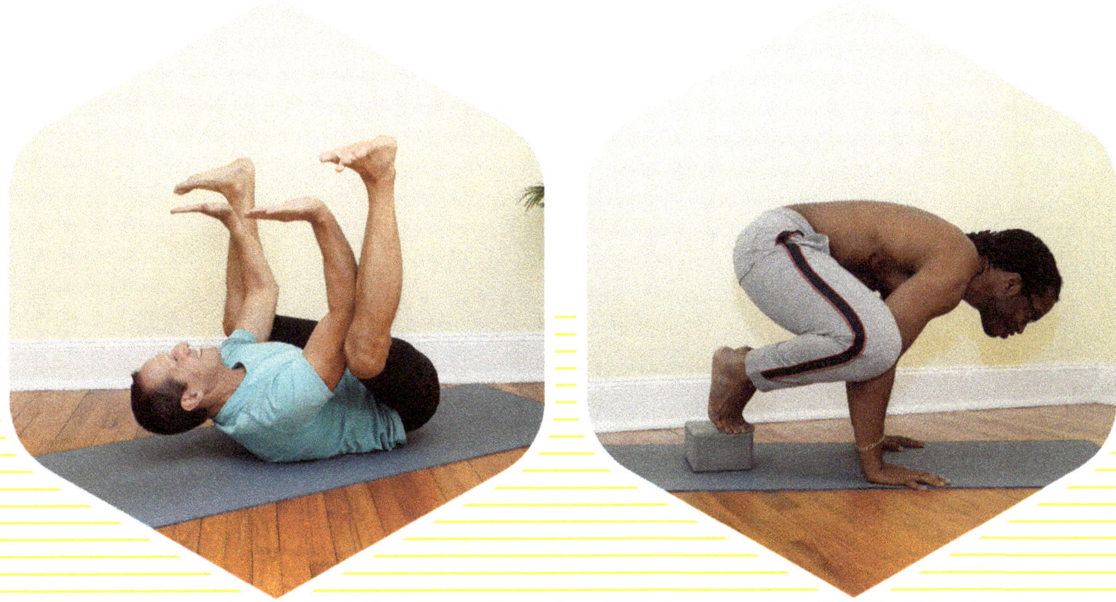

Crow Pose, supine variation

Upright variation with block

Ear Pressure Pose

ALSO CALLED: Karnapidasana

WHAT IT DOES FOR YOUR INNER HIPS: This is a physically and mentally challenging pose that requires both strength in the groins and flexibility in the neck, shoulder, and back muscles.

TUNE IT UP: It's important that you press the backs of your shoulders very firmly down into the floor to support the weight of your torso and hips off of your neck, which is in full flexion. The groin strengthening action is, as the name implies, from pressing your knees in against your ears. If your knees reach the floor in this pose, touch your big toes and press your heels together.

Do not try to do this pose until you're very comfortable in both Plow Pose (Halasana) and Shoulder Stand Pose (Salamba Sarvangasana). (See chapter 5, pages 254 and 257, respectively.) It's a terrible idea to roll onto your upper back and try forcing your way into this pose. That will most likely leave you injured and frustrated. First do other poses that will help you build sufficient strength and flexibility in the shoulders, neck, and back.

If it feels scary, painful, or extremely difficult to do this pose, stop. Come out and work on a variation of Plow Pose or Shoulder Stand, which use these same muscle groups. Remember to adjust the intensity of these alternate poses with tools like blocks, bolsters, and straps to ensure you are working in the best variation for your body today. The most damaging fitness advice ever given was, "No pain, no gain." I shudder to think how many injuries those words have caused.

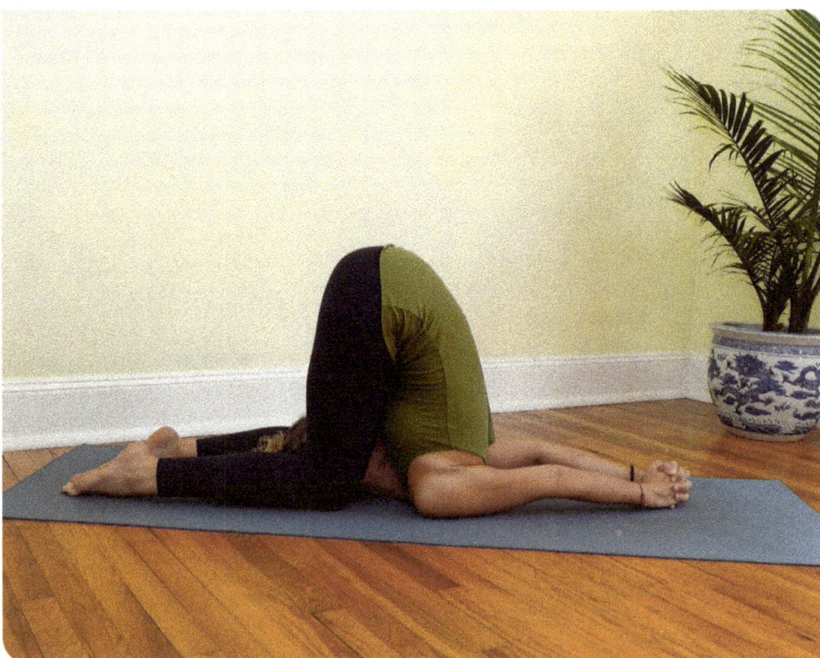

Ear Pressure Pose

MECHANIC'S NOTE:
Build a Sustainable Practice

The mark of a mature, sustainable yoga practice is knowing how to get the most benefit from your practice on any given day without harming your body. Unfortunately a lot of people insist on learning this the hard way, by pushing too hard and getting injured, and only recognize the ignorance that led to their injury after the fact. This is an immature and unsustainable way to practice yoga.

My hope is that this book will help you avoid some of those painful, distressing experiences. Learn what you need to do in each pose by listening closely to your body. Don't look at what anyone else is doing. Keep your focus on your own mat and inside your own body. Every day is different inside your body. Something that was a good idea yesterday may not be within reach today. Don't worry about it. Do a different variation. Be as honest and humble as you can be. I promise, that's the path to real progress.

CHAPTER 4

CORE

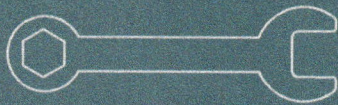

Your core isn't what you think it is. Many people mistakenly think that their core is just the "six-pack" of abdominal muscles (rectus abdominis) on their belly. In fact, your core includes *all* of the muscles in your torso, from your hips to your shoulders. Think of your arms, legs, and head as spokes on a wheel, and your core as the hub.

Yoga is great for building core strength, because it includes both *isotonic* and *isometric* muscle work. Isotonic work is when your muscles resist weight while moving, either contracting (*concentric* isotonic work) or extending (*eccentric* isotonic work). In a yoga class, your core muscles do both.

Isometric exercise happens when you hold still with your muscles engaged. There's a lot of isometric core work in yoga, because muscles all around your torso must stabilize your middle against the position of your arms, legs, and head: to hold Plank Pose, raise your arms in Warrior One, or keep your legs up in Boat Pose.

So yoga gives you isotonic exercise as you move, and isometric exercise when you hold still. Using your torso muscles in all of these ways at once is very effective for building core strength.

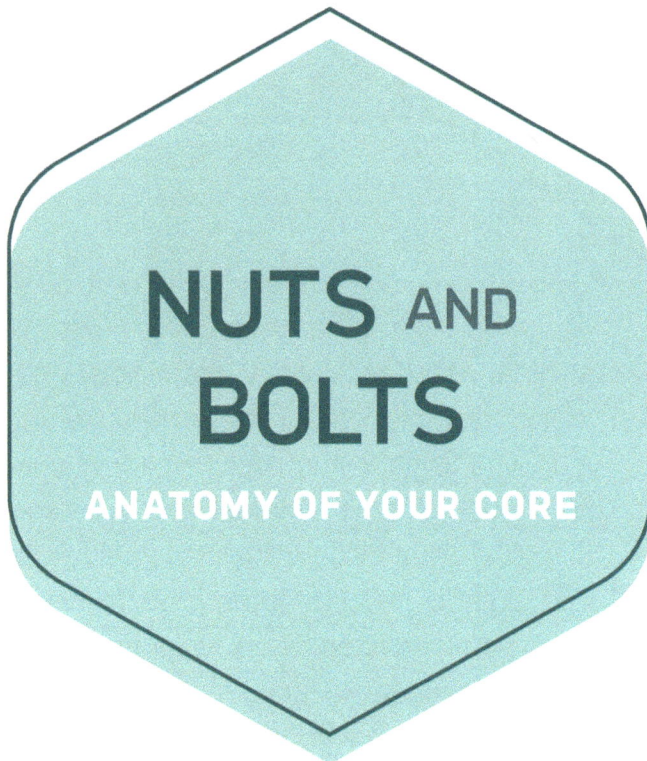

If your torso is the core of your body, your spine is the core of your core. It runs right through the middle, bounded at the base of your lower back by your pelvic girdle. That's the two large, curved bones that make up your hips, plus the flat plate of bone between them, your sacrum. Your tail bone (your coccyx) is a little nub at the bottom of your sacrum. Despite what some yoga instructors say about moving your tail bone, you actually cannot voluntarily move it. Your coccyx just goes along for the ride when you change your pelvic tilt.

The upper end of your core is where your spine passes through your shoulder girdle. It's a structure that's like a scaffolding, made up of the heads of your upper arm bones (humeri, or humerus if singular), collarbones (clavicles), shoulder blades (scapulas), and breast bone (sternum).

Let's take a closer look at this remarkable structure that provides your whole body with strength and support.

Bones and Joints

Though it's sometimes called your "backbone," your spine is actually made up of 24 separate bones, called vertebrae, stacked in a curving column. Your spine sits on top of a flat, boney plate at the back of your pelvis: your sacrum, which is five vertebrae fused together. Your spine has two main jobs: to protect your spinal cord (which is an extension of your brain) and the peripheral nerves that emerge from it; and to facilitate moving your torso and head freely while distributing the forces this movement creates.

You have 24 ribs (12 pairs) that attach to your spine between the vertebrae. Since the rib cage encloses your lungs, which move as you breathe, your ribs have to move too. Every time you inhale, your ribs expand out and backwards toward your spine. And on the exhale, the rib cage releases, with your ribs shifting inwards and slightly away from your spine.

Although your ribs have a range of complex movements, for our purposes it will be easiest to think of the connections between your ribs and spine (your costovertebral joints) as moving like a swinging door (although, technically they are not hinge joints). When you inhale, the door swings open–the front of the hinge (your chest) gets wider and the back of the hinge (your costovertebral joints) gets narrower. When you exhale, the door swings shut, making the front

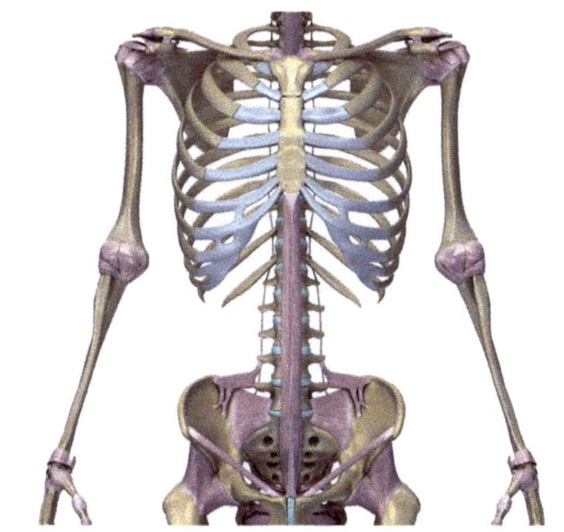

Your pelvis and your shoulder girdle form the lower and upper ends of your core, respectively.

MECHANIC'S NOTE: BEWARE OF COPYCATS

Your pelvis and shoulders are copycats. They want to move the same way. They're like BFFs. It's not that they *can't* move differently from each other—they just don't like to. When you slump your shoulders and chest forward, your pelvis also tucks under. By the same token, when you pull your shoulders back and lift your chest, your pelvis tips forward and puts a little arch in your low back. Knowing how to correctly position your pelvic and shoulder girdles is the key to finding proper alignment in every yoga pose.

Try this: Sit up straight, close your eyes, and slowly slump. Do this a few times in a row, paying close attention to what your shoulders and hips are doing in relation to each other. See? They're copycats! When your shoulders round, your pelvis tucks under. When you draw your shoulders upright and lift your chest, your pelvis follows suit. So when you're doing yoga, remember this default setting in your body and work with it. When you let your shoulders and chest fall forward, your pelvis is going to round under as well. When you draw your shoulders back and lift your chest your sitting bones will swing back behind you. Use this as a tool to adjust your alignment as you practice.

of the hinge close while the back of the hinge opens.

Yoga promotes spinal health by preserving the normal full range of motion between your vertebrae. This requires both strength and flexibility throughout your entire core. To understand how yoga affects your spinal column, it's important to know that your spine is made up of three sections: your neck (cervical spine), your mid-back (thoracic spine), and your lower back (lumbar spine).

Each section of your spine is designed to move differently, with vertebrae to match. Every one of your spinal vertebrae has little foot-like structures on it, called facets. The way these facets fit together determines the direction and degree of movement at each vertebral joint. Because the facets are positioned differently in each of your three spinal sections, the normal range of movement for each section of your spine differs. You don't want to change this. It's the way your spine is made.

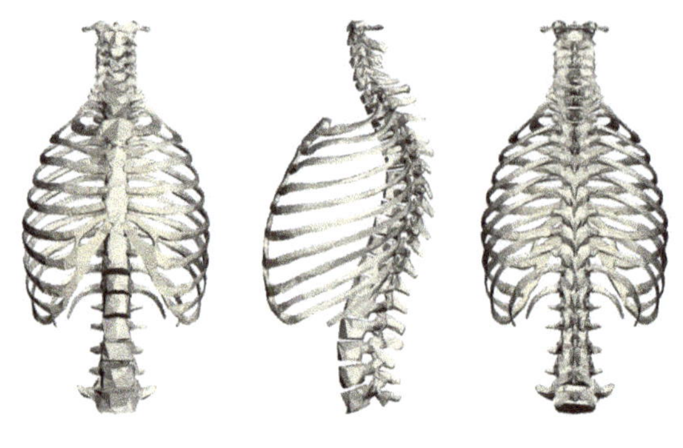

Your ribs attach to the spine between your vertebrae.

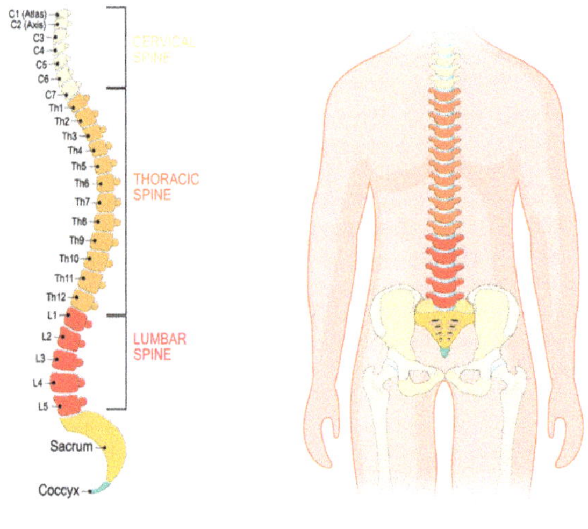

Your spine is described in three sections: cervical, thoracic, and lumbar.

Your Cervical Spine

Your neck—anatomically speaking, your cervical spine—has seven vertebrae that carry a natural backward (lordotic) curve. The facets in your cervical spine are pretty flat; they stand on top of each other sort of like plates stacked in your kitchen cabinet. With the facets in this position, your neck can easily bend forward (flex), bend backward (extend), and turn (rotate). But your neck cannot bend very far to the side. When you tip your ear toward your shoulder, it soon feels "stuck" and won't go any further. That's the point where one facet has slid as far as it can over the other, and has met the edge of the one below it. This is the normal, natural limit of side-bending in your neck. Pulling on your head to try to make it go further sideways risks injuring it. Be gentle. Don't yank on your lovely neck.

The smallest vertebrae of your spine are in your neck. They're small because unlike lower vertebrae, they don't need to support the weight of your entire body. That's why it's so important not to rush into poses like Shoulder Stand (Salamba Sarvangasana), Head Stand (Sirsasana), Plow (Halansana), and Ear Pressure Pose (Karnapidasana). These poses invert your body, putting your torso, hips, and legs above your neck. So it's essential that you build enough strength and flexibility to support this weight off of your cervical vertebrae *before* you try these poses—not *while* trying them. If your chest, arm, shoulder, back, and neck muscles cannot support most of this weight off of your neck bones (the vertebrae), you risk injury. It's not worth it. Be patient. Remember, yoga should heal and strengthen your body, not harm it.

Your head is heavy. The average human head weighs eight to twelve pounds; for reference, a full gallon jug of water weighs eight pounds (an apt comparison, since your brain is mostly water—and no, smarter people don't have heavier heads). Your neck vertebrae and your head have a special relationship that enables you to bear that weight. The natural backward curve (lordotic curve) of your neck acts like a shock-absorber, distributing the weight and movement of your heavy head. When we consider how our bodies handle this load, it becomes clear that the human muscular and skeletal systems function most effectively with your ears positioned over your shoulders, shoulders over hips, hips over knees, and knees over ankles. Yes, your ears should be carried over your shoulders—not out in front of them!

Unfortunately, many of us have developed a misaligned default position that we walk around in most of the time. To witness this for yourself, check out your own posture: Stand with your back against a wall, and your heels near the baseboard (they don't have to touch it). Close your eyes and put the back of your head and your shoulders against the wall. Relax your arms and hands, with your palms facing your thighs, and touch the sides of your pinky fingers to the wall. Gently pull your low back a little bit toward the wall, and pull your ribs in a bit. Welcome to vertical! Take a few breaths and notice how you feel. Do you feel like you're leaning backward? You're not. Is it hard to stand up straight? That's all you're doing.

MECHANIC'S NOTE: TWISTING POSES

Some instructors use the term "wringing" to describe the rotating action of your body in twisting yoga poses. I *intensely* dislike using this term in yoga instruction. Your spine is not a dirty dishcloth or an old mop. You should not be squeezing and grinding your vertebrae as this word suggests. The purpose of twisting poses is NOT to "wring toxins" (or anything else) out of your spine. Many instructors say this sort of thing in class, but what a terrible thing to do to your beautiful, wonderful, amazing spinal column! Your body already knows how to eliminate any unneeded metabolic byproducts that are inside you. And even if you ingest toxic substances, cranking your spinal column around in circles will not help get rid of them. But it will damage your vertebral joints, and the tissues that stabilize and protect them.

Intensely twisting one vertebra over the next does not support spinal health. In fact, it's quite the opposite. If you twist too intensely (too far, too fast, too hard), you risk damaging your discs, ligaments, cartilage, and other structures that support your spine, and degrading your spinal health. Please, do not think of twists as "wringing out your spine". That's not the purpose of rotated or revolved poses and using this "wringing" terminology in class encourages students to move in a harmful, not a healthful, manner.

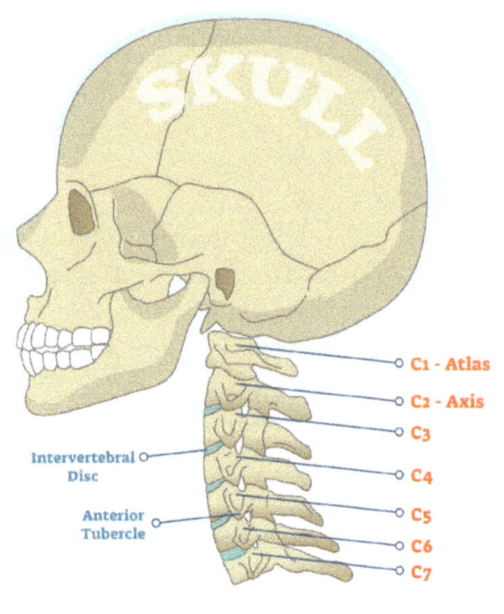

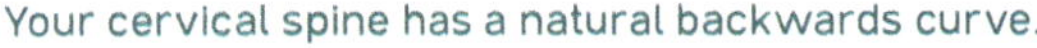

Your cervical spine has a natural backwards curve.

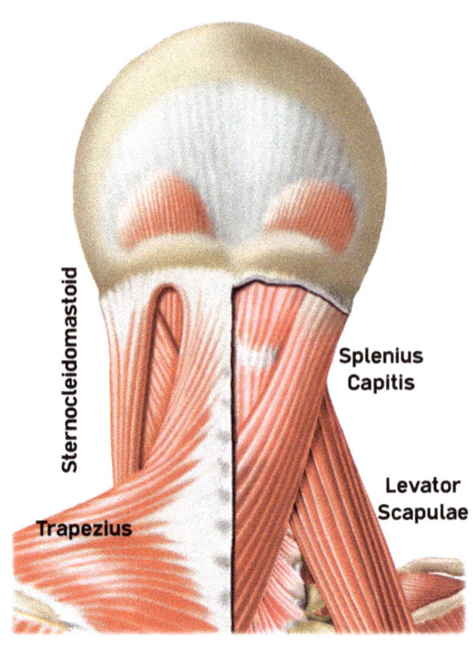

The muscles of your neck are meant to hold your head over your shoulders.

Next, keep your eyes closed and slowly relax back into your regular stance—the way you stand around every day. Notice what part of you peeled off the wall first, and how far. Did your weight drop into one foot? Did one knee bend? Take a breath or two here, and then draw your head, shoulders, and pinkies toward the wall, and stand up straight again. (No judgment.) The wall is not leaning backwards, even though you may feel like you are. This exercise is a great way to become aware of your own posture habits, so you can make changes that will help you maintain normal function in your bones, joints, and muscles.

Here's another major contributor to throwing our posture out of whack: Many of us habitually look down at the ground while we walk. For many people, especially if we're older, part of this habit comes from a fear of falling. Or it may be a way of avoiding eye-contact, and withdrawing from the outside world. And of course, many of us walk around this way while constantly looking at down at our phones. Whatever the cause, the problem is that over time, this head-down posture gets hardened into your body, and triggers a cascade of other issues. Looking down puts your head in front of your spine (out of correct/central alignment), and hangs all eight to twelve pounds of its weight on only one or two neck vertebrae (mostly cervical vertebrae six and seven).

This habitual forward head carriage can cause chronic neck inflammation, abnormal boney changes in your vertebrae, and uneven wear on the discs between your vertebrae. Those problems cause a domino effect down your spine, making your shoulders and mid-back slump forward as well. As we mentioned earlier, the copycat effect is going to make your pelvis tuck under too. Which in turn shortens your hamstrings and affects the movement of your hips and knees.

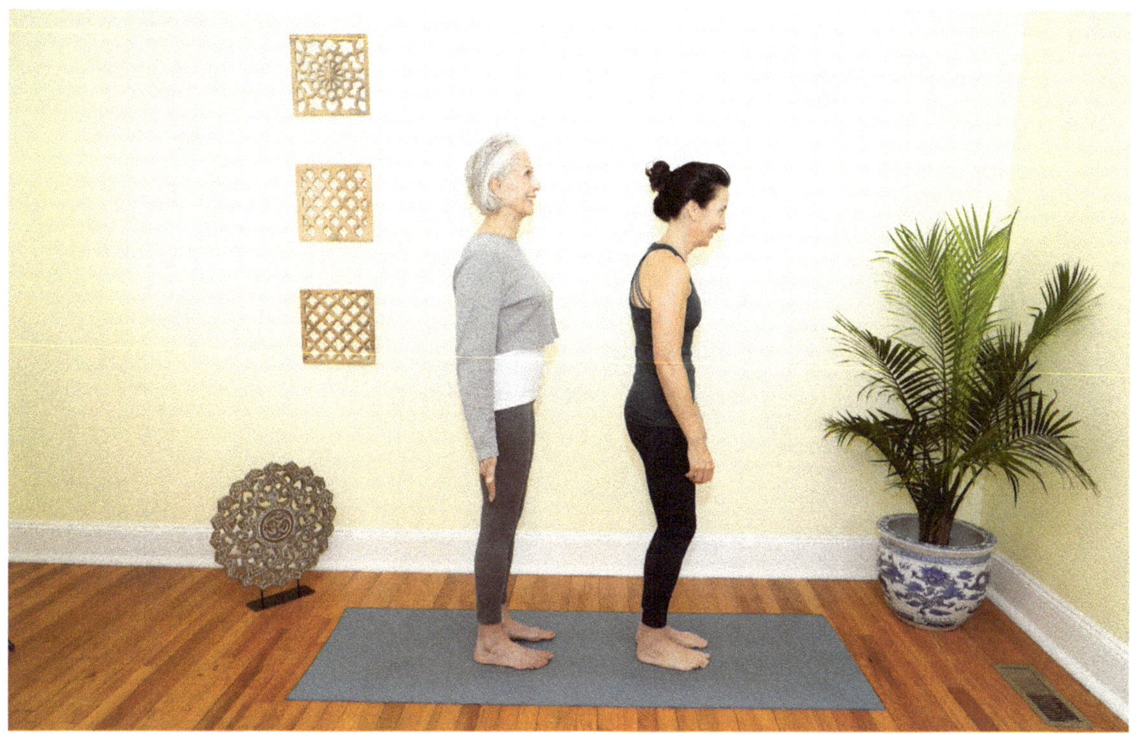

Standing up straight (left), vs. forward head carriage (right). Don't be a downer. Hold your head up with your ears over your shoulders.

It doesn't have to be that way. You don't need to constantly look at the ground. In most everyday circumstances, when walking indoors or on smooth pavement or a sidewalk, most people can walk safely by just glancing down every now and then as necessary. Upright head carriage (central/correct alignment) distributes the weight of your head more evenly onto all seven neck vertebrae. And isn't it safer to look at what's in front of you as you walk, than to be scrolling through your social media feed?

A regular yoga practice can help you start reforming your posture. To maximize this, be certain not to have slouchy posture while you practice, and pay attention to where you're looking during class. When you're standing upright, look directly forward or slightly upward. Don't look down at the floor—that will pull your shoulders and chest down into that slumped position you're trying to get rid of. This might be challenging to change, but remember, everything takes practice—both good habits and bad habits take time to establish. Be patient, and use your yoga practice to build good posture habits.

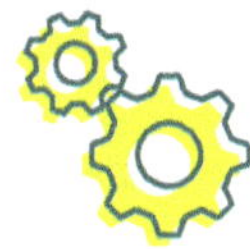

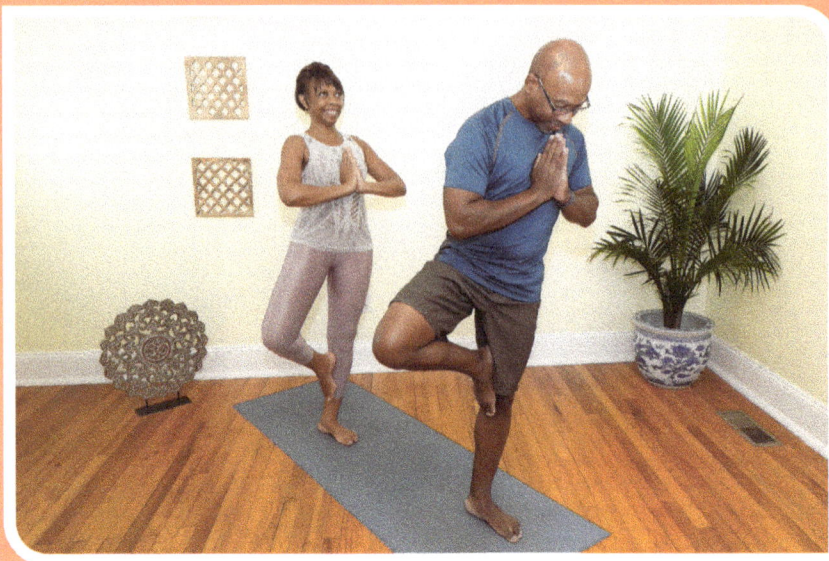

Tree Pose
Correct alignment at left; don't be a downer.

MECHANIC'S NOTE: Don't Look Down

Some yoga instructors tell students to look at the floor if they're having trouble keeping their balance. I disagree with this instruction. Although looking down does make balancing a little easier by letting your eyes focus on something nearby, it reinforces bad posture and forward head carriage. It also means you're learning to balance while out of correct alignment. Which means muscles throughout your entire body will adjust to the weight of your head being in front, instead of on top of your spine where it belongs. That's just one more thing you'll have to correct later. Students sometimes tell me that they only look down with their eyes, that they don't tilt their head downward. I'm skeptical. Eventually your head will follow your gaze; it's nearly impossible to resist this natural tendency. If you look down with your eyes, you'll eventually end up with forward head carriage and shoulder slump.

If balancing is a challenge during your yoga practice, put your mat near a wall and steady yourself by lightly touching the wall as needed. No matter what, keep your ears over your shoulders. Lightly touching a wall to help balance (instead of looking down at the floor) strengthens an essential component of balance called your proprioception (which you may remember from chapter 1). At the same time, this positive habit reinforces correct/central alignment throughout your body, and reforms your posture to be more upright.

Your Thoracic Spine

As we move down the spine from your neck to your mid-back (the thoracic spine), we find that the vertebrae become bigger and sturdier. This part of your back carries a heavier load than your neck. To more effectively distribute the increased weight and greater forces of movement, the twelve vertebrae in your mid-back form a natural, forward curvature (a kyphotic curve).

The facets in your mid-back sit at a slightly upward angle, unlike your cervical facets, which are flatter. This upward tilt of the thoracic facets allows your mid-back to bend forward (flex), turn (rotate), and bend sideways fairly easily. But with the facets shaped that way, your mid-back does not bend backward (extend) very far. Of course, the natural forward curve also works against back-bending in the thoracic spine. Because of those structural realities, your mid-back can't contribute much to backward-bending yoga poses.

Which is why it's important to understand that the vertebrae of your spine should not be the focus when you try a back-bending pose. If you're having trouble with backbends, please understand that your spine is not the problem. Approaching these poses by cranking on your spinal skeleton is misguided, and puts you at risk for injury.

So, what should you focus on? The two biggest restrictions to back-bending are:

- **Tight muscles and soft tissues** on the front of your body (your quads, hip flexors, abs, and chest).
- **Weak muscles** on the back of your body (your shoulders, upper back, glutes, and hamstrings).

So when you're working on back bending poses, focus on building flexibility in the muscles on your front, and strength in the back. To see this more clearly, observe your yoga teacher demonstrating the pose, or simply search online for pictures of people doing yoga backbends, like Wheel Pose. Notice how the mid-back (the thoracic spine) is usually pretty flat. Even with the thoracic vertebrae in full extension, because that section of the spine normally bends slightly forward, it looks flat during the backbend. You'll never make your spine into a rainbow or horse-shoe shape! If you did, it would be a terrible injury. (Note: Pictures of people doing extreme back-bends in the mid-spine most often reflect abnormal vertebral anatomy that may be genetic or surgically altered, or damage to the vertebral joints that allows abnormal movement.)

Be patient. Be careful. Plan on making gradual progress that's sustainable. Remember, yoga is not a war with your body. Ask it to change little by little, and it will.

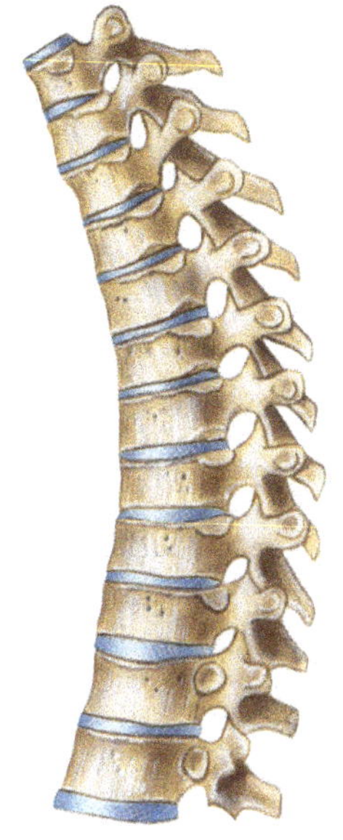

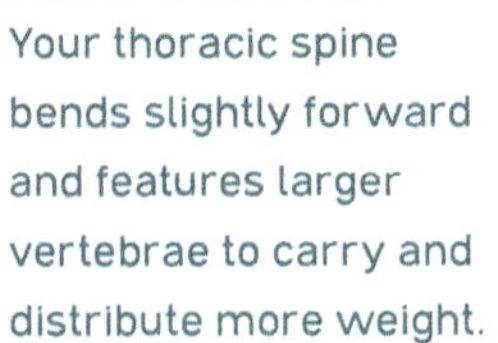

Your thoracic spine bends slightly forward and features larger vertebrae to carry and distribute more weight.

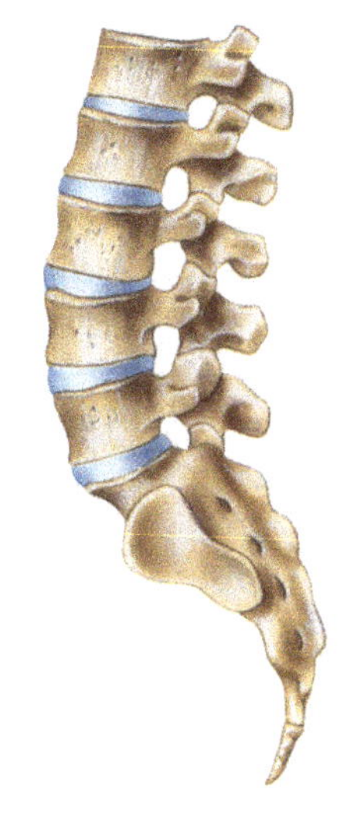

The lumbar spine consists of five large vertebrae that bend slightly backward.

Your Lumbar Spine

Your body's largest spinal vertebrae are in your low back, aka your lumbar spine. This makes sense, because these bones handle the weight and movement of your entire upper torso. Your low back has five vertebrae, and together they create a natural backward (lordotic) curve—like the curve in your neck.

The facet joints of your low back (lumbar) vertebrae are, essentially, vertical. This means that your low back can pretty easily bend forward (flex) and backward (extend). But because of the facet position, for all practical purposes your low back cannot rotate or side bend. Technically speaking, your low back vertebrae do have approximately four-millimeters of rotation and side-bending movement. That's less than half the width of a standard pencil eraser! So, when doing yoga poses, it's best to think of your lumbar spine as having no ability to rotate or side-bend.

Twisting yoga poses are widely misunderstood, and often taught incorrectly with regard to the lumbar spine. It's common to hear a yoga instructor tell students to "rotate from the base of your spine." Please understand that this is anatomically impossible to do without damaging your low back. The only way to safely turn your low back in a revolved yoga pose is to turn your hips and pelvis. Remember, your lumbar spine sits on top of your pelvis at your sacrum. If you don't let the pelvis turn in the direction you're twisting, then you can only rotate your mid-back and neck.

The last place in your spine where one vertebra can rotate over the next is where your last mid-back vertebrae (thoracic vertebra number 12, or T-12) meets your first lumbar vertebra (L-1). If you do not move your pelvis in the direction of the turn, you can only rotate from your thoracic-lumbar junction (T-12/L-1) upward. There's nothing wrong with doing that, as long as you don't force the twist further by using your arms to crank yourself around. That's a good way to injure your low back.

Understanding how your spine works will enable you to avoid injury: If your pelvis is held in place and not allowed to turn with your torso and shoulders, your low back cannot turn. Period. To involve your lower back in a revolved pose, you must turn your pelvis. Never force your vertebrae into unnatural movements. Move the three sections of your spine the way each is designed to move. And, remember, they're designed to move differently.

Core Muscles

The muscles of your core are essential for doing every position and movement in your yoga practice. For our purposes, I think it makes most sense to look at yoga poses that stretch and strengthen your entire core, and the actions in each pose that do this.

Of course, central alignment is key. That means sending your weight, or the force of a movement, through the centers of your bones and joints. When you learn to hold your shoulders and pelvis in central alignment during yoga practice, you'll begin building much more core strength. The core muscles of your waist (rectus abdominus, transverse abdominus, and your obliques) and back (latissimus dorsi, rhomboids, erector spinae, serratus anterior, serratus superior, serratus posterior, quadratus lumborum, and your trapezius) become very strong and flexible when you practice with correct alignment.

You should stretch and strengthen the front and back of your torso (your entire core) evenly, to avoid imbalanced muscle groups that can contribute to misalignment and injury.

Because the muscles of your body work together in groups, we can't really isolate yoga poses that stretch or strengthen just one muscle in the core. Generally speaking, yoga poses that

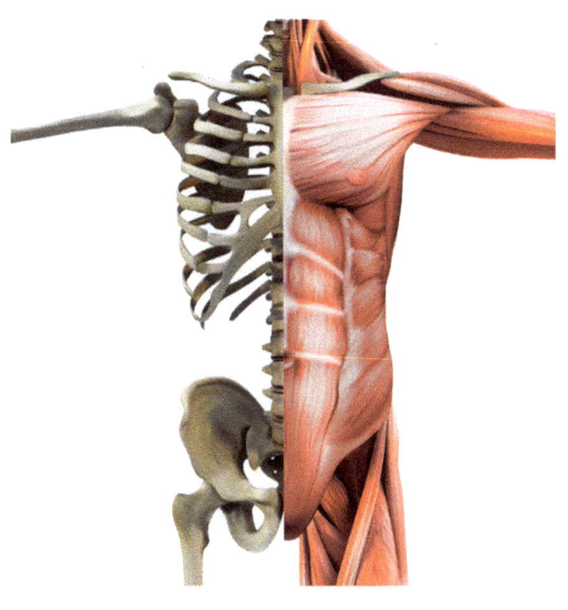

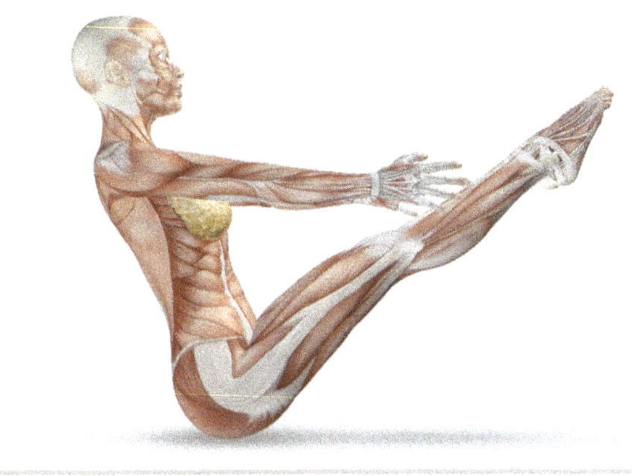

Your entire torso is your core, not just your belly.

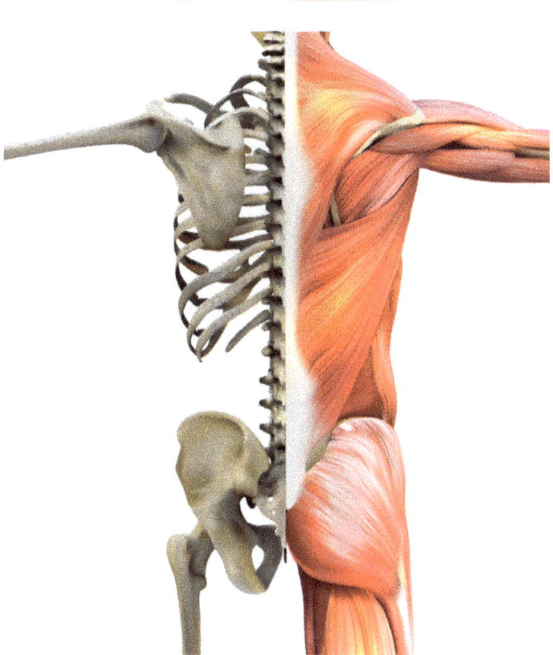

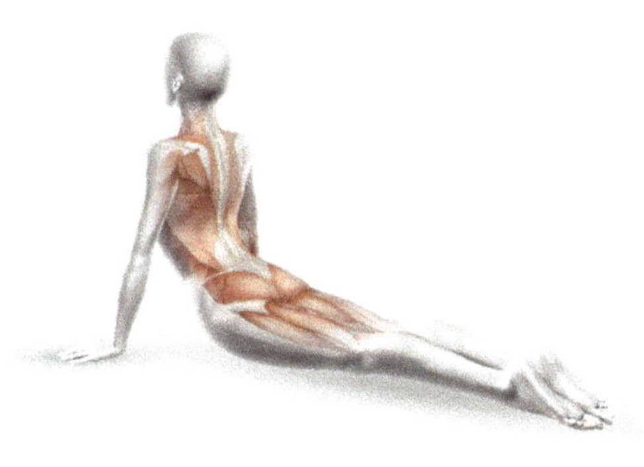

A yoga pose that stretches your core in front will strengthen the muscles in back and visa versa.

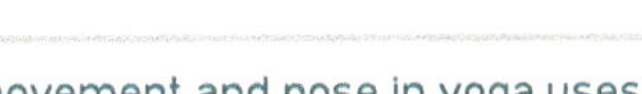

Every movement and pose in yoga uses the muscles of your core

stretch your back muscles build core strength on your front body (for example, forward folds). And poses that stretch the core muscles on the front of your body build strength on your back body (backbends, for example). This is because opposing muscle groups contract to pull your torso in either direction. Notice how the opposing muscle groups work while you practice. Don't just focus on the strongest physical sensation—investigate how all your muscles are feeling.

For sure, some muscles feel like they're working harder than others in a pose. But understand that many other muscles are also working. It's hard to notice all the other, more subtle muscles at work, because your weakest or tightest muscles are crying out so loudly. The same pose can feel very different to two people who have different sets of weak or tight muscles. This is the value of holding still once you've gotten into a pose. Now you have a few breaths to draw your attention inward, and scan each part of your body. What are your legs and feet doing? What do they feel like? Your waist and back? Your shoulders, arms, and neck?

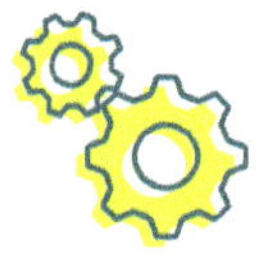

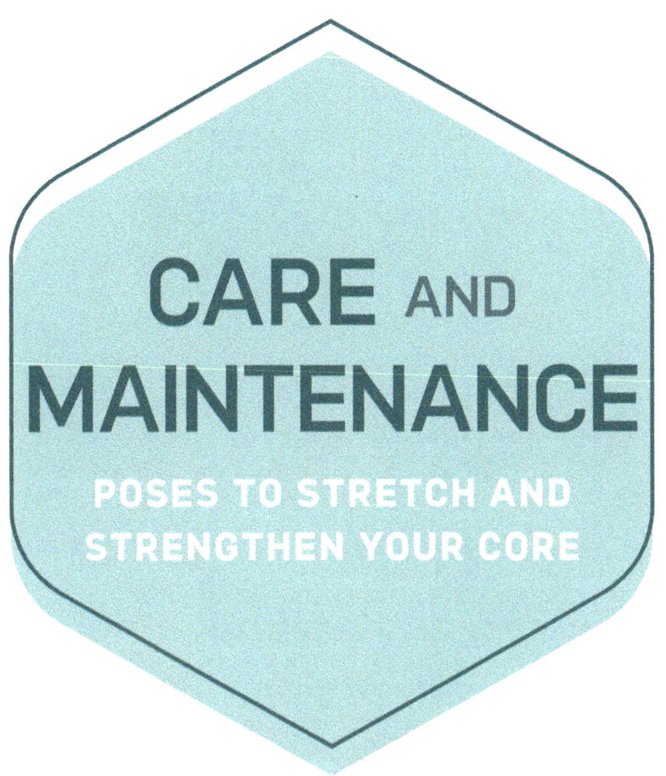

CARE AND MAINTENANCE

POSES TO STRETCH AND STRENGTHEN YOUR CORE

Now that you have a good understanding of how your spine is put together and what your core really is, let's apply that knowledge. In the next section, we'll explore a variety of poses that strengthen and stretch your core. Remember, poses that stretch and extend your front core muscles will strengthen and contract your back core muscles. By the same token, poses that stretch your back, strengthen your front.

Opposing muscles groups work together to create movement and to hold a position in stillness. Keep this in mind while you practice and try to become aware of the many muscle groups at work in each pose. This is a great way to discover new insights and make your yoga practice more effective. Start at the hub of the wheel, so to speak, at the center of your core and scan outward from there. Be curious about what every part of your body is doing all the way to your fingertips and toes.

Cat and Cow Pose

ALSO CALLED: Bitilasana

WHAT IT DOES FOR YOUR CORE: Some yoga poses stretch and strengthen your core from all angles: front, side, and back. The two-position sequence of Cat and Cow Pose does this by alternately flexing and extending your spine. Cat and Cow Pose is often used as a warm-up at the beginning of a yoga class, because it also helps focus your mind on your breathing by following your inhales and exhales as you move.

TUNE IT UP: On an exhale, draw your chin toward your chest and round inward (flex) to Cat Pose. On an inhale, look upward and extend your spine into Cow Pose. Focus on connecting your breathing with your movement. Pay attention to moving your eyes as well as your body; look up with your eyes more than your face in Cow Pose, and look in toward your belly in Cat. In both Cat and Cow, pause for a second to draw your knees slightly inward toward each other (they won't actually move much). Making an inward action with your thighs activates the muscles of your low belly (transverse abdominus) and your pelvic floor. This is a good place to start finding an awareness of something we call the root lock (mula bandha). This is a contraction of the deep low belly and pelvic floor muscles that you can use to help you move further in many poses.

Traditionally, Cat and Cow Pose is done on all fours, but it can also be done seated. If your back is grumpy at the start of class, elevate your hips by sitting up on a block, bolster, or folded blanket. If you're seated, keep your elbows as straight as possible, and press your hands away from your chest.

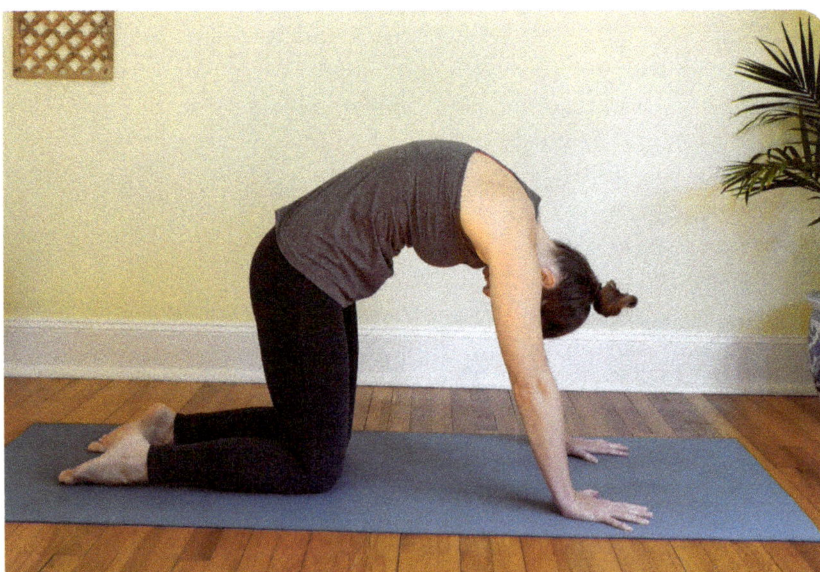

Cat Pose (Spinal Flexion)

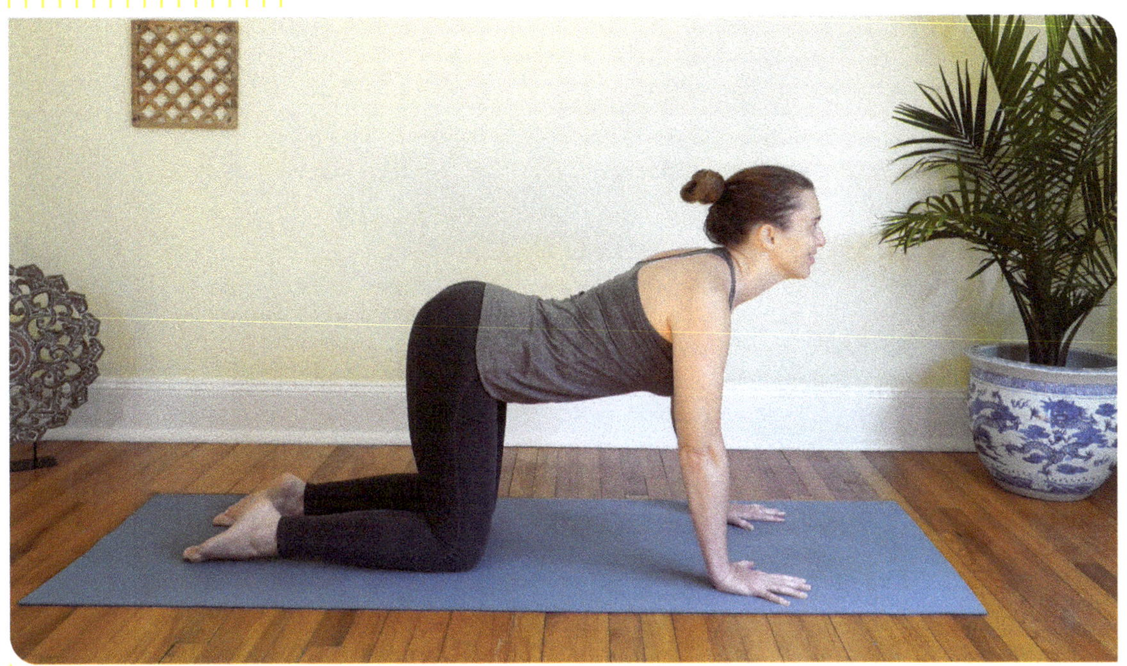

Cow Pose (Spinal Extension)

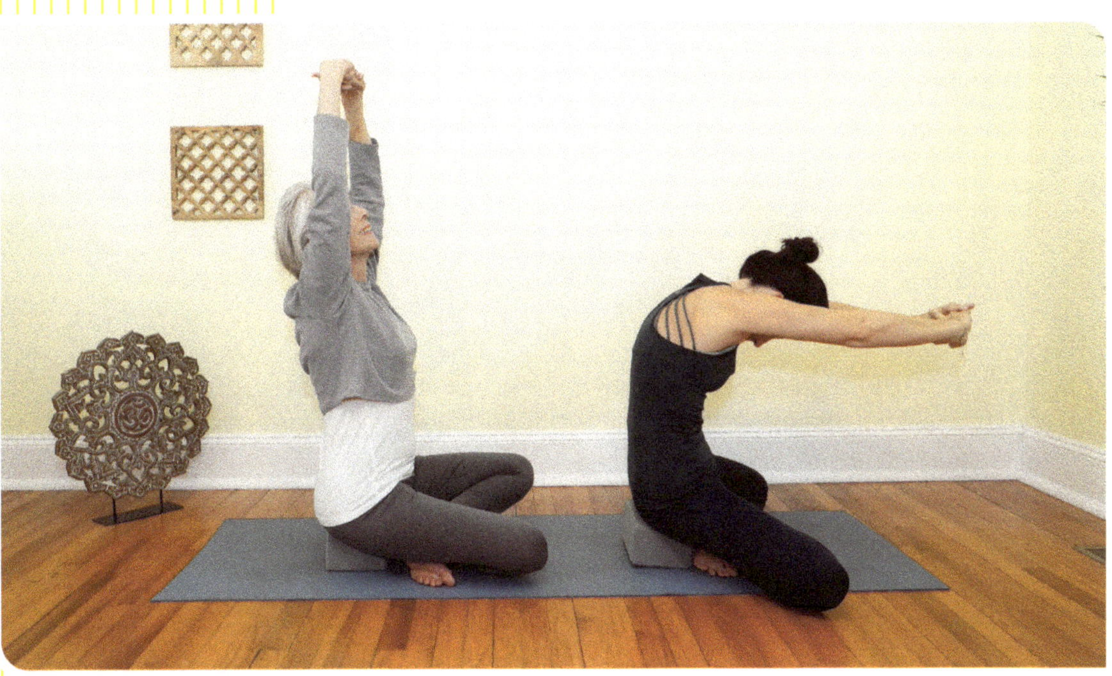

Cat and Cow Pose, seated variation

Extended Mountain Pose

ALSO CALLED: Utthita Tadasana

WHAT IT DOES FOR YOUR CORE: Extended Mountain Pose is one of the foundational poses in yoga. It takes a lot of core strength—front, back, and sides—to stand evenly on both feet and raise your arms up with straight elbows.

TUNE IT UP: It's very important to have straight elbows here, since bending them substantially reduces the work in your abdominal and back muscles. To experience this for yourself, stand with your hands by your sides, press your heels slightly outward, pull your sitting bones down a bit toward your hamstrings, and lift your chest. Raise your arms on an inhale with straight elbows, moving your hands as wide apart as needed to get your elbows straight. Notice how hard all the muscles of your core are working. Now let your elbows bend, and feel how most of that muscle-work turns off. Take a breath and straighten them again. Feel the difference.

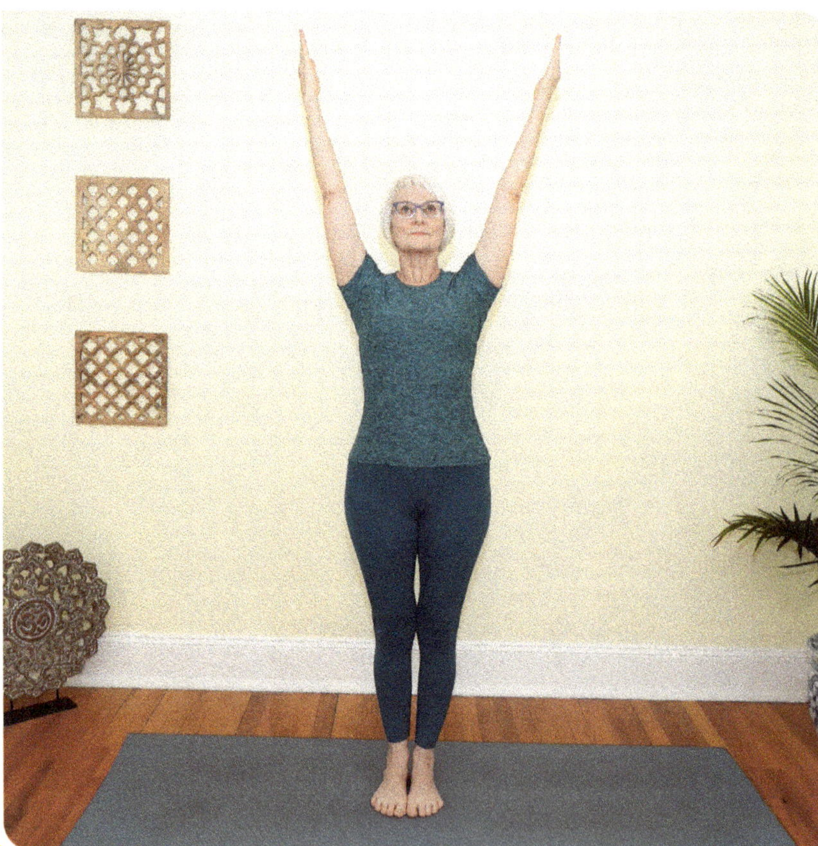

Extended Mountain Pose

MECHANIC'S NOTE:
Straight Elbows for Strength

Over time, you might build enough strength to bring your hands closer together overhead with straight elbows in Mountain Pose. Eventually your palms might touch, but don't worry about that. It's not the goal. What matters is that you don't practice the pose with bent elbows. No matter where your hands are, get those elbows straight to be sure you don't miss the core and upper back strengthening benefits of this pose.

The reason it's so tempting to bend your elbows when you raise your arms is because the core muscle-work needed to keep them straight makes breathing more difficult. A lot of people are unaware that when they raise their arms, they automatically hold their breath. It's a natural tendency you can overcome by paying close attention to the flow of your breath in practice.

The anatomical reason is that all of the muscles that move your arms are on the walls of your chest (your front, side, and back chest-walls). That means the same muscles that raise your arms are also involved in moving your rib cage when you breathe. Raising your arms with straight elbows asks these muscles to do both at once—to straighten and hold up your arms, while also moving your rib cage to breathe.

Extended Mountain Pose may look easy, but it really takes a lot of strength and focus. Just the act of breathing deeply with your arms extended will make your core stronger.

Staff Pose

ALSO CALLED: Dandasana

WHAT IT DOES FOR YOUR CORE: This is another foundational yoga pose that's surprisingly difficult. It takes a lot of strength in all sides of your core to hold your spine upright with your legs extended.

TUNE IT UP: If your hamstrings are tight, sit on a bolster or folded blanket. Put your hands flat against the mat or bolster by your hips, and press them down and slightly outward to help lift your chest. Pull your shoulder blades together and slightly down your back during this pose, like you've got a $100 bill tucked in the back of your armpit on a windy day. Keep your thigh muscles (your quads) very firm, and turn the upper inner thighs a little bit inward. Push your heels forward to flex your feet, and look forward or slightly up. Another option is to draw your chin down toward your chest while lifting your breast bone (sternum) up toward your chin. This variation gives you a nice stretch on the back of your neck.

Remember, you'll tend to hold your breath in this pose, because your core muscles are working hard to both hold your body up and move your rib cage to breathe. Focus on taking slow deep breaths.

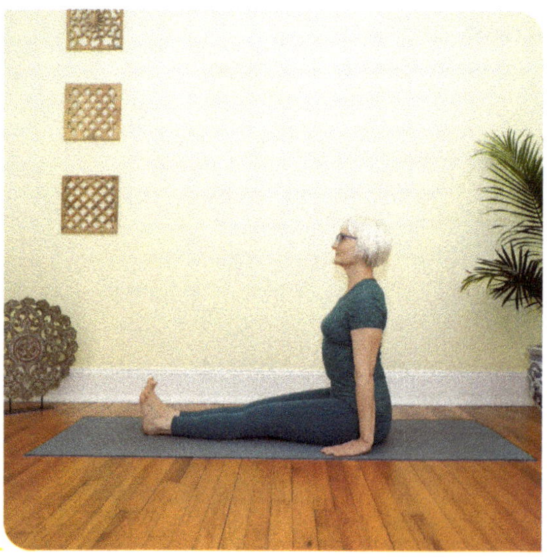

Staff Pose

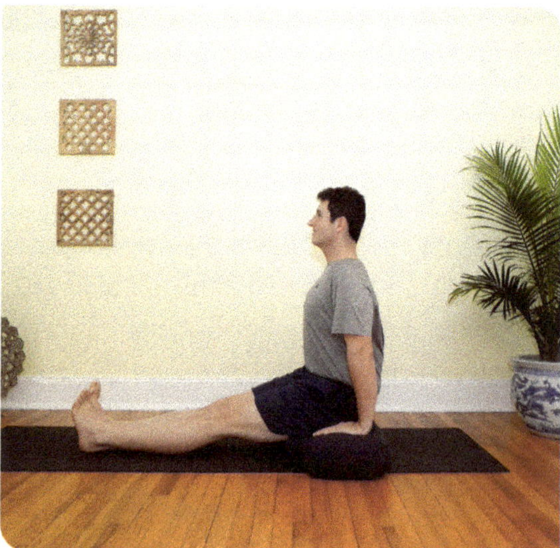

Variation with bolster

Boat Pose

ALSO CALLED: Navasana

WHAT IT DOES: Another great, all-around core-strengthener.

TUNE IT UP: When learning this pose, start with your toes on the floor and your hands behind your knees. Slowly build strength by lifting one foot at a time. Eventually, you'll lift both feet and hold your shins parallel to the floor. Then you can work on letting go of your legs and reaching your arms forward with straight elbows. One day, your legs might straighten with your toes pointed toward the ceiling. Don't worry—you have nothing to prove here. You're just doing this to develop symmetrical strength and flexibility across your core muscle groups to help keep your body fully mobile.

In any variation of Boat Pose, you can increase the strength challenge for your core by extending your arms up toward the ceiling. If you're holding behind your knees, start by raising one arm at a time. Look forward or slightly upward, and breathe deeply. And remember to keep your elbows as straight as possible.

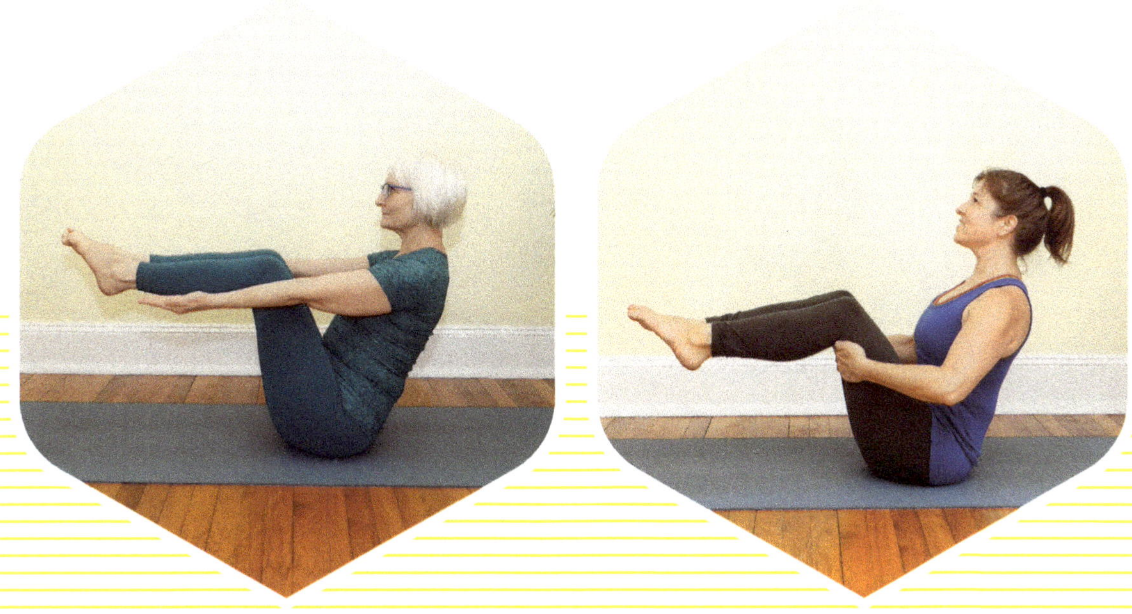

Boat Pose

Variation holding the legs

Gate Pose

ALSO CALLED: Parighasana

WHAT THEY DO FOR YOUR CORE: I prefer these variations where you lean away from the extended leg instead of side-bending toward it (the traditional way to do Gate Pose). Both the original pose and the variations strengthen your entire core. I find there is less risk of straining your low back in this "leaning away" variation, because one hand is on the floor to help support the weight of your torso. The muscular action in both versions is similar.

TUNE IT UP: In the leaning away variation, focus on lifting your upper rib cage and hip toward the ceiling. Don't let your hips sag down or drop back behind you. Put a block under the lower hand if you have difficulty reaching the floor, or if putting your hand on the floor makes your chest drop forward and your butt stick out.

Start by raising your top arm toward the ceiling with a straight elbow. Eventually, you'll be strong and flexible enough to reach the top arm out over your ear. You can increase the strength challenge even more by bending the lower elbow and resting that forearm on a block. Breathe.

To stretch your upper hip, keep the back foot (on the extended leg) flat on the floor, with your toes pointed forward (toward the long edge of your mat). Do not let your toes turn toward the back (short edge) of your mat.

To build even more core strength and balance, lift the back (extended) leg so your heel is level with your hip. Flex the lifted foot and push outward with your heel. Steady your thoughts by holding your eyes still. Gaze softly at one point and breathe deeply.

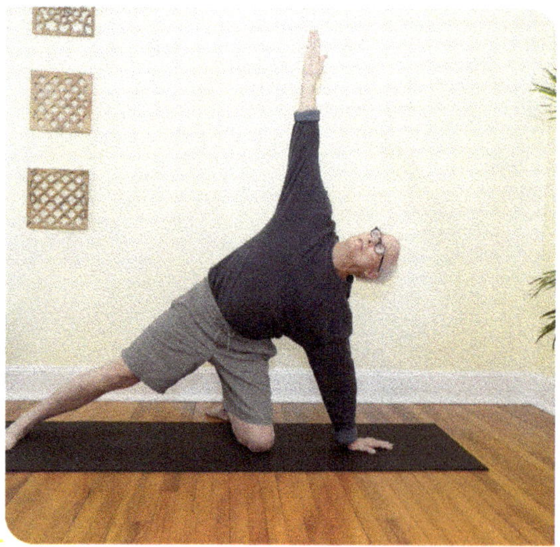

Gate Pose, variation

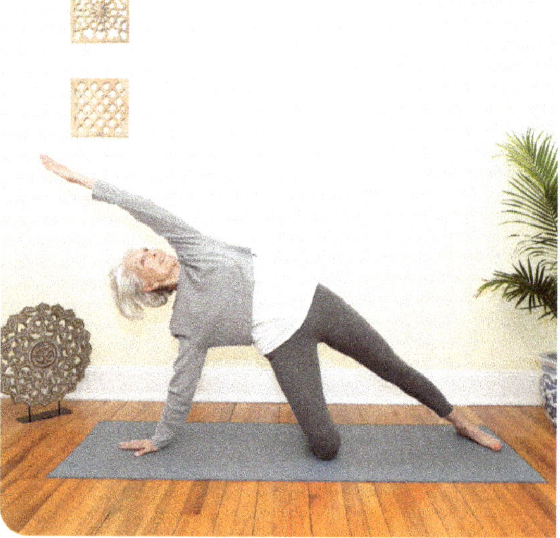

Gate Pose, variation

Side Plank Pose

ALSO CALLED: Vasisthasana

WHAT IT DOES FOR YOUR CORE: This pose is similar to the Gate Pose variation above, but with both legs extended.

TUNE IT UP: If your core is weak or tight, start by reaching the top arm toward the ceiling. Once you build enough core strength and flexibility, you can begin reaching the lifted arm over your ear. Do not bend your elbow. Remember, all the muscles that move your arm are connected to your chest wall, so reaching your arm over your ear with a straight elbow may be more difficult than you might expect. Moving the arm will also challenge your ability to breathe deeply. This is the subtle, inner-strengthening work of yoga. Try to notice it. Take your time.

If balancing is a challenge, put your lower forearm on the floor or a block. But be aware that while this makes balancing easier, it makes lifting your hips harder. When most people first try this pose, the top foot tries to "grip onto" the lower foot. Work over time to push your heels out, and stack your flexed feet side-by-side as if you're standing on the floor. It's harder than you might think. Be patient. Small adjustments like getting your feet flexed and stacked evenly take a lot of body awareness. But these are the small tweaks that help you build more strength, focus, and flexibility. These types of subtle adjustments are what propel your practice forward over time.

Mechanic's Note: Take a Broad View Notice what all the parts of your body are doing in a pose. Investigate any muscle that's struggling. Is that because it's weak or because it's inflexible? Both? Take your time. Breathe steadily. It takes a long time to develop functional strength and flexibility. Keep getting on your mat and practicing at your own pace. Your body will adapt. Have faith. No judgement.

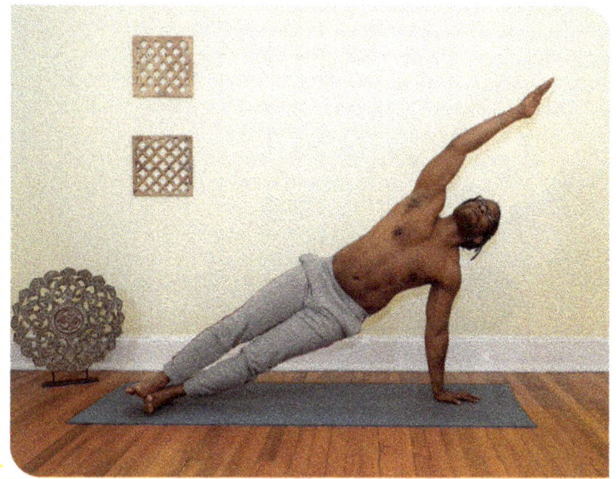

Side Plank Pose

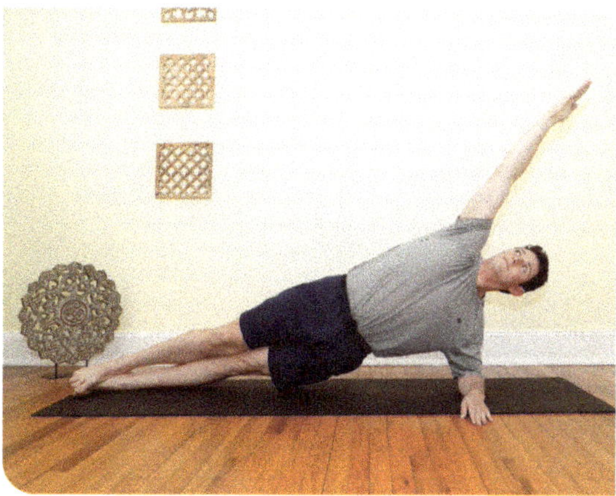

Variation with forearm on floor

Warrior Three Pose

ALSO CALLED: Virabhadrasana Three

WHAT IT DOES FOR YOUR CORE: Builds a lot of all-around core strength, particularly in your back muscles.

TUNE IT UP: Putting blocks under your hands in this pose lets you focus on lifting your chest and rib cage up away from the floor. Your torso should be stretching forward, not curling down, in Warrior Three.

Spend several months using blocks before you start bringing one hand at a time back beside your hip, alternating sides each time. Keep your elbows straight. Eventually, you'll be strong enough to have both hands reaching back beside your hips.

From there, bend your elbows and bring your palms together in front of your chest (prayer hands, or anjali mudra). With your hands at your chest, focus on pulling your shoulders up onto your back. Don't let your shoulders sag toward the floor.

From there, you can increase the core-strengthening benefits of this pose by extending the arm on the lifted-leg side forward. When you feel steady, try reaching both arms forward. Straighten your elbows. Be patient. It takes a long time to build this much strength.

When learning difficult standing balances, start near a wall to focus on your alignment, strength, and breathing.

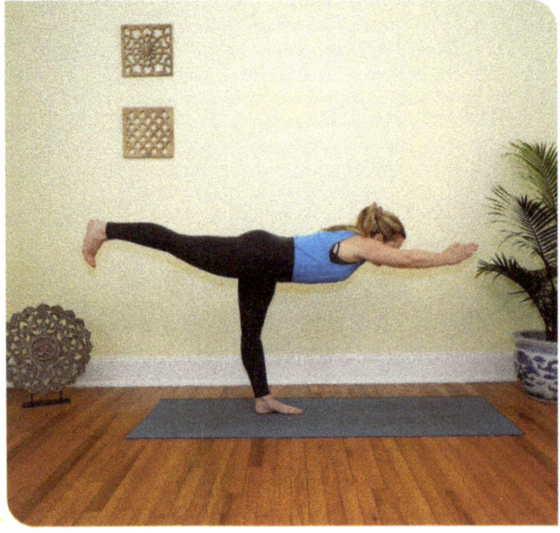

Warrior Three Pose

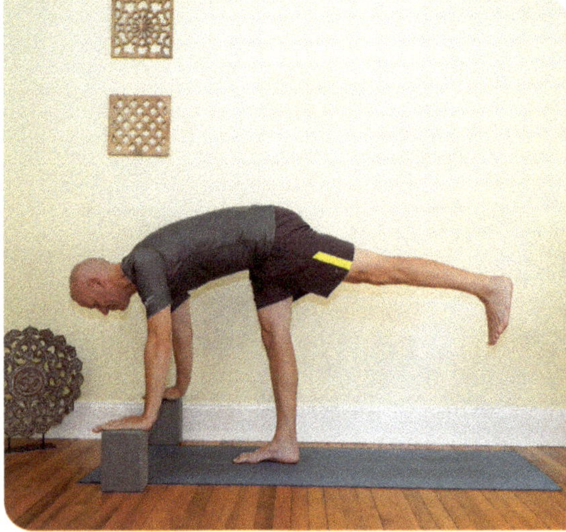

Variation with blocks

Revolved Hand to Foot Pose

ALSO CALLED: Parivrtta Hasta Pandangustasana

WHAT IT DOES FOR YOUR CORE: Like most standing poses that are revolved or turned, this pose builds a great deal of core strength. Your abdominal muscles work to turn your torso toward the lifted (front) leg, while your back muscles hold your torso upright. If your abdominal muscles are weak, turning toward the lifted leg will be quite difficult. If your back muscles are weak, your chest will tend to curl forward over the lifted leg.

TUNE IT UP: Revolved, standing balance poses also strengthen your mental focus. Do not let your eyes jump all around the room. Set a soft gazing point and hold your vision there. After you feel steady and balanced in the pose, you can begin shifting your gaze toward your back hand. This is the last thing to work on in this pose. Moving your gazing point is done by shifting your eyes back, one half-inch at a time. Stop moving your eyes when you get wobbly.

This complex balancing pose takes a great deal of patience and strength. If you're new to this pose, don't waste your time trying to get into the position while hopping around on your mat. Instead, I recommend standing sideways by a wall, with the leg you'll lift closest to the wall. Then:

- Put your fingertips (on the lifted leg side) on the wall behind you at about chest height.
- Lift the leg that's by the wall with a bent knee, and hold across the thigh, knee, shin, ankle, or foot with your free hand.
- Now walk your fingers backward on the wall until your elbow is straight and your palm is flat on the wall. Your face and chest will turn toward the wall as you walk that hand back. Keep the lifted knee bent while you get your torso turned and your back arm in place.
- Focus on turning your torso with the strength of your core and holding your spine upright with the strength of your back. Breathe.
- Eventually you will start to straighten the lifted leg and move your gaze toward your back hand. When you start to shift your gaze, do it a little at a time. When your balance falters, stop shifting your eyes there and firm up your foundation. Focus on feeling steady and secure.

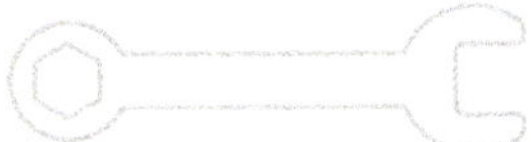

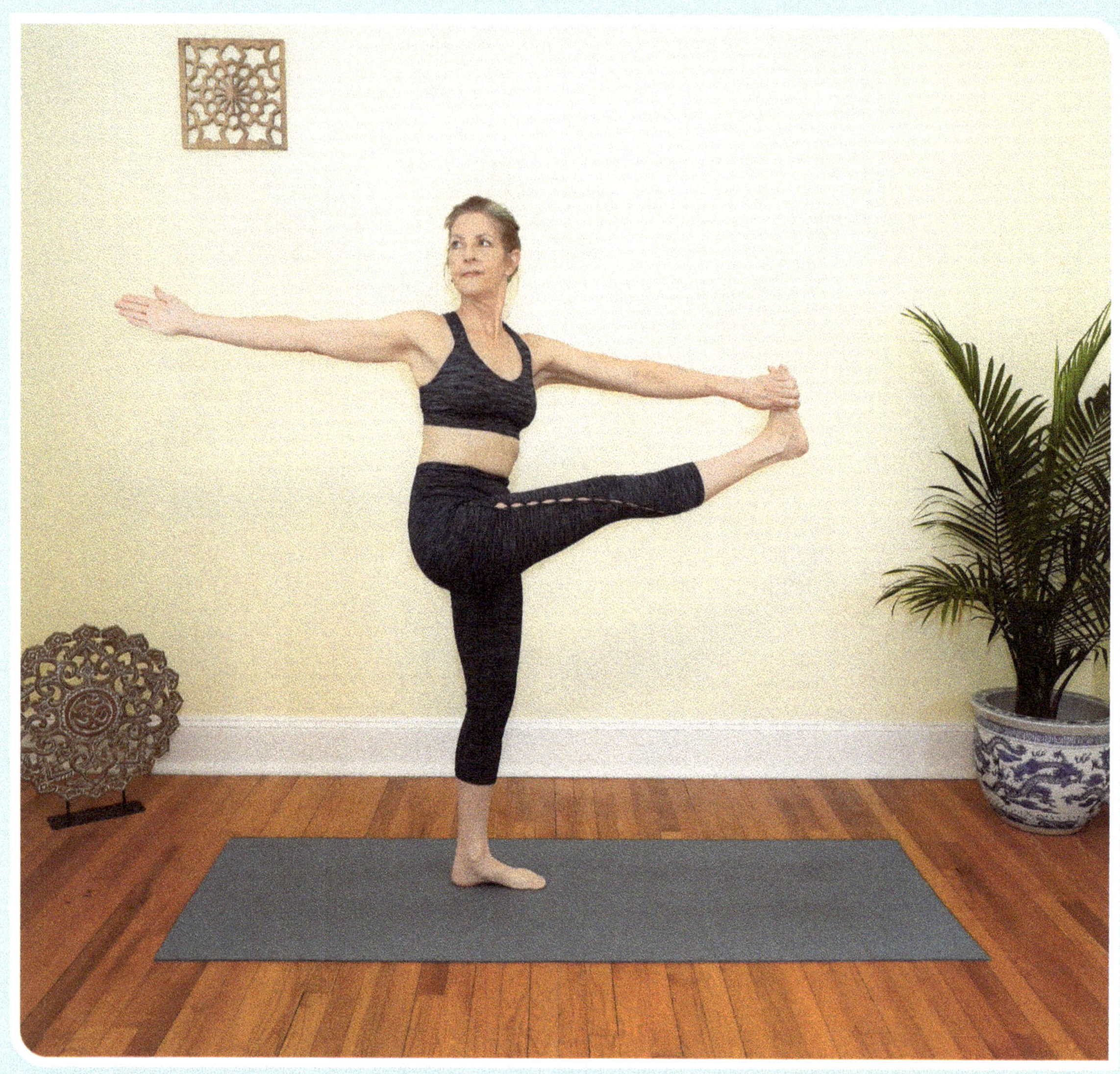

Revolved Hand to Foot Pose

Both Big Toes Pose

ALSO CALLED: Ubhaya Pandangustasana

WHAT IT DOES FOR YOUR CORE: Yet another all-around core strengthener. Because it's tricky to balance on your butt, Both Big Toes Pose also builds a lot of mental focus.

TUNE IT UP: If you can't get your knees straight holding both big toes (by hooking your index and middle fingers around your big toes), use a strap around the balls of your feet. Either way, start with your knees bent and your heels hovering just off the floor. Lean back and find a place to balance on your seat just behind your sitting bones. Then, slowly straighten your legs by pushing with your feet and pulling back against that action from your shoulders. Work from the center of your upper back to pull back on your feet. Do not bend your elbows and use your biceps.

Your elbows and knees should stay completely straight, whether or not you're using a strap. Working with bent elbows and bent knees is an ineffective way to stretch your hamstrings and strengthen your core.

Focus on extending yourself up and away from your hips. Lift your chest and raise your rib cage away from your pelvis. Push your heels forward and look slightly up past your toes.

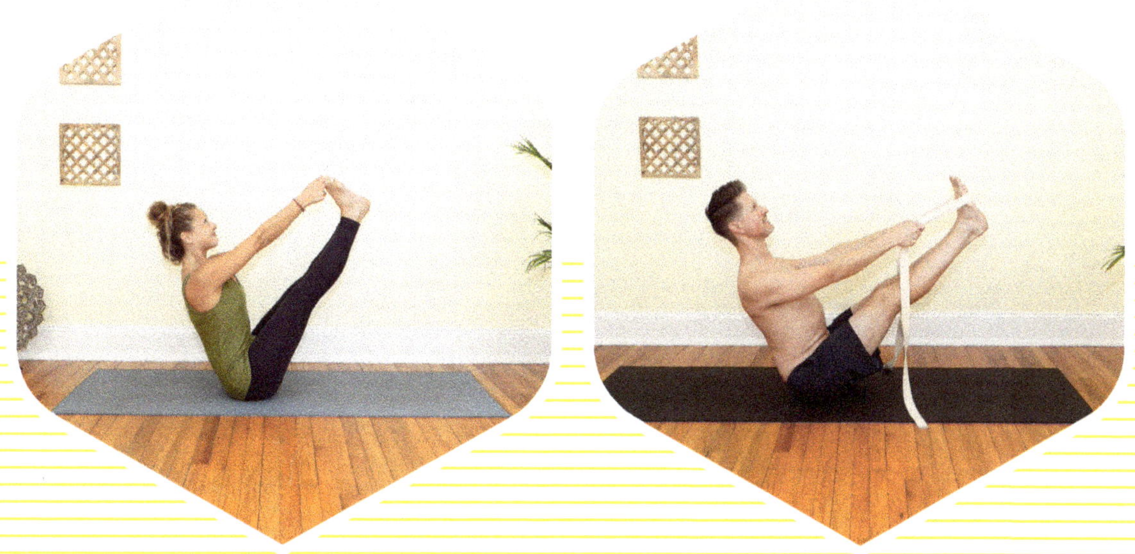

Both Big Toes Pose

Variation with strap

Upward Facing Lotus Pose

ALSO CALLED: Upavistha Padmasana

WHAT IT DOES FOR YOUR CORE: This pose is considered an "advanced" pose because it requires a great deal of strength in all sides of your core, as well as intense mental focus. This unsupported pose is entered from Shoulder Stand (Salamba Sarvangasna), so you should feel comfortable and steady in Shoulder Stand before trying it. (Shoulder Stand is discussed in chapter 5.)

TUNE IT UP: From Shoulder Stand with your arms supporting your back, bend your right knee and use one hand to help tuck it into half Lotus Pose (Padmasana). Then switch and use the other hand to move your left leg into full Lotus. If you can't put your legs into full Lotus, cross your shins or ankles (right leg crosses first). At this stage, your shins are near your chest.

Carefully bring one hand at a time onto each knee, and slowly lift your legs and hips upward, coming to balance on the tops of your shoulders.

Eventually, your arms will be completely straight, although they do not actually bear much of the weight of your legs. That work is primarily done by your core, back, and shoulder muscles. You may find that gently pressing your knees into your hands provides some resistance, to help activate your upper back and press your shoulders more firmly into the floor.

Focus on drawing your shoulder blades toward the center of your back, to help protect your neck (cervical vertebrae).

The three balancing points in this pose are the tops of each shoulder and the back of your head. Do not balance on your neck. It helps to press your chin firmly into your chest. This is a big stretch for the muscles in the back of your neck.

As in every unsupported shoulder balance, first spend time developing a very strong (vertical) Shoulder Stand Pose with correct alignment. Do not attempt Upward Facing Lotus Pose unless your core, shoulder, back, and chest muscles are very strong. Remember, in this pose you lift the weight of your hips and legs using only your core strength. Don't worry if it seems out of reach. You'll have a happy and fulfilled life even if you never attempt this pose!

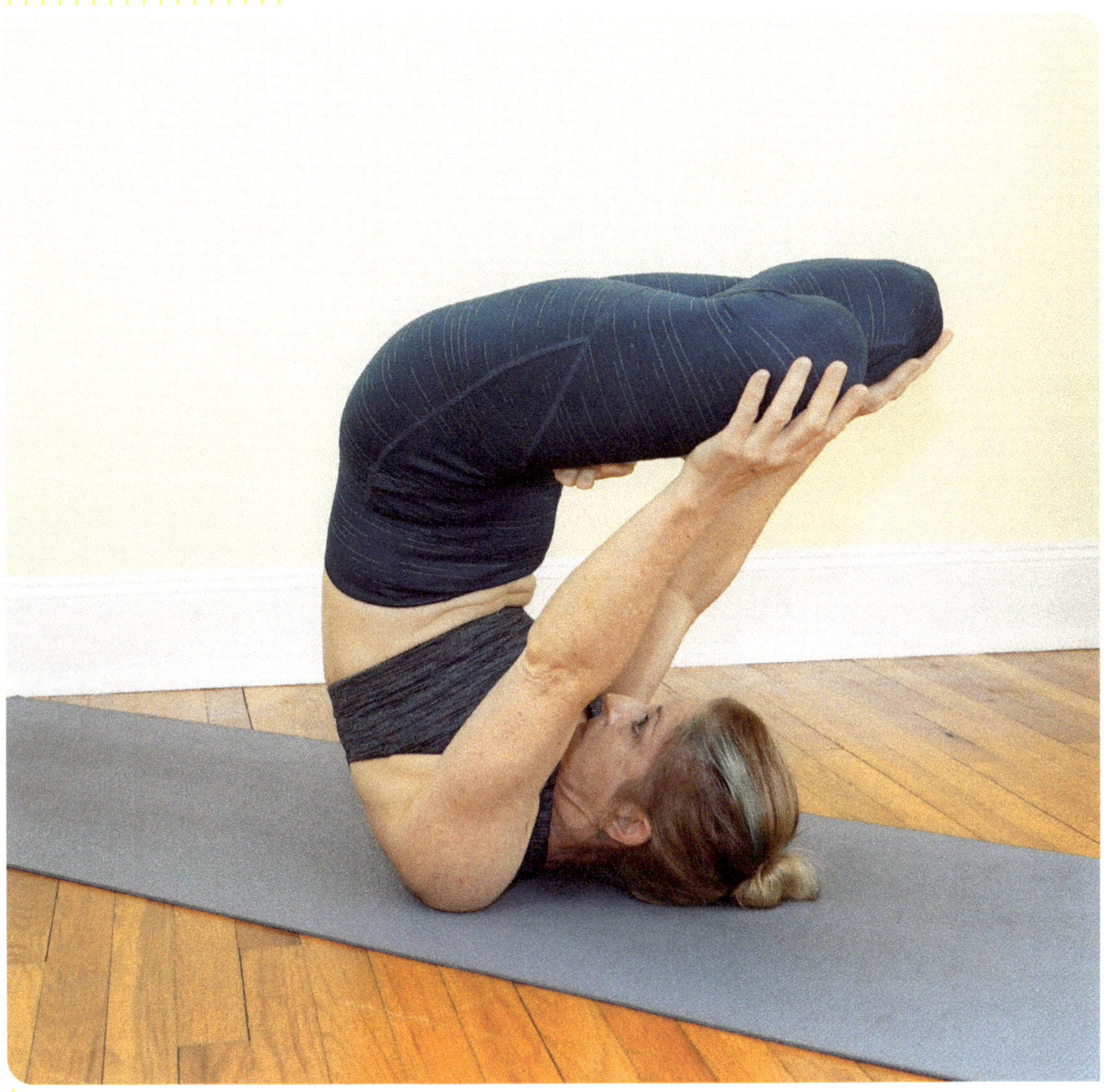

Upward Facing Lotus Pose

Reclining Angle Pose

ALSO CALLED: Supta Konasana

WHAT IT DOES FOR YOUR CORE: Builds strength in all sides of your core. Your back, abdominal, chest, and shoulder muscles work hard to lift the weight of your hips up off of your neck (cervical spine).

TUNE IT UP: It's important to hold your big toes in this pose, because you need that resistance to activate your shoulder muscles and press them down into the floor. It's OK to bend your knees in order to reach your toes. Pull back with your shoulders to help lift your hips.

Important: Most of your weight should be on the tops of your shoulders, not on your neck. If your knees are bent, be very careful not to let your shoulder blades slide apart, rounding your upper back. If your back rounds, the weight of your hips and legs will fall into your neck. Keep squeezing your shoulder blades together on your back, to put the weight up on top of your shoulder points.

To protect your neck in this pose, you must take the weight of your hips and legs up onto your shoulder tops. If you cannot do this, spend more time building strength in similar poses that don't put so much weight above your shoulders. For example, in Plow Pose, Bridge Pose, and Shoulder Stand, you can use your arms and hands to support some of the weight of your legs and hips. You can also use blocks, a bolster, or the wall to support even more weight in these poses.

Work in supported, preparatory poses until you have enough strength and flexibility in your shoulders, core, and back to remove your tools and do the unsupported version. Make sure you are quite comfortable in supported variations of other, similar poses before trying Reclining Angle Pose. Do not rush into this pose before your body is ready.

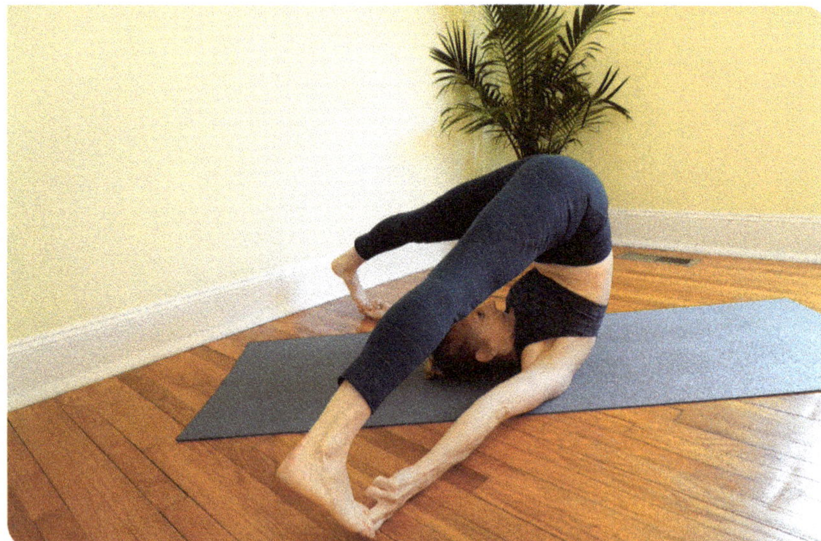

Reclining Angle Pose

Upward Facing Dog Pose

ALSO CALLED: Urdhva Mukha Svanasana

WHAT IT DOES FOR YOUR CORE: Back-bending poses stretch your abdominal muscles while strengthening your back.

TUNE IT UP: If you're tight or inflexible in the front of your core (your abs), this pose can put pressure on your low back. To reduce this possibility, simply lower your knees to the floor.

If your knees are lifted off the floor, firm up your thigh muscles (your quads). Regardless of whether your knees are on the mat or lifted, keep your hamstrings and glutes (your butt muscles) engaged to help protect your low back.

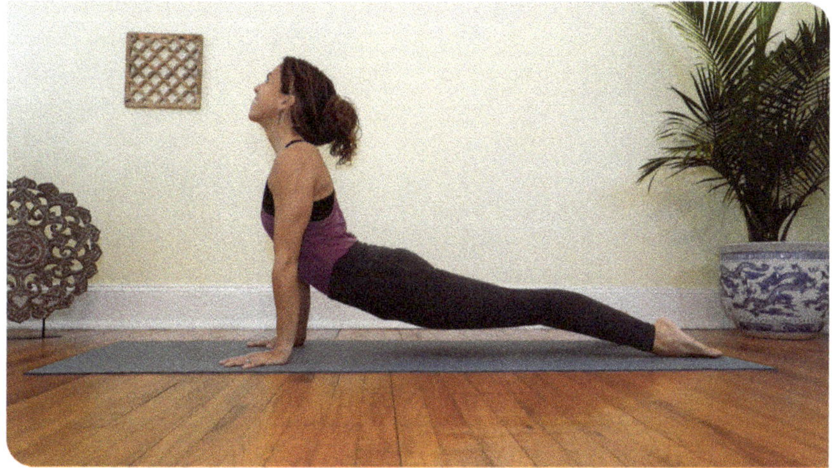

Upward Facing Dog Pose

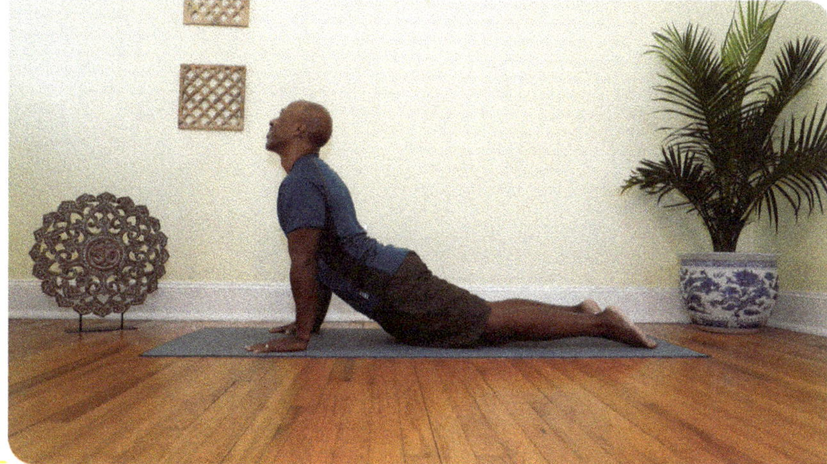

Variation with knees on floor

Baby Cobra Pose

ALSO CALLED: Bhujangasana

Locust Pose

ALSO CALLED: Salabhasana

WHAT THEY DO FOR YOUR CORE: Both Locust and Baby Cobra strengthen your entire core—front, sides, and back. The primary difference is that Baby Cobra is less strenuous because your arms and legs are on the floor, whereas in Locust Pose all of your limbs are eventually lifted. That said, in the preparatory position for Locust and Baby Cobra keep your head and legs down to allow you to focus on pulling your shoulders up off the floor by themselves. It's harder than you might think. Baby Cobra Pose draws the heels of your hands back beside your upper ribs. Unlike full Cobra Pose, you do not straighten your elbows to lift your chest in Baby Cobra. Instead, you lift the weight of your head and chest using only the strength of your back and core abdominal muscles.

TUNE IT UP: If your back and abs are weak, keep your forehead and feet on the floor and draw your shoulder blades together on your back, lifting only your shoulders and stretching across your chest. At the same time, tighten your leg muscles to lift your knee-caps off the floor, but not your feet.

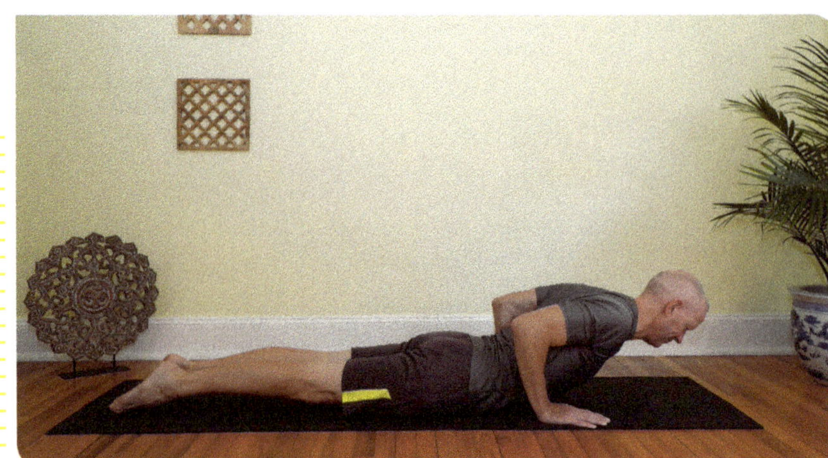

Baby Cobra Pose

This is also an option in locust pose, which has a similar action in the core and back muscles, but with your arms extended back alongside your hips. Again, if your back and abs are weak, or your chest muscles are tight, start practicing the actions of this pose with your forehead on the floor.

Lifting your head adds a lot of work for your back and abs; remember, your head weighs eight to twelve pounds.

If you do lift your head and chest, resist the natural tendency to stick your chin forward. Jutting your chin forward shifts the work out of your core abdominal muscles and into the trapezius muscles on the back of your neck and shoulders. Most people have weak abs and tight trapezius muscles, so most folks will tend to stick their chin out in these poses. In both poses, focus on keeping the back of your neck lengthened by looking at the floor just in front of your face.

Keeping your chin tucked in a little bit will make your abs and mid-back do the lifting work.

The tiny movement of bringing your chin one inch closer to your throat makes a huge difference. Try it: Come into either Baby Cobra or Locust Pose and stick your chin forward. Feel how your abdominal muscles turn off when you do this. Slowly draw your chin in toward your throat, just a little. Feel how your abdominal muscles turn back on. Interesting, right? It's these small adjustments that come with better body awareness which really move your yoga practice forward.

As in all back-bending poses, firmly engaging your leg muscles helps protect your low back from strain. In Locust Pose, spend time developing strength and flexibility by doing the pose with your head, chest, arms, and legs on the floor (lifting only your shoulders, as described above) before you move on to the more intense version. Keep your elbows and knees straight, and draw your legs together as you lift to strengthen the ab muscles in the pit of your belly. Don't let your legs drift apart. Keep your heels together and touching. Do not stick your chin forward; that only crimps your neck and reduces the work in your back and abdominal muscles. Be patient. Strengthening and stretching your core is slow work, but surely worth it.

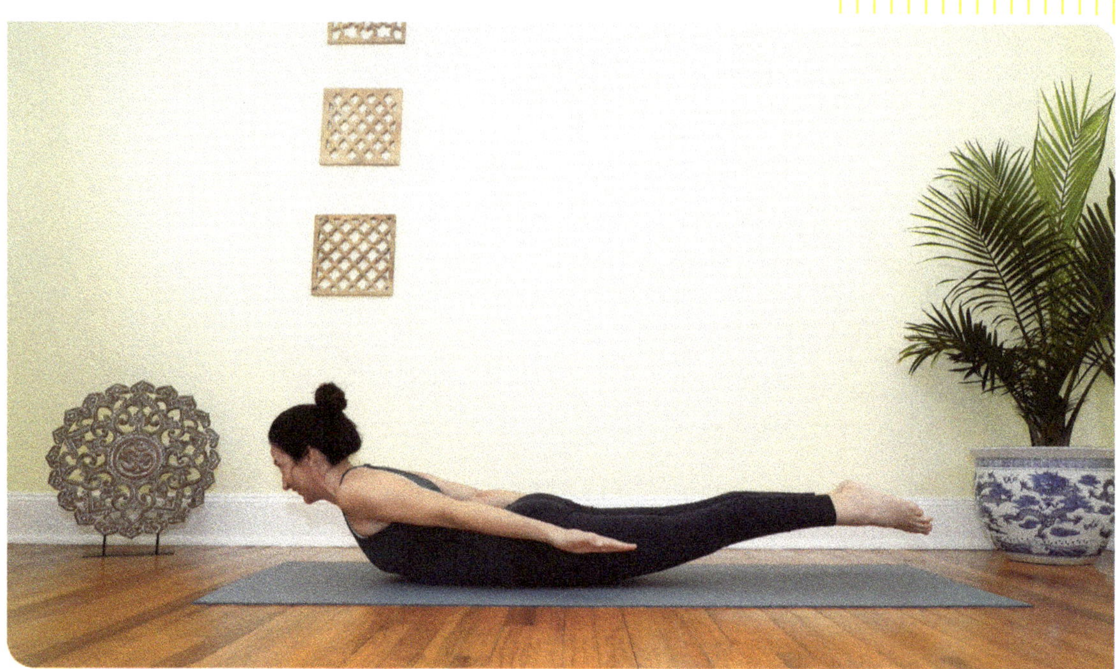

Locust Pose

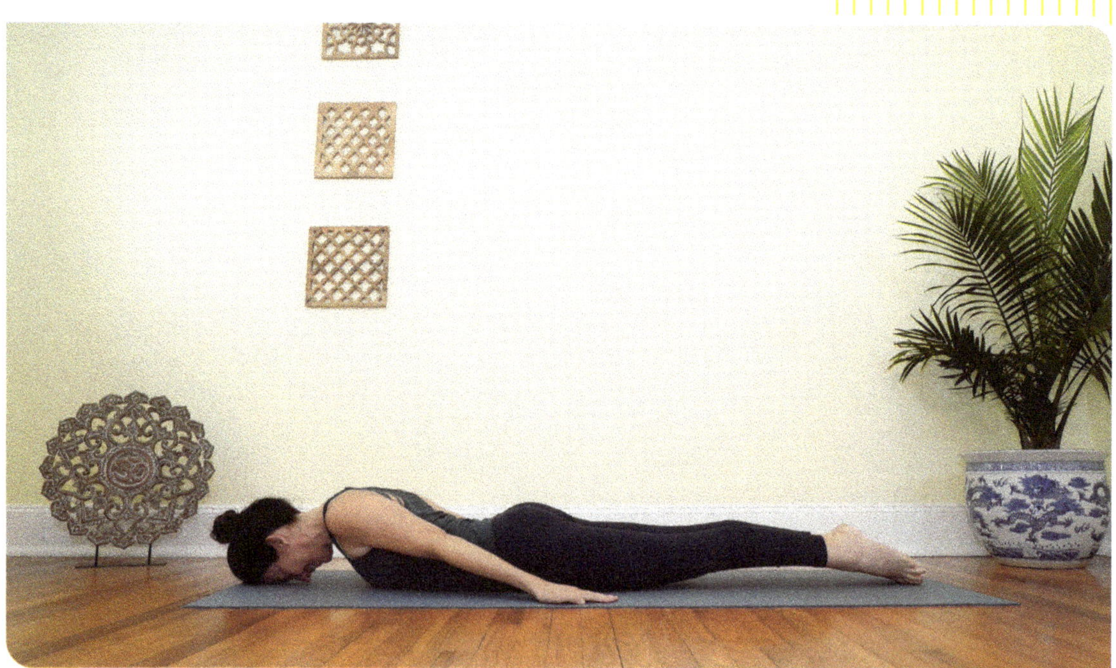

Locust Pose, variation with forehead on mat

Fish Pose

ALSO CALLED: Matsyasana

WHAT IT DOES FOR YOUR CORE: Fish Pose is a supine back-bending pose that requires a lot of back strength to support the weight of your torso off of your neck and head. This pose also calls for chest and ab flexibility. Approach Fish Pose in stages to help protect your neck, while building the strength and flexibility you need to do it effectively.

TUNE IT UP: When starting to learn this pose, use a block under your shoulders to support some of your torso weight. With your chest lifted on a block, look forward at your feet and bring your hands behind your head to support its weight. Next, shift your gaze to look up at the ceiling, letting your head rest back into your hands. Keep your hands behind your head, and look further back by tilting your head further back. Or, if you have neck issues, simply look back with your eyes but don't move your head any further back. In either case, move your eyes as if trying to see the wall behind you. If your head touches the mat, release your hands and bring your palms together in front of your chest (anjali mudra). If your head does not touch the floor, put a folded blanket under the back of your head to support it. Do not let your head hang free in space. That risks straining your neck.

After you build some back strength and frontal flexibility, you can remove the block and use a strap to support some of the weight off of your head and neck. Sitting upright, run a strap from hand-to-hand under your butt. Hold it in each hand with your palms facing up. Pull outward on the strap and press your elbows down into the floor to lift your chest. Your hands (your knuckles) will be off the floor while your elbows press very firmly down. First, just lift your chest and look at the ceiling. Then, slowly, begin looking for the wall behind you. Keep pulling up on the strap and pressing down with your elbows. Maybe the top of your head will come to the floor. If not, sit up and put a folded blanket where it will support your head, and enter the pose again.

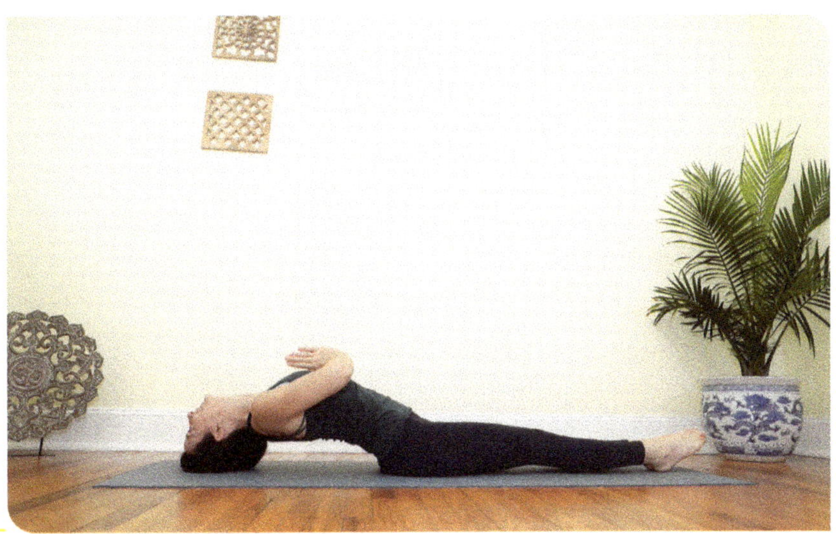

Fish Pose

In all variations of Fish Pose, your legs must be very active and your shoulder blades must draw firmly together on your back. Do not lay back and go limp, that's a recipe for injuring your neck. Press your heels and calves down and keep your thighs firm. If your hands are together in front of your chest, lift your elbows up to the ceiling while pulling your shoulder blades together on your back.

As in all back bends, your gazing point makes a big difference. Once you are settled into whatever variation is most appropriate for your body, and your head is at the best angle for your neck (tilted slightly back, or all the way back, on the floor), move your eyeballs upwards, as if you're trying to see your eyebrows. Don't move your face or your head any further, only move your eyes in their sockets. This eye position (called a gazing point, or drishti) tells your brain that you're moving backward. Conversely, looking at the ceiling or down at your nose tells your brain that you intend to sit up. Your brain has to know where you want to go in order to fire the right muscles to get you there.

Try it: Get into your favorite version of Fish Pose and slowly alternate where your eyes are looking. Look back toward your eyebrows, and then down toward your nose. As you do this, notice how the small muscles in your throat and neck either relax to help you bend backward, or contract to help you sit upright. Crazy, right?

So where you take your eyes can be an important help or a big hindrance when moving into backbends. You don't need to move your entire head or face—just move your eyeballs in their sockets toward the direction you want to go.

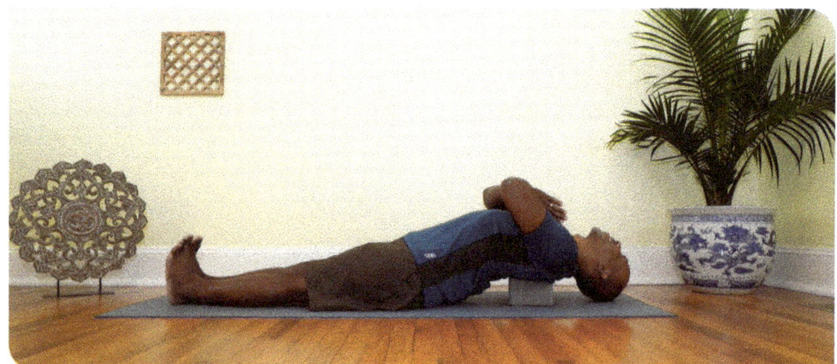

Variation with block

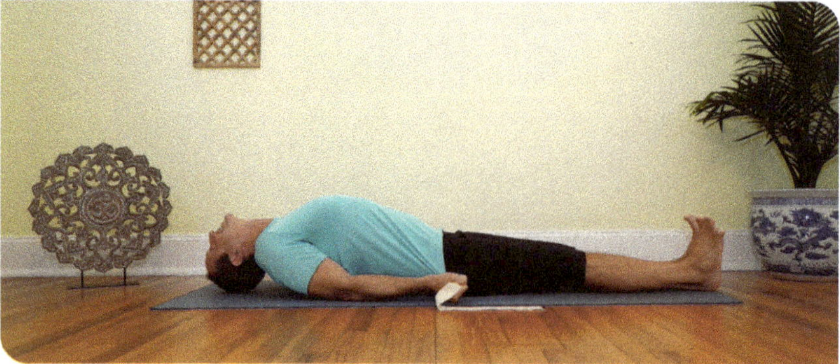

Variation with strap

Upward Facing Bow Pose

ALSO CALLED: Urdva Dhanurasana, Wheel Pose

WHAT IT DOES FOR YOUR CORE: This pose strengthens your back, core, and shoulders while stretching the entire front side of your body. It's very challenging to breathe in intense back bends like this one. You build tremendous core strength in all of the preparatory stages, as well as in the full pose, simply by breathing deeply while the muscles in your back are contracting to lift and the muscles on your front are extending to stretch.

TUNE IT UP: This is a very challenging back bend. Fortunately, there are lots of preparatory variations to start building the strength and flexibility you'll need to eventually do it (or not; Remember, no pose is mandatory). It's important to understand that doing the preparatory variations for this and all poses is not something to avoid, or be ashamed or embarrassed about. The preparatory variations (called kramas) provide essential strengthening and stretching benefits to your body.

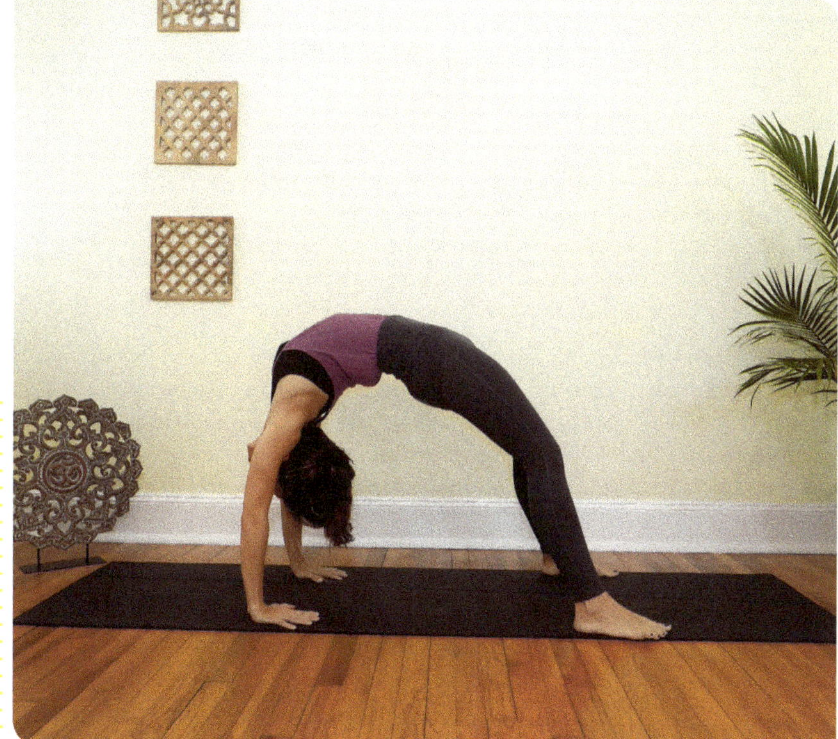

Upward-Facing Bow Pose

Stage One: The first stage of Upward-Facing Bow Pose is to lie on your back with your knees bent and put your palms flat on the floor by your shoulders, with your elbows pointing up to the ceiling (not out to the sides). Placing your hands in this position can be very challenging. Don't strain. Keep your hands there and shift your focus to the rest of your body. Draw your low back (lumbar spine) down toward the floor and press your feet forward. Breathe.

Stage Two: Once you can get your palms flat with your elbows pointing up, you can try the next krama. For stage two, lift your hips, but keep your shoulders on the floor. This begins building the leg strength and awareness you'll need to protect your low back. Press your feet strongly down and forward while tilting your sitting bones slightly toward your heels. Don't let your knees fall outward. Keep your thighs parallel. Breathe.

Stage Three: Once you can lift your hips high and keep your breath moving steadily, you're ready to try stage three. In this step, you can use blocks to support the weight of your hips, and start using your arms to lift some weight off of your shoulders and upper back. To enter this variation of Wheel Pose, lie on your back holding a block in each hand. Bend your knees and put your feet on the floor. Then lift your hips and slide both blocks under the back of your pelvis (your sacrum). Note: the higher you're able to set the blocks in this stage, the easier the next step will be.

Stage Four: Once you can breathe fully with the blocks under the back of your pelvis, and your hands by your head, you're ready for the final preparatory stage. Press down with your hands and lift your shoulders off the floor until you can slide up onto the top of your head. Do not force your head underneath you—forcing this step can injure your neck. If you cannot put the crown of your head on the floor, keep the back of your head and shoulders on the floor and breathe deeply here to build more flexibility across your front core.

Tight muscles on the front of your body (primarily your core abdominals and hip flexors) are what prevent you from getting the crown of your head on the floor. That tightness prevents you from getting the blocks set up high enough to tuck your head under. Again, do not force your head underneath you. This is a process that depends on becoming more flexible across your front core muscles. Be patient. Focus on pointing your elbows directly up at the ceiling and pressing your feet down and forward. Press your palms down and breathe deeply to increase the stretch across your front.

Stage Five: Eventually, you may become strong and flexible enough to lift all the way up in one motion from lying flat on your back. Upward-Facing Bow (or Wheel) Pose only becomes possible little by little. Progress in this pose is incremental. It usually takes many months or years to press fully up into it. No hurry. No worries.

As you're working on this pose, it's important to understand that you are not trying to make your spine arch like a rainbow or a horse-shoe. Remember, your mid-spine vertebrae don't naturally back-bend very much at all. That's the way your spine is designed. To do back-bending movements, you must develop flexibility across the entire front of your body—your throat, shoulders, chest, abdominals, hip flexors, and quads. At the same time, you must build strength across your back body—neck, shoulders, back, glutes, hamstrings, and lower legs.

First stage

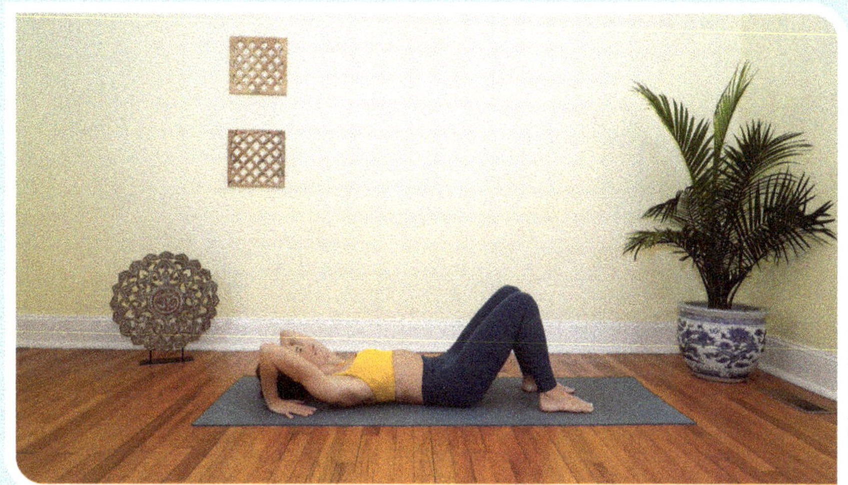

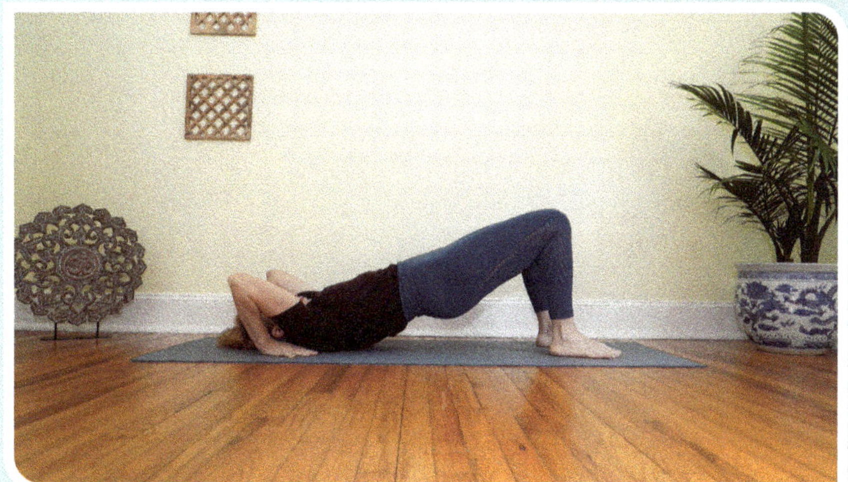

Second stage

Third stage

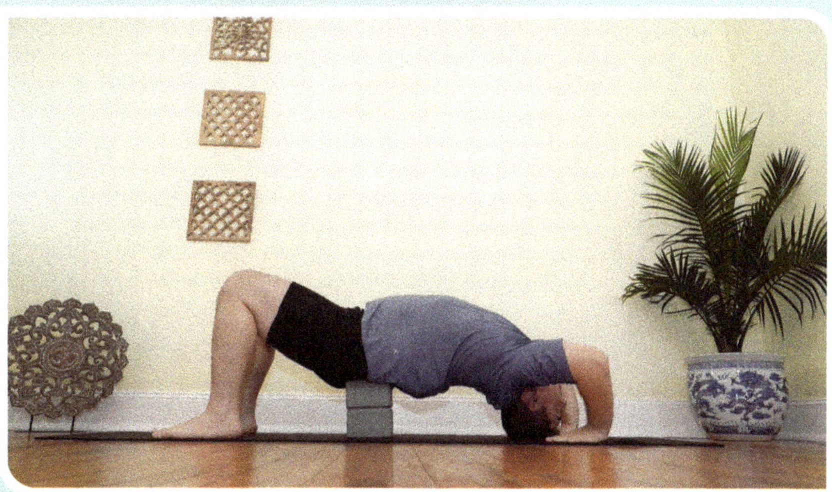

It's misguided to focus on the vertebral joints of your spine when you're working on Wheel Pose. And the mistaken perception that the bones of your spine are what's holding you back can lead to injuries. What restricts your back-bending ability is muscular tightness in the front of your body, and/or muscular weakness in the back of your body. Your spine can only extend to the specific degree that each of its three sections is designed to allow. You do not want to change how the vertebrae of your spine are constructed. As in any other pose, focus on changing your muscles, not your bones, cartilage, or ligaments.

In Upward-Facing Bow Pose, and all of its preparatory variations, your leg strength pressing down and forward is what shifts your chest and shoulders back over your arms. Before your shoulders arrive above your hands, this pose creates a very intense stretch (extension) for your wrists. Be aware that this extreme wrist extension is greatest in the early stages, and decreases as you become flexible and strong enough to get your shoulders above your hands.

When you come down from whatever variation of Wheel Pose you're doing, take a moment to press the backs of your hands against each other (flexing your wrists) as a counter-movement to the stretch (extension) they got in the pose. Making circles with your wrists is also a nice counter-action to that extension.

Building wrist flexibility and shoulder strength are important benefits that take time. You may spend months or even years doing the preparatory variations of this pose. Be patient. Commit to working with your body where it is today. Breathe. Don't give up. Work hard, but don't force it.

Take your backbends slow and steady.

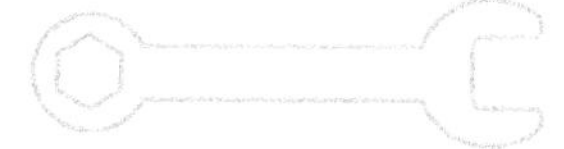

MECHANIC'S NOTE: Get Comfortable with Discomfort

For some poses, you may spend months or years practicing each preparatory stage or krama. Don't worry. You get tremendous benefits from doing the preparatory variations; it doesn't matter if you ever do the full version of any pose. Choose the variation that's most appropriate for your body today, and apply yourself to doing it correctly and with a focused mind, that's all that matters.

Remember, your yoga practice should be therapeutic. It's meant to build balanced strength and flexibility across all of your muscles. But the benefits of a regular yoga practice are not just physical. Some of the most significant benefits are mental and emotional. Challenging poses like Upward-Facing Bow Pose build humility, patience, courage, and persistence. Difficult poses make us confront that part of ourselves that wants to run for the hills as soon as the going gets tough. It's the variations and stages (or kramas) that help us to balance comfort with discomfort. And after all, finding comfort with discomfort—easefulness during anxiety or effort—is one of the most important things that doing yoga poses can teach us.

King Dancer Pose

ALSO KNOWN AS: Natarajasana

WHAT IT DOES FOR YOUR CORE: Builds a lot of core strength and flexibility, as well as mental focus.

TUNE IT UP: Start by standing up straight on one foot while holding your other foot behind you. Try to have your knees side by side. Bring your free arm out in front of your shoulder, palm facing up. Look forward or slightly up.

Begin lifting your back foot up behind you. Do not look down at the floor; keep your eyes aimed forward or slightly upward. As your foot comes up, your chest will naturally shift forward to counter-balance. Focus on lifting your foot, your chest, and your gaze. Your front hand will also slowly rise up, until it is slightly higher than your shoulders. Breathe.

As in most standing balances, one of the most common mistakes is to look at the floor during this pose. Do not look down! Looking at the floor drops your chest and shoulders down when they should be lifting up. If balance is a problem, stand next to a wall with the back of your out-stretched hand against it. Keep your elbow straight; don't bend your elbow or put your palm on the wall. Instead, slide the back of your hand up the wall with a straight elbow. Tilt slowly forward and lift your foot behind you. Look up. Lift up. Reach up.

You can also use a strap to do a variation of King Dancer Pose that creates a more intense stretch for your abdominal muscles, and more strengthening for your back and shoulders.

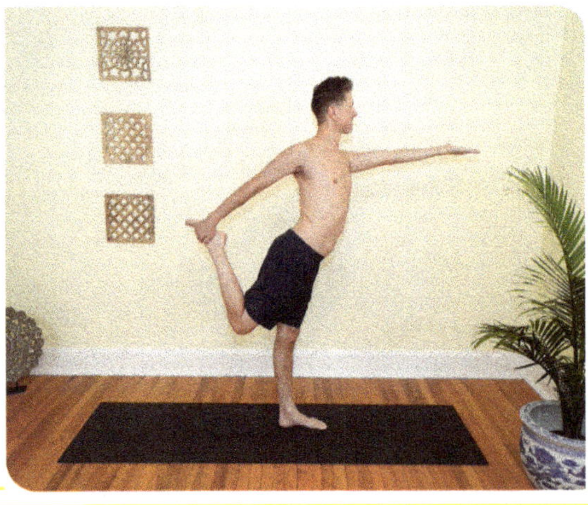

King Dancer Pose

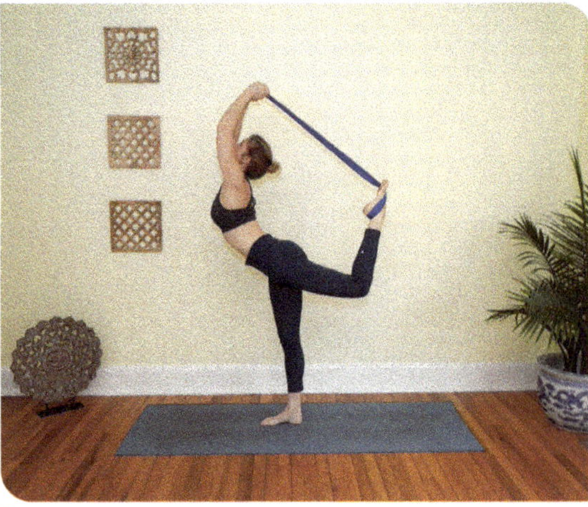

Variation with strap

HERE'S HOW IT WORKS:

To get the strap on the lifting foot, you'll have to make a little sandal out of it. Bend both knees and lean forward. (It's not very graceful, but don't worry.) If you're near a wall, you can lean against it for support while you get the strap in place. Put the middle of the strap around the back of your ankle. Then, bring both sides forward to the top of your foot and hold them together. Thread both sides between your big- and second-toes (where the thong on your flip-flops goes). From there, run both sides under the bottom of your foot. Now you have a little strap-sandal.

Hold both ends of the strap together in the hand on that same side, and stand up straight. Reach the free arm forward at shoulder height with your palm up. Put the side of your free hand and/or your shoulder against the wall. Bend your knee to lift the strapped foot behind you and bring the hand holding the strap onto your shoulder. The other hand is on the wall. Pause to point your bent elbow on the strap side forward (not out to the side) and get your balance.

The next step is to hold the strap on top of your head with both hands. Pause, point your elbows forward (not out to the sides) and get your balance with your shoulder or upper arm touching the wall. Breathe. Slowly begin straightening your elbows by reaching your knuckles to the ceiling, and lift the strapped foot up behind you. Pause. Find your balance. Breathe. Move your hands upward in small increments, pausing often to steady your balance. Do not look down at the floor.

If you lose your balance, let go of the strap. Do not hop around, especially if you're not beside a wall to help you balance.

Eventually, you may have the strength and flexibility to begin walking your hands down the strap toward the lifted foot behind you. This is less important than simply building flexibility across your front belly muscles and strength across your upper back. You may never reach your foot. Don't worry, that isn't important. It's just your foot, after all. Whether you're using a strap or not, focus on lifting your hand(s) and your foot up to the ceiling during this pose. Do not let your chest and shoulders dive down toward the floor. Your chest will automatically move forward to counter-balance the lifting leg behind you. Think up—not down—to stretch your abdominal muscles. Get your elbows as straight as possible. Smile. It's only yoga.

Intense Stretch Pose

ALSO CALLED: Uttanasana, Standing Forward Fold

WHAT IT DOES FOR YOUR CORE: Builds strength in your abdominal muscles through the action of drawing your torso and head toward your legs. At the same time, this pose stretches your back muscles (and, of course, the hamstrings on the backs of your thighs).

TUNE IT UP: Most of us tend to look forward when we bend over. It's an automatic reaction to help keep your balance. But lifting your head to look forward creates tension in the back of your neck (your trapezius muscles), and prevents you from getting the full benefits of this pose—strengthening your abdominals and stretching your back.

Remember, your head weighs eight to twelve pounds. Pulling it in and up toward your belly instead of looking forward is like doing an abdominal crunch. At the bottom of your forward fold—with your knees bent or straight—draw your chin into your chest and look up toward your hips. As you curl your forehead into your legs, you will feel your abdominal muscles contract firmly.

Put your hand on blocks if they don't easily reach the floor. Even though you are bent forward, do not let your shoulders sag down. Instead, strongly pull your shoulder blades up onto the middle of your back.

To exit the pose, look slightly forward of your feet and press your feet outward, using your leg muscles to stand up, not your lower back. This action of pressing your feet outward as you bend forward and stand back up will help prevent low back strain. Because we do Standing Forward Fold Pose over and over in a yoga practice, it's important to learn to use your legs—not your back—to enter and exit it. Your low back will thank you, and your legs will get very strong.

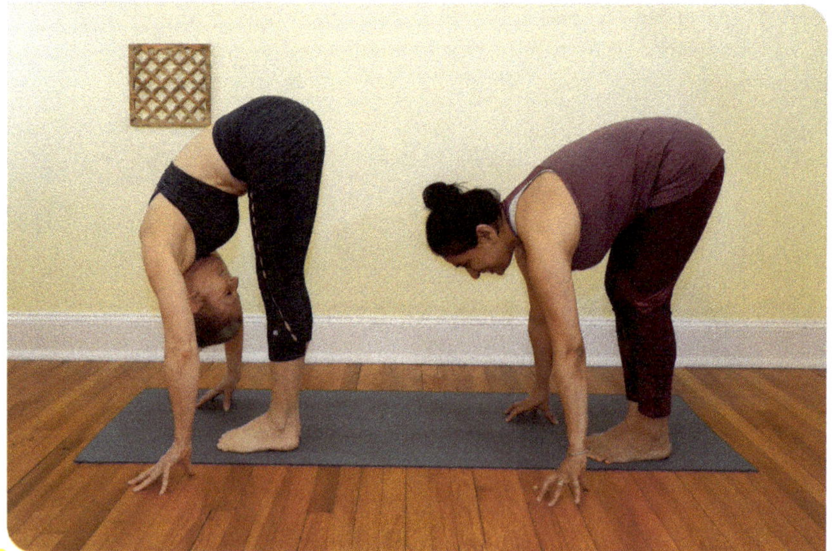

Intense Stretch Pose. Tuck in your chin and look up at your hips (left) instead of looking forward (right).

Child's Pose

ALSO CALLED: Balasana

Yogic Seal Pose

ALSO CALLED: Yoga Mudrasana

WHAT THEY DO FOR YOUR CORE: These are basic forward-bending yoga poses that are often used to begin and end class. You can also use Child's Pose as a resting pose during class. While the focus in these poses is on your breathing and cultivating an inner sense of calm, some physical actions still apply. Draw your abdominal muscles gently inward in both. These poses also provide a big stretch for your back muscles.

TUNE IT UP: Put a very tiny flex in your toes during these poses to keep a little energy in your feet. If your hands are on the floor, gently press your fingertips down into the mat. If your back or neck muscles are tight, you can rest your forehead on a block in either of these poses. In Child's Pose you can put your elbows on the floor and let your head hang down to stretch the back of your neck and shoulders.

Yogic Seal Pose requires more abdominal and back strength, because the weight of your torso comes forward without the support of your arms. Press your forearms against your back for support when entering or exiting this, or any other, unsupported forward bending pose. Do not let your shoulders round down. As in all forward folds, draw them up onto your back, away from the floor.

You can hold one wrist with the opposite hand behind your back in Yogic Seal Pose. If your chest and shoulders are more flexible, you might hold opposite elbows. If you are able to sit comfortably in Lotus Pose (Padmasana), with your feet tucked into your hip creases, you might eventually hold your big toes with opposite hands in this pose (arms crossed behind your back). Gently squeeze whatever you are holding with your hands.

As always, choose the variation that is best for your body today. All forward folding poses build strength in your front and stretch your back.

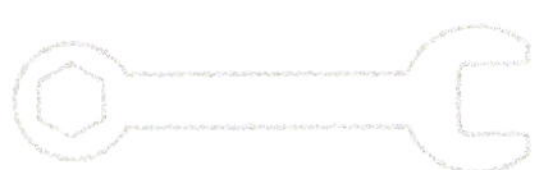

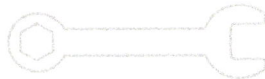

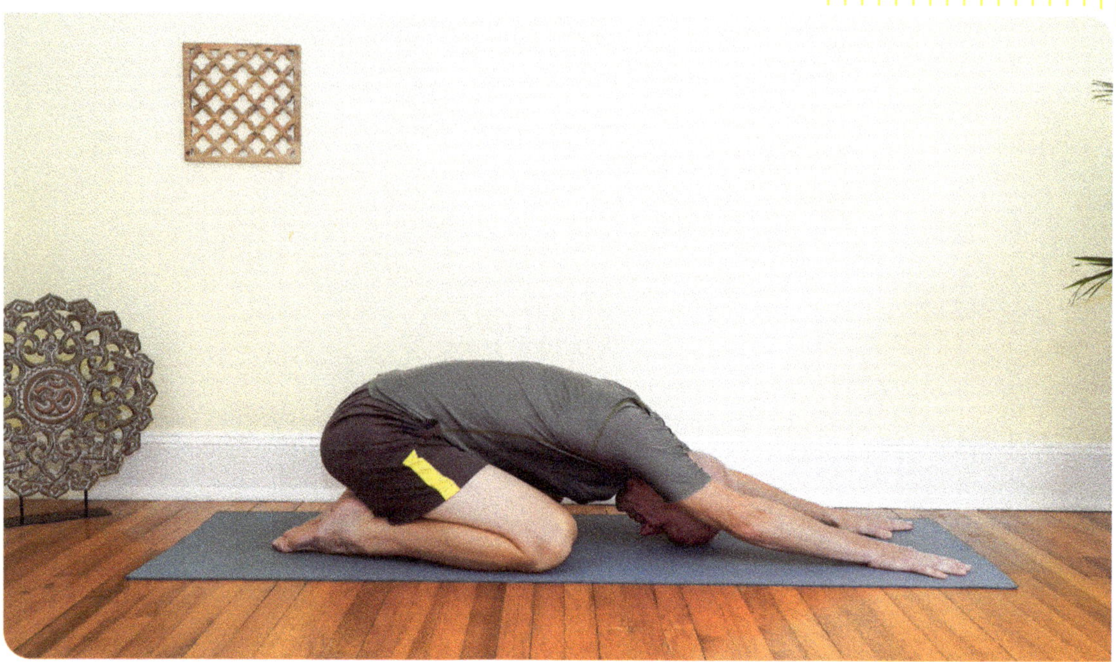

Child's Pose

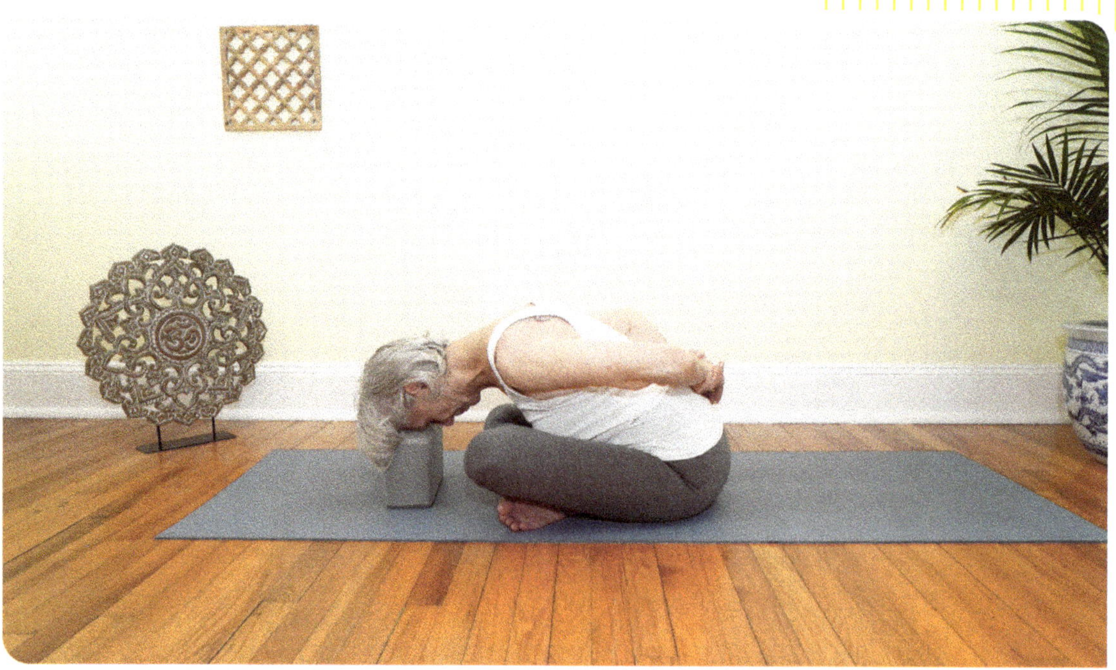

Yogic Seal Pose, variation with block

Head of Knee Pose, A

ALSO CALLED: Janu Sirsasana, A

WHAT IT DOES FOR YOUR CORE: Another good strengthener for your front core muscles, and a good stretch for your back core muscles.

TUNE IT UP: I prefer the translation Head *of* Knee Pose, rather than Head *to* Knee Pose, because it describes an essential muscular action in this pose: to draw the head of the bent knee forward. This subtle action engages your lower abdominal muscles (transverse abdominus), and helps protect your low back from strain and overstretching. It is incorrect to focus on bringing your head to your knee, because that motion rounds your back and shoulders down to the leg.

Keep the knee of the extended leg straight by pressing your heel forward and flexing your foot. As in all forward folds, focus on lifting your shoulder blades up onto your back as you lean forward. Do not let your shoulders round down.

If pulling your shoulders back means you can't reach your foot, so be it. Tuck your hands, palms-up, under your thigh or your calf, and focus on hinging from your hip crease (not curling your spine down).

All three versions of Head of Knee Pose (Janu Sirsasana, A, B, and C) are big stretches for your low back. Go slow. Breathe. Progress in yoga is incremental. Have patience and respect your body.

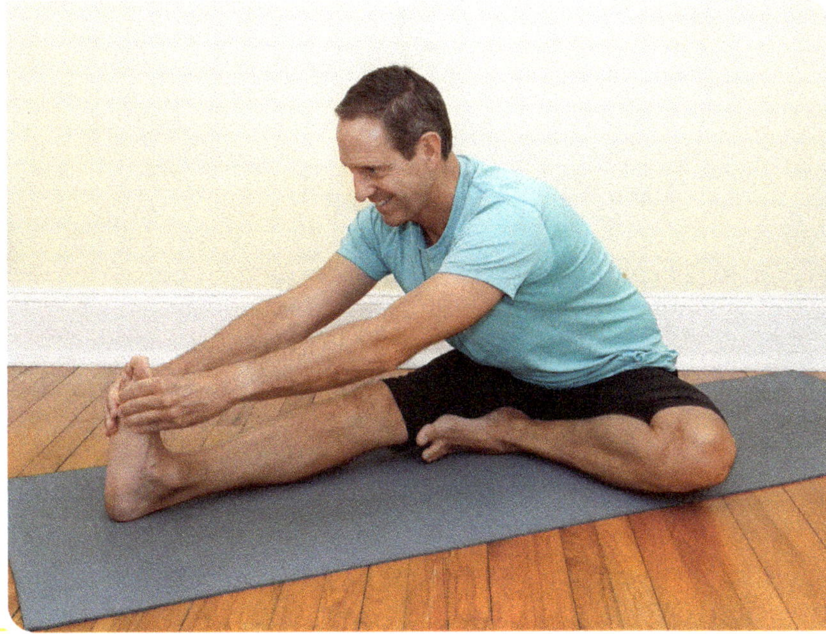

Head of Knee Pose, A

Wide Angle Seated Forward Bend Pose

ALSO CALLED: Upavistha Konasana

WHAT IT DOES FOR YOUR CORE: This pose requires a lot of strength in the core abdominal muscles, to support the weight of your torso as it leans forward. Your hands are not out in front so they can't support much of your torso weight. You have to rely on core strength. As you lean further and further forward, the stretch for your lower back muscles increases.

TUNE IT UP: Remember, there are forward folds but no downward folds in yoga. Keep your spine as straight as possible. Do not round your back and shoulders. One day, your chest might touch the floor. Maybe. Who cares? The focus is on patiently building strength and flexibility.

Extend your chest as if you are lifting your ribs up and forward away from your hips. Keep your leg muscles very firm, and press your heels firmly outward to keep your knees straight.

Your fingertips can be on the floor behind your hips, or you can put your hands on your thighs or shins. If you can easily reach your feet, hold onto your big toes. Eventually, as you build more strength and flexibility, you can hold the outer edges of your feet (the pinky toe sides). No hurry to reach them, though. They're just feet.

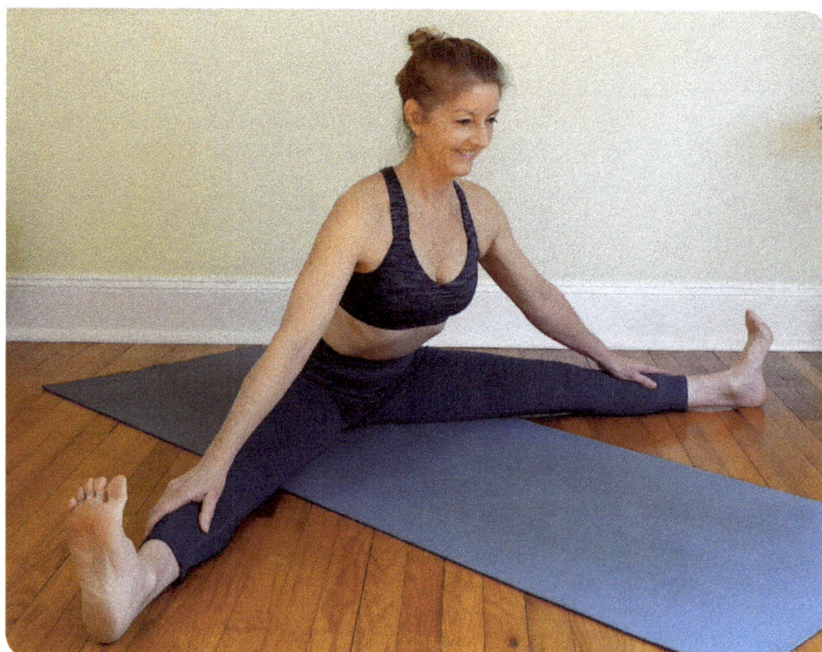

Wide Angle Seated Forward Bend Pose

The Sage's Pose, A and B

ALSO CALLED: Marichyasana, A and B

WHAT THEY DO FOR YOUR CORE: This series of poses builds strength in your front core muscles, while stretching your back, shoulder, and outer hip muscles. Your abdominal muscles must work very hard to support your torso while your hands are clasped behind your back.

TUNE IT UP: Do not let your shoulders sag toward the floor. Instead, draw your shoulder blades together on your back and lift your ribs up, away from your hips. These lifting actions help your hands eventually reach far enough behind your back to clasp.

In versions A and B, if your hands don't clasp yet, hold the back of your heel on the leg you arm is wrapping. Do not crank yourself into these positions before your body is ready. Injury is the only reward you'll find for that behavior. Don't disrespect your body.

Tools are very helpful in the Marichyasana poses. Holding a strap from hand to hand behind your back will help you start finding the muscular actions needed to extend your chest forward while simultaneously pulling your hands down and back behind you.

Note that versions A and B are the same, except in version B the leg that was extended is now tucked up into your hip crease (in Half Lotus Pose, or Ardha Padmasana).

Be patient with the Marichyasana family. It takes a long time to build the front core strength and back flexibility needed to do them. Don't let your ego injure your body.

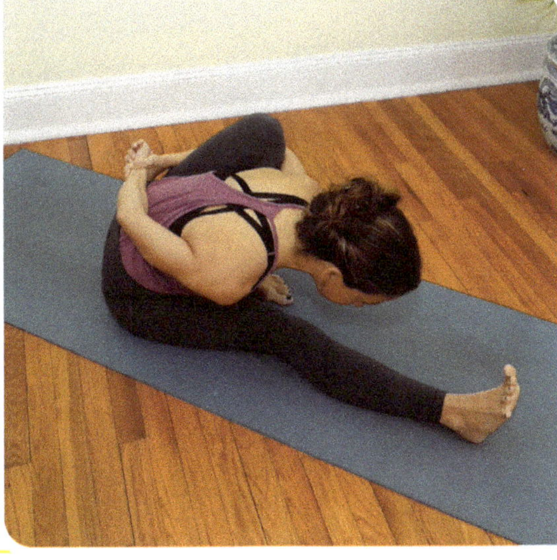

The Sage's Pose, A

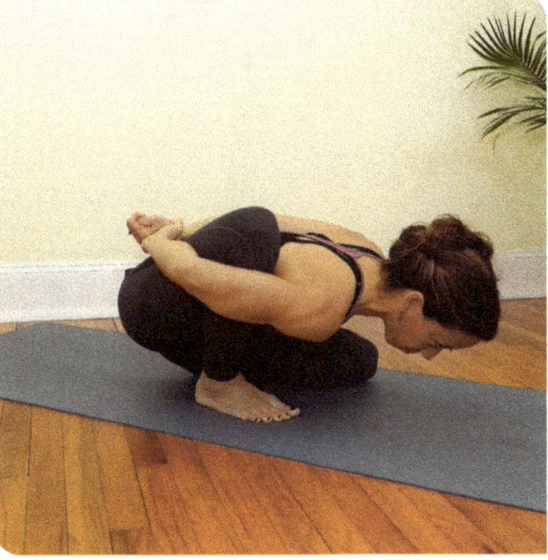

The Sage's Pose, B

Reclined Hand to Big Toe Pose, C

ALSO CALLED: Supta Padangustasana, C

Extended Hand to Big Toe Pose, C

ALSO CALLED: Utthita Hasta Padangustasana, C

WHAT THEY DO FOR YOUR CORE: Both build strength in the front core abdominal muscles, while stretching your back muscles. The standing pose also builds a lot of mental focus as you try to maintain your balance while folding forward over your lifted leg. As always, if you feel unsteady, stand by a wall and let your elbow lightly touch it.

TUNE IT UP: Focus on using your core strength to draw your torso toward your leg. At the same time, think about pulling the lifted leg up—as if you're trying to pull it over your head. Even though you're using your arms to pull your leg up, keep your shoulder blades settled down on your back. Do not let your shoulders climb up toward your neck.

Draw your upper thighs slightly in toward each other to engage your low belly muscles, and help protect your low back from strain.

There's a tendency is to hold your breath when you lean toward your leg. This does not help. In fact, holding your breath only makes these poses harder. Try to keep breathing, and focus on inhaling deeply.

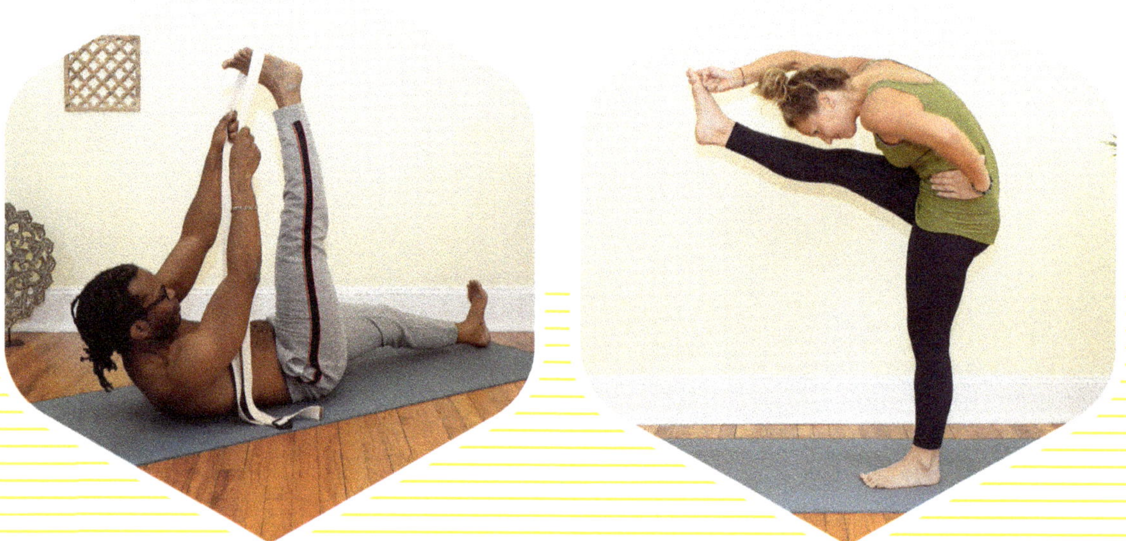

Reclined Hand to Big Toe Pose, C

Extended Hand to Big Toe Pose, C

Upward Facing Intense Stretch Pose

ALSO CALLED: Urdhva Mukha Paschimottanasana

WHAT IT DOES FOR YOUR CORE: Stretches the back muscles and hamstrings, while using the front core muscles to draw your torso toward your legs. Unlike the seated version (Seated Forward Bend Pose), in this upward-facing version you hold your heels and use your arms to pull your chest to your legs. In the seated version, you avoid using your arm strength to get closer to your legs, and instead focus on extending your chest forward. When you're balanced on your butt in this upward facing version, there's less risk of overstretching your lower back muscles by using your arm strength to move your chest toward your legs.

TUNE IT UP: To enter this pose, sit with your knees bent and the tips of your toes resting lightly on the floor. Get a good grip on your heels and rock back to lift your toes just a few inches off the floor. Pause and find a balancing point just behind your sitting bones.

Once your balance feels steady, slowly begin straightening your legs. It may take several months or years of practice before you can get your knees completely straight; until then, use a strap around your feet. It will take even longer to start closing the gap between your torso and your legs. There is a delicate balance between lifting your chest and drawing your torso and legs closer together.

Wherever you are in the process of learning this pose, look slightly upward and breathe.

Remember, incremental progress is still progress. Be patient.

Resist the natural tendency to lift your shoulders. Instead, focus on drawing your shoulder blades down your back. Your arm and shoulder muscles should pull slightly downward on your heels or the strap—as if you're trying to slot your thigh bones deeper into your hip sockets. If you're using a strap around your feet, bend your elbows to pull down on your feet.

This pose requires a lot of mental focus to stay balanced on your seat.

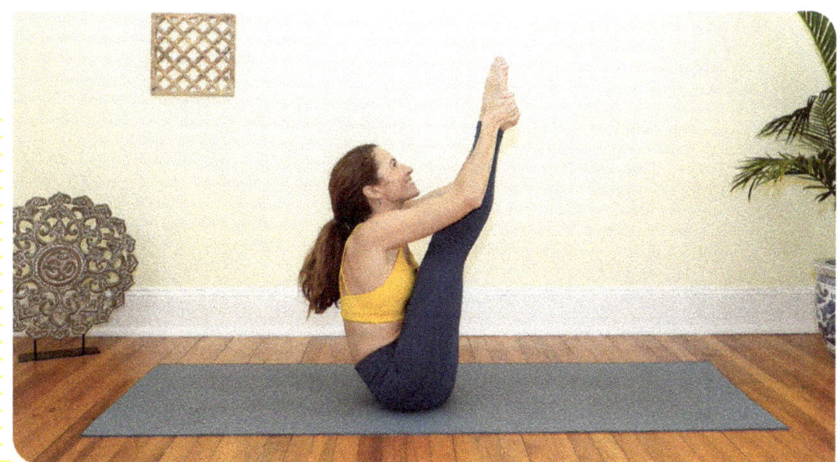

Upward Facing Intense Stretch Pose

Intense Three-Limbed Forward Folding Pose

ALSO CALLED: Triang Mukhaikapada Paschimottanasana

WHAT IT DOES FOR YOUR CORE: This pose helps build a lot of strength in your side waist (oblique) muscles, because you must press down on the sitting bone and hip of your bent-leg to keep from tipping over toward the straight leg. The further you lean forward, the more this hip wants to lift up.

TUNE IT UP: If your knee is irritated in this fully flexed position, or if you have tight hips or hamstrings, put a block under the hip on your straight leg side to relieve pressure in your bent knee, hip, and low back.

Do not let your shoulders sag down, or drop your head toward your knee. Instead, look at your front foot and reach your chest forward away from your hips. Focus on hinging at your hip crease, and not rounding your back.

Don't worry if your hands do not easily reach your foot. Just tuck your hands (palms-up) under your thigh or shin. As the name states, this is an intense pose. Go slow. Be patient. Breathe.

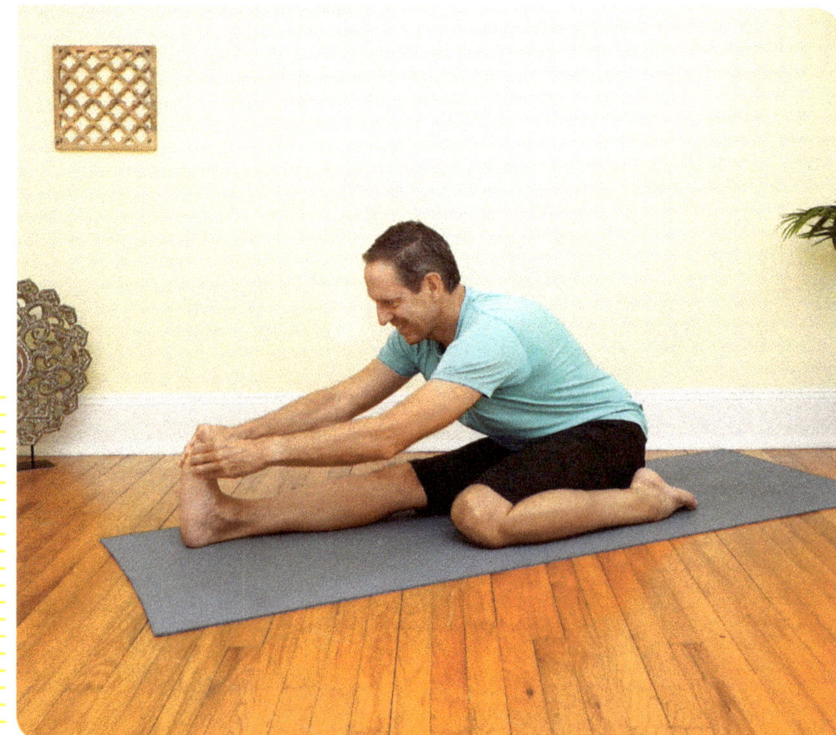

Intense Three-Limbed Forward Folding Pose

Half-Bound Lotus Intense West Stretch Pose

ALSO CALLED: Ardha Baddha Padma Paschimottanasana

WHAT IT DOES FOR YOUR CORE: This is another great pose for building core abdominal strength while stretching your back muscles. As in many other poses that provide these two benefits, your abdominal muscles must draw your torso forward. Meanwhile, your back muscles must lengthen and stretch.

TUNE IT UP: If your hips are tight, you may have difficulty safely tucking one foot up in your hip crease (in Half Lotus Pose, Ardha Padmasana). Be very careful not to introduce rotational force into your knee, which is a hinge joint. Do not force your foot into your hip crease. Instead, either keep your foot on the floor with the sole against your inner thigh (as in Head of Knee Pose, A), or support your bent knee on a block.

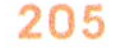

If the arm wrapping behind your back does not reach your foot, just use a strap. Also, don't worry if you can't reach your toes on the extended leg side. Just rest your fingertips on the floor or tuck your fingers (palm-up) under your extended thigh or shin. Do not strain or round your back to reach your foot. Keep your extended knee straight and your thigh muscles (quadriceps) very firm. Breathe.

Remember, in forward folds the focus is on lifting your shoulders up onto your back as you lean forward. This action of drawing your shoulder blades together will help the hand behind your back to reach your foot. Rounding your shoulders actually makes reaching your foot more difficult. If you're using a strap around the tucked foot, pull back and down with the hand holding it to send your chest forward.

Regarding the name of this pose, it's interesting to note that in yoga, your back is considered the "west side" of your body and your front is considered the "east side" of your body. This is because yoga was traditionally practiced in the morning, facing the rising sun to the east.

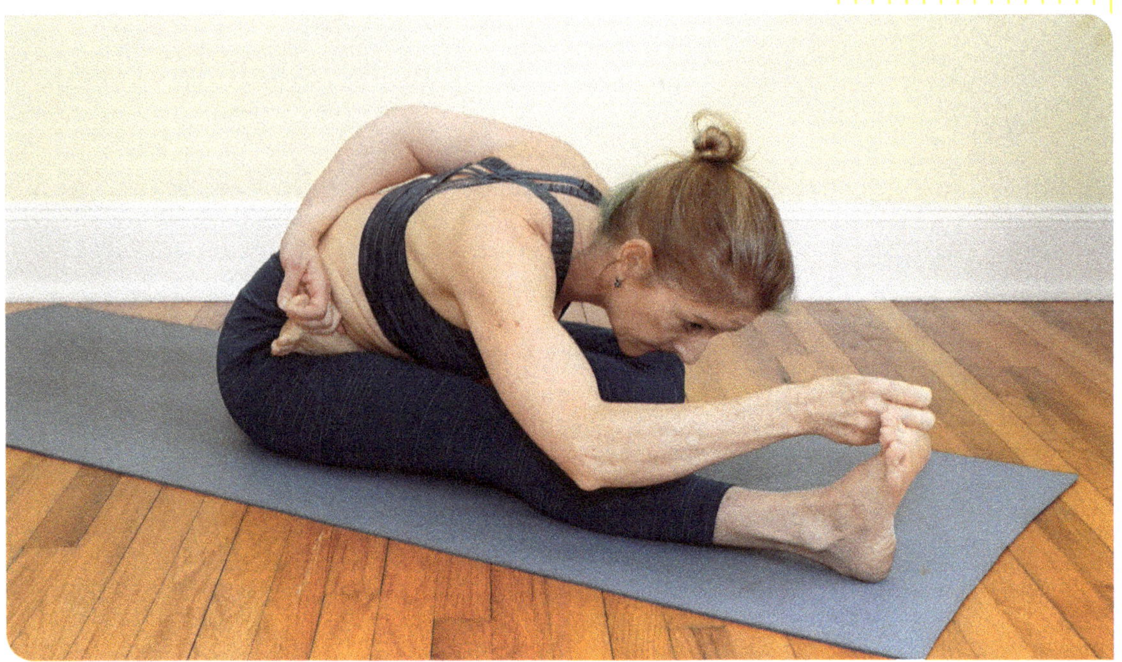

Half-Bound Lotus Intense West Stretch Pose

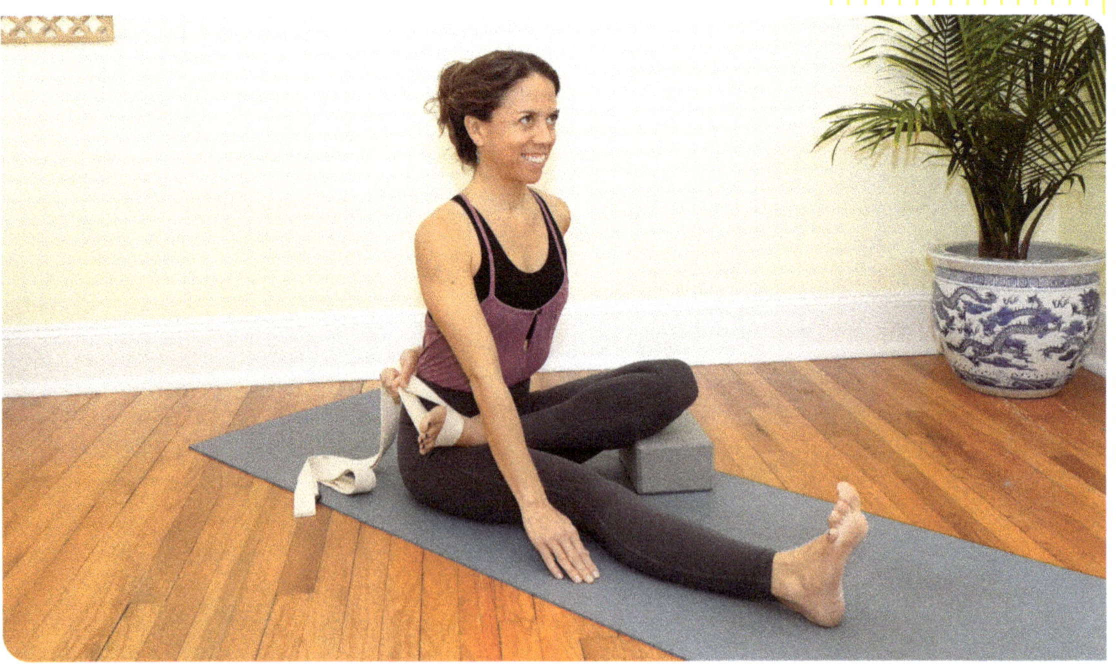

Variation with block and strap

Bound Angle Pose, B

ALSO CALLED: Baddha Konasana B, Butterfly Pose, Cobbler's Pose,

WHAT IT DOES FOR YOUR CORE: Uses your core abdominal muscles to draw your torso in and down toward your feet. Eventually the top of your head might touch your feet, but do not drop your shoulders to get there. This pose also gives your neck muscles a nice stretch.

TUNE IT UP: Tuck your chin to your chest and roll down your spine, folding forward while at the same time drawing your shoulder blades up onto your back. Drawing your shoulders up, away from the direction of forward folds, is counter-intuitive and will take some time to get used to. Just keep trying, you'll figure it out. Use your abdominal muscles to curl inward in this pose. It's helpful to pull slightly up or forward with your hands on your ankles or feet.

Press your thigh bones (your femurs) firmly down. Your elbows can also help press your thighs down.

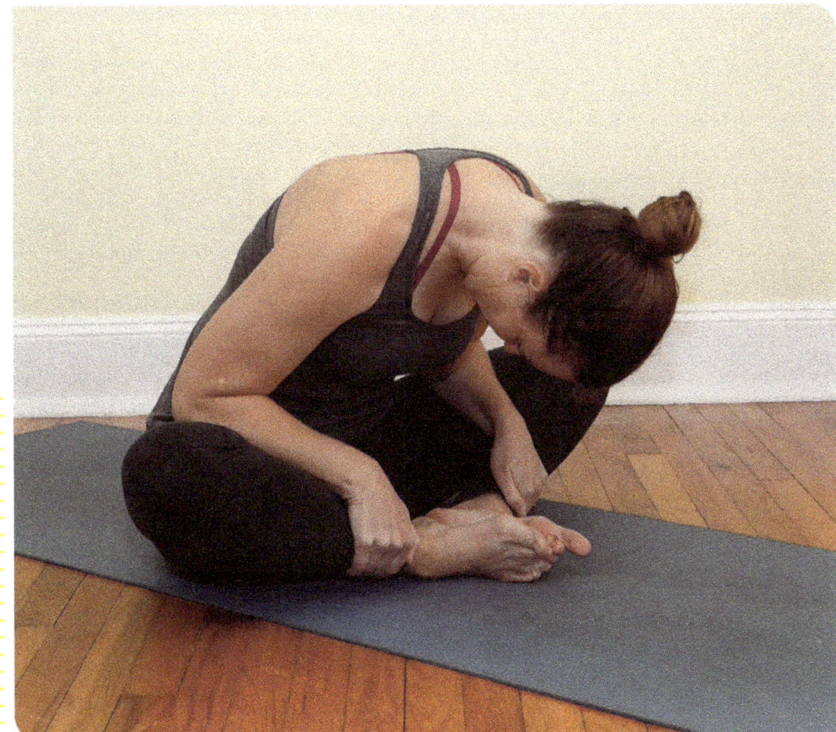

Bound Angle Pose, B

Turtle Pose

ALSO CALLED: Kurmasana

WHAT IT DOES FOR YOUR CORE: This pose builds a tremendous amount of core abdominal strength at every step of preparation, and in the full version. It's a very intense back stretch, so be careful as you are learning it. Pushing or forcing your way into Turtle Pose will strain your low back.

TUNE IT UP: This is an "advanced" pose because it requires so much abdominal strength and back flexibility. To start, stand or sit with your knees bent deeply. Thread your arms, one at a time, behind your knees, working your shoulders as far behind your legs as you can without causing too much strain across your back.

If you start from a standing position, place your feet slightly wider than your hips, lean forward and bend your knees deeply to hold onto the backs of your ankles. Pause and look through your legs at the ceiling behind you to help work your shoulders further through your legs. Plant your palms flat on the floor behind your heels and lower your hips to the floor with your arms threaded under. Once you are seated, slowly extend your legs by sliding your heels forward. Most people have to keep their knees bent until they've been practicing this pose for a long time. Eventually, your back muscles become more flexible and your heels slide further forward, letting letting your chest come closer to the floor. Don't force or hurry this pose.

Kurmasana is a long journey that takes many years. Pushing yourself into this pose can strain your low back. Go slow. Remember, it's just yoga. Breathe.

No matter how bent your knees are, keep your elbows straight, reaching your arms out to the sides or slightly back toward your hips. If you feel that there's too much pressure in the front of your shoulders, try rolling your arms very slightly inward by pressing your thumbs and index fingers down harder than your pinky-fingers. Press your heels firmly outward, even if your knees are bent.

Having your heels on hard flooring, off your sticky mat, will help them gradually slide out as your knees straighten. This is an inch-by-inch process. One day your knees might be straight with your heels lifted off the floor. But don't worry about all that. Focus on reaching your chest forward and listening closely for where your body tells you to stop.

The first thing that touches the floor in this pose, for most people, is their forehead. As your back muscles elongate, you can stretch your chest further forward and your chin may reach the floor.

Approach Turtle Pose with patience and humility. It takes years of practice to do this intense pose safely and effectively. You can live a long and happy life even if you never attempt this pose.

Mechanic's Note: Slow and Steady Wins Remember, yoga is a therapeutic practice for your body and mind. You'll pay a high price for forcing your way into poses your body isn't prepared for. So, practice wisely.

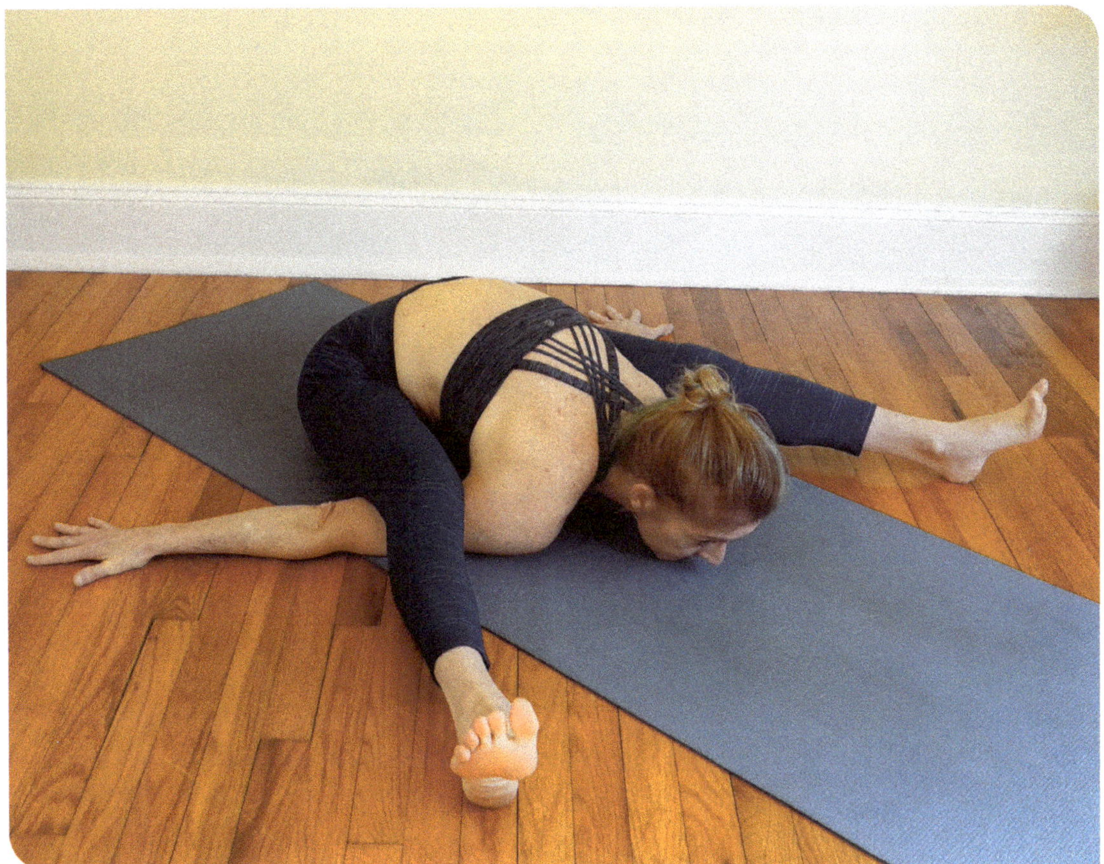

Turtle Pose

Embryo Pose

ALSO CALLED: Pindasana

WHAT IT DOES FOR YOUR CORE: This pose asks your abdominal muscles to pull your torso inward, and stretches your back muscles at the same time.

TUNE IT UP: The easiest way to enter this pose is from Shoulder Stand Pose (Salamba Sarvangasana, chapter 5). You must have a comfortable Shoulder Stand practice to start trying out this pose. Beginning in Shoulder Stand, fold your legs one at a time (right foot first) into a crossed position. Eventually, your hips may be flexible enough to tuck your feet into your hip creases for Lotus Pose (Padmasana).

After your legs are in position—either crossed or in Lotus Pose—wrap your arms around your thighs as tightly as you can, and draw your knees into your chest while staying balanced on the tops of your shoulders. If your hands do not reach one another to clasp, just hold your shins or thighs. Use your arms to pull yourself into a tight ball. Focus on staying as high on your shoulder tops as possible. Press your shoulders strongly down into the floor to help lift some weight off of your upper back and neck.

This inward-looking pose compresses your body, your breathing, and your thoughts. Look at a single gazing point (your drishti), and steady yourself from the inside using your breath.

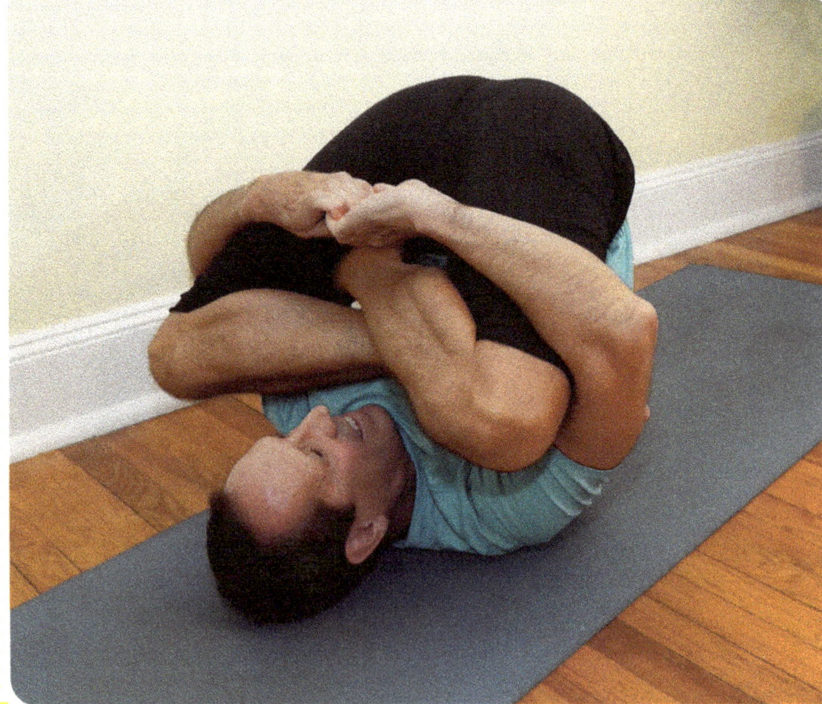

Embryo Pose

CHAPTER 5

SHOULDERS, ARMS, AND WRISTS

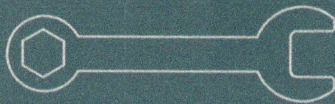

Yoga creates a lot of upper body strength because so many poses are supported by your arms, such as Downward Dog, Upward Dog, Shoulder Stand, Bridge Pose, and, obviously, arm balances like Crow Pose, Headstand, and Handstand. But a lot of people don't realize that poses requiring you to raise your arms overhead, bind them behind your back, or hold them extended straight outward also require a lot of upper body strength and flexibility. That's because all of the muscles that extend and move your arms are connected to your front or back chest wall. In this chapter, we're going to explore how your arms are integrated into your torso, and what that means for building upper body strength and flexibility by doing yoga.

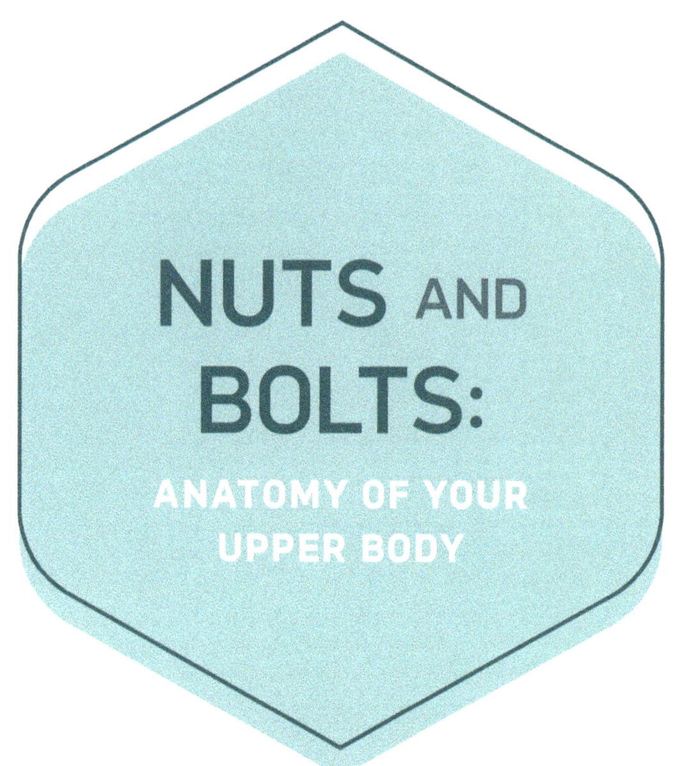

NUTS AND BOLTS: ANATOMY OF YOUR UPPER BODY

As we discussed in chapter 4, your body's core includes your entire torso—not just those washboard abdominal muscles on your belly. We've talked about your pelvis, which anchors the base of your core, and your spine, which runs through your core from top to bottom. Your "upper body" is the top third of your torso, where your shoulders and arms on either side are bound to your core by the muscles of your chest and back. Your shoulder girdle echoes your pelvic girdle in that it's a circular complex of bones and muscles that create a stabilizing hub of strength. So in this chapter we'll focus on the upper end of your core, namely your shoulders, and the arms that they support.

The Shoulder Joint

Your shoulders are the most mobile joints in your body which also makes them the easiest joints to injure. Like the hip, the shoulder is a ball-and-socket joint. But there are some important differences. Unlike your hip, your shoulder does not have a deep, boney socket that limits its range of motion. Instead, your shoulder joint is wrapped by soft tissues—muscles,

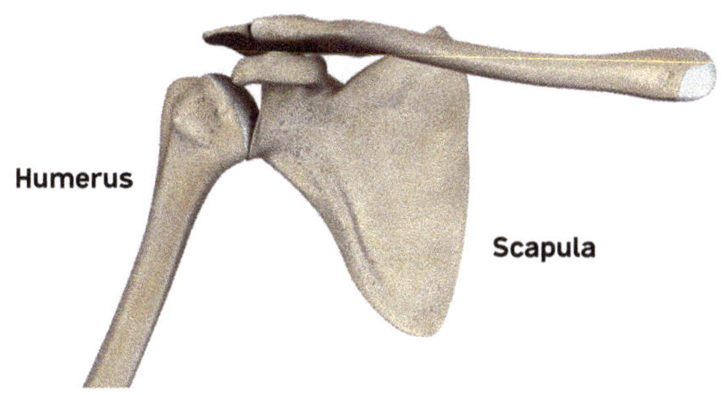

There are 2 bones at your primary shoulder joint, but there are 7 bones in your entire shoulder girdle.

ligaments, and tendons—that form what's called your rotator cuff.

This network of muscles and connective tissues moves your upper arm bone (your humerus) in the socket of your shoulder joint, which is located on your shoulder blade (your scapula). Your shoulder socket isn't much of a socket, really; it's simply a small, flat area (called the glenoid) on the outer edge of your shoulder blade. While your upper leg bone (femur) fits deeply into the hip socket, the main thing holding your humerus in its socket is the network of muscles, tendons, and ligaments that make up your rotator cuff.

Anatomy of the Shoulder Girdle

The main bones of your shoulder joint are the upper arm bone (humerus), and your shoulder blade (scapula), which is on your upper back. A lot of people think their shoulder joints are the boney points at the top of their arms. In fact, the shoulder joint itself is behind what most people think of as their shoulders. It's the whole outer section of your upper chest and back. This is important to understand when you're doing yoga poses.

Seven separate bones form your shoulder girdle, making it less stable than your pelvic girdle.

MECHANIC'S NOTE

Doing yoga with incorrect alignment can injure your rotator cuff and other shoulder structures. Remember, correct alignment—keeping the weight or force moving through the centers of your bones and joints—is critical for avoiding injury. Take extra care not to over-stretch the structures that stabilize your shoulders, such as ligaments and tendon attachments.

Remember, endless flexibility is not the goal of practicing yoga poses. The goal is to keep your joints moving smoothly within their normal full range of motion, no more and no less.

To get aligned correctly in any yoga pose, it's important to understand that the position of your arms affects your whole upper chest and back, not just your shoulder joint.

All seven of these bones influence the movement of your shoulder joint. They are your: breast bone (sternum, the center of your chest); two collarbones (left and right clavicles); two upper arm bones (humerus, plural humeri); and two shoulder blades (left and right scapulae).

Your clavicles across your upper chest, and your breast bone, form the front of your shoulder girdle. The inner end of each collarbone connects to your breast bone, in the center of your chest. That juncture is called the sternoclavicular joint. The outer end of each collarbone is connected to your shoulder blade by ligaments (this is called the acromioclavicular joint).

Collarbones

The joint where your collarbone meets your breast bone is a partial spinning joint. It rolls slightly back and toward your throat when you lift your arm in front of your body, and rolls slightly forward and down when you extend your arm directly behind you. You can feel this for yourself. Put your left finger tips on your right collarbone, and place your right palm against the front of your right thigh. Then raise your right arm straight up and over your head, as if you were hailing a cab. Notice how your collarbone rolls back toward your throat. Now, bring your right arm down and straight back behind your hip. Notice how your collarbone rolls forward. The position of your arm affects your entire upper chest and back, not just your shoulders.

Arms

If you stand with your arms at your sides and your palms facing your hips, turning your palms to face forward is *outward* or *external* rotation; this motion rotates your arms away from your body. If you turn your palms backward to face the wall behind you, that's *inward* or *internal* rotation. In yoga, we emphasize external rotation of the upper arms to help protect your rotator cuff and other soft tissues around your shoulders.

The "ball" of your shoulder's ball-and-socket joint is not symmetrical like a tennis ball. Instead, it's smooth on the inner half and very bumpy on the outer half. These bumps are attachment points for the many muscles and

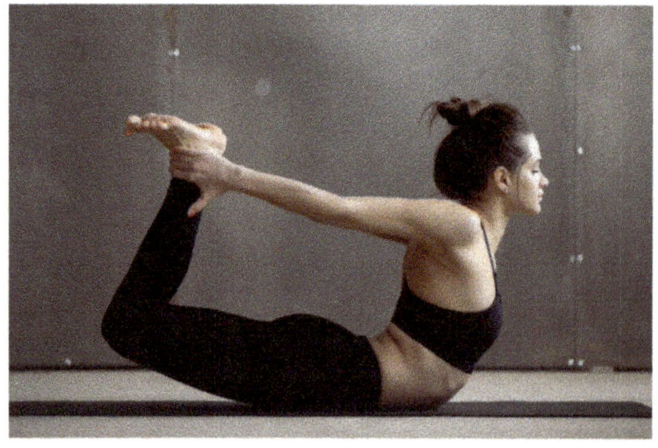

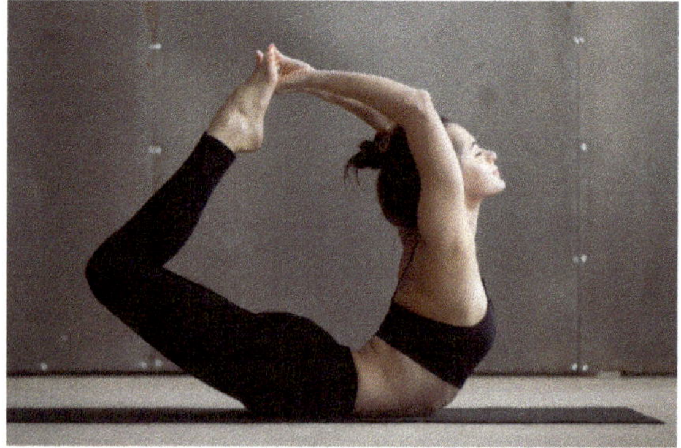

With the thumbs facing down in Bow Pose (left), the arms are internally rotated and shoulder movement is more restricted. With the thumbs facing up (right), the arms are externally rotated which allows maximum range of arm movement.

rotator cuff tissues that control your shoulder movements. One of these bumps, called the greater tubercle, can cause problems if you don't maintain outward rotation of your upper arm bone during yoga practice. Try this: Stand up with your hands out at about waist height. Keep your elbows straight and turn your palms up toward the ceiling. This will rotate your upper arm bones outward. Now, raise your arms overhead and touch your palms. Easy, right? With your upper arm bones rotated outward, that bump (the greater tubercle) passes behind the end of your shoulder blade (your acromium).

Now, bring your arms back to waist height with straight elbows and turn your palms down toward the floor. Your upper arm bones are now rotated inward. Try to raise your arms up and over head. Impossible, right? Notice how your arms get stuck just above shoulder height. That's because the greater tubercle bump is hitting the end of your shoulder blade (your acromium), and stopping the movement of your arm at your shoulder joint. (If you can raise your arms much higher than your shoulders with your palms facing down, you're cheating.)

What's important to understand is this: internal rotation of your upper arm bone—that is, turning your arms inward toward the centerline of your mat—limits shoulder and arm movement. In weight bearing poses, for example Downward Dog, if your upper arms are turned inward (internally rotated), you risk injuring the soft tissues of your rotator cuff because the joint will not be in correct central alignment, and your upper arm bone (humerus) will pinch against the end of your collarbone. With outward rotation (drawing your outer armpit down toward the floor), you will be able to engage all the muscles of the rotator cuff to hold the joint in correct central alignment. In other words, the forces being put on your shoulder joint will be centrally stabilized. This is why good yoga instructors are always reminding you to turn

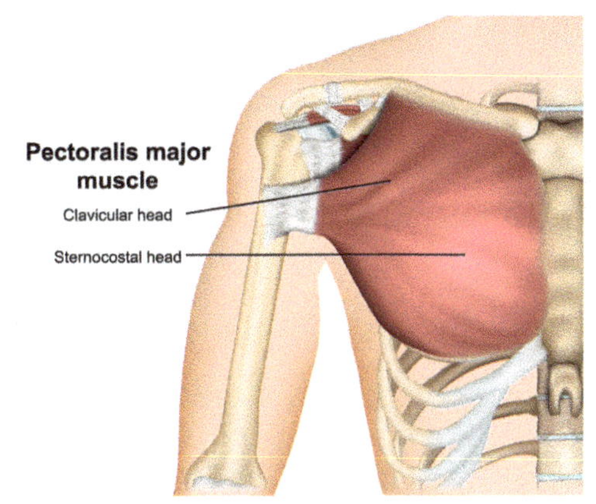

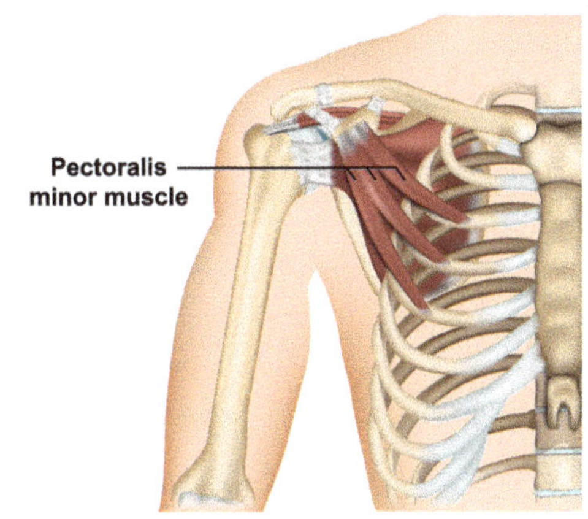

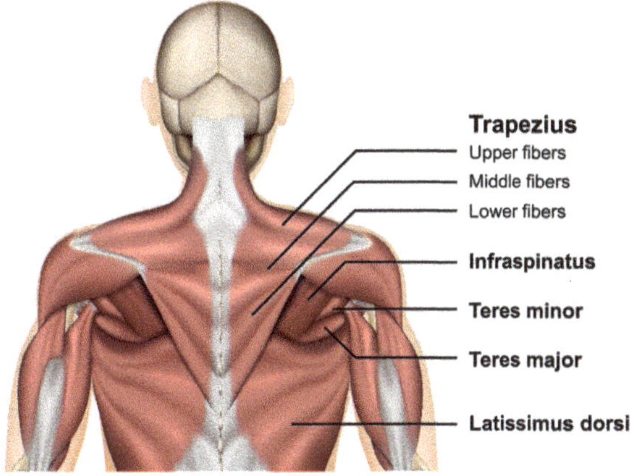

Muscles that move your arms, from the front (top, center) and back (bottom).

MECHANIC'S NOTE: Beware of Dinosaur Arms

Some people develop develop dinosaur arms or what I call "T-Rex Syndrome" without noticing it. They stop fully extending their arms for routine tasks, and instead use only their forearms and hands. When people fall into this T-Rex habit, their shoulder and upper back muscles almost never have to do any work. T-Rex Syndrome weakens your upper back, core, and chest muscles, and limits shoulder mobility. Slouching over a cell phone or computer keyboard, or while watching TV or driving, is a big contributor. Over time, this pattern of contraction (especially in the elbows) hardens, and these folks lose the ability to fully straighten their arms.

It's a disturbingly common situation. Look around next time you're at the grocery store, and watch how rarely some of your fellow shoppers fully extend their arms as they reach for items on the shelves or push their carts. Because of the way your arms are tied into your torso by muscles on your front and back chest wall, keeping your hands close to your torso also contributes to weakening your core abdominal and back muscles.

T-Rex syndrome is an example of a muscular imbalance—meaning some muscle groups are doing too much work, while others aren't doing enough. A muscular imbalance plays havoc with your range of motion, and it's a common cause of restricted shoulder mobility. But muscular imbalances aren't just a problem for couch potatoes. They're also common in people who lift weights or do other intense, repetitive exercises. This can build up certain muscle groups while ignoring the small, deep muscles that stabilize and support these movements. A steady, sustainable yoga practice can help unravel muscular imbalances—both those caused by too little muscle work, and those caused by too much.

your upper arms outward (external rotation). External rotation protects your shoulder joint, and allows your arms and shoulders to have maximum range of motion.

There's a lot going on when you move your arms. All of the muscles that move your upper arm bones are connected to your chest wall and upper back—including your shoulder blades. To take your arms through their full range of motion, you need flexibility and strength in your chest muscles (your pectorals), neck (sternocleidomastoids), shoulders (deltoids), and upper back (trapezius, rhomboids, serratus, teres). To have full range of motion in your arms, your shoulder blades must be able to slide freely across your upper back. A lot of people lose normal range of movement in their shoulders because they have tight, weak upper back and chest muscles.

Very flexible people and very strong people can have different challenges in the same yoga pose. A steady, regular yoga practice can help straighten out your own particular muscular imbalances. Remember, you won't be aware of the habits that cause imbalances in your own body. So you can avoid injury by always approaching your yoga practice with questions, not demands.

Yoga and Your Shoulders

It is important to understand the strengths and limitations of your own shoulder girdle in order to practice yoga safely and effectively. People with a lot of upper body flexibility have very different challenges than people who are very strong in their upper body.

Very flexible people are often muscularly weak, and need to focus more on building muscle strength to support the weight or force of movement out of their shoulder, elbow, and wrist joints. In other words, they need to resist "hanging" in their joints. This means sagging your weight down into the bones of the joint itself rather than asking your muscles to do their job—which is to lift the weight and direct the force out of the joints. Flexible, weak people must work hard to engage their muscles and lift out of their joints in Downward-Facing Dog Pose (Adho Mukha Svanasana), Table Top Pose (Bharmanasana), and Plank Pose. By contrast, strong, inflexible people, who have overbuilt muscles in their upper body, need to focus on restoring flexibility in their large muscles and often need to strengthen their smaller, deep muscles.

And that brings up an important principle to remember in your yoga practice: We each have our own unique challenges. The same pose may be difficult for everyone, but in a different way. Some will struggle to make their muscles contract to do more work, while others will struggle to extend tight, overbuilt muscles. Whichever situation applies to you, be patient.

Aggressive stretching and strengthening only leads to injury. Gently and persistently ask your muscles to grow longer and stronger, a little bit at a time. Approach your practice with curiosity—not demands. Remember, slow and steady wins the race.

Elbow, Forearm, and Wrist Bones

You have three primary bones in your arms: your humerus, radius, and ulna; just like you have three primary bones in your legs (your femur, tibia, and fibula). Your upper arm bone (your humerus) meets the larger lower arm bone (the ulna) at your elbow joint. The smaller bone (radius) runs beside the ulna and connects to it just below your elbow. Your wrist joint is formed in a similar way as your ankle joint. Your two forearm bones (one larger and one smaller) each make up one side of your wrist

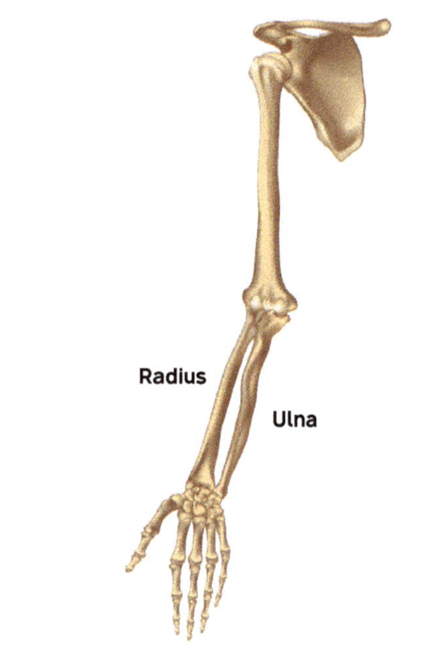

Bones of your forearm, elbow, and wrist

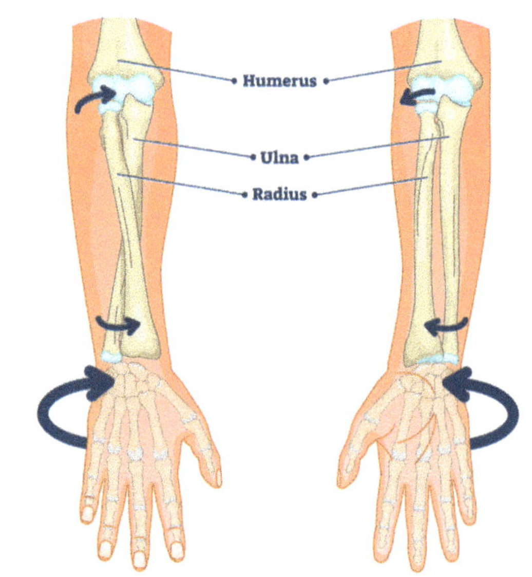

Your radioulnar joint is a spinning joint, which allows your forearms to rotate.

joint. So the two bumps you feel on your inner and outer wrist are the ends of two different bones. Just like the two bumps on your inner and outer ankle are the ends of two different shin bones (tibia and fibula).

The most interesting thing about your arms is that they have two joints in the middle. One, your elbow, is a hinge joint (like your knee) that opens in one direction, like the hinge of a door. The other, more interesting joint, is just below your elbow, where your two forearm bones meet each other. We don't think of this joint very often—it doesn't even have a common name, like "elbow." But this radioulnar joint would be hard to live without. It's a spinning joint. Your radius (the smaller bone) rolls across your ulna, so that the two bones cross over each other and make an X when you rotate your forearm (what you think of as turning your wrist).

This ingenious arrangement of the forearm bones allows you to turn your lower arm while holding your upper arm still. It may not seem like it but that's a big deal! The ability to rotate your lower arm is crucial for doing many activities of daily life.

Check this out: Pick up an imaginary car key and put it into the ignition. Now, try to turn on your car without rotating your lower arm. It can't be done. Reach out and grab an imaginary door knob; open the door without rotating your lower arm. Nope, can't be done. Pick up a soup spoon, get some soup into your mouth without rotating your lower arm. Grab the tab on a soda can and open it without rotating your lower arm. In every case, you'll fail, or maybe spill something all over yourself. All of these tasks—and many more—rely on that unique spinning action of your lower forearm joint (your radioulna joint).

In yoga, the most obvious place we use this spinning joint is in Downward Facing Dog Pose (Adho Mukha Svanasana). Sit up or stand up and hold your arms out in front at shoulder height. Turn your palms and your inner-elbows up to face the ceiling. Hold them here and feel how your upper arm bones (your humeri) have rotated outward, in the same direction as your forearms did. Now, keep your arms straight out, and your upper arms turned outward (imagine you're holding a $100 dollar bill in each armpit), but rotate your palms down toward the floor. Flex your wrists back, pulling the backs of your hands towards you with palms out as if you were pressing against a wall. The insides of your elbows should still be facing up. This is the position your hands would be in if they were pressing against the floor in Downward Dog.

These two opposing actions of the forearms and upper arms are the basis of Downward-Facing Dog Pose (Adho Mukha Svanasana). Feel the challenge of these arm motions in your upper back muscles? And here you don't even have any weight on your arms. Take a few breaths, and try to remember the feeling of this muscular action for reference the next time you're in the pose.

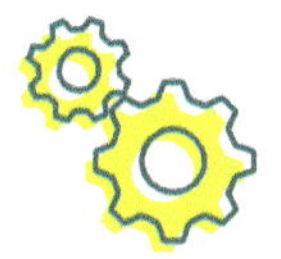

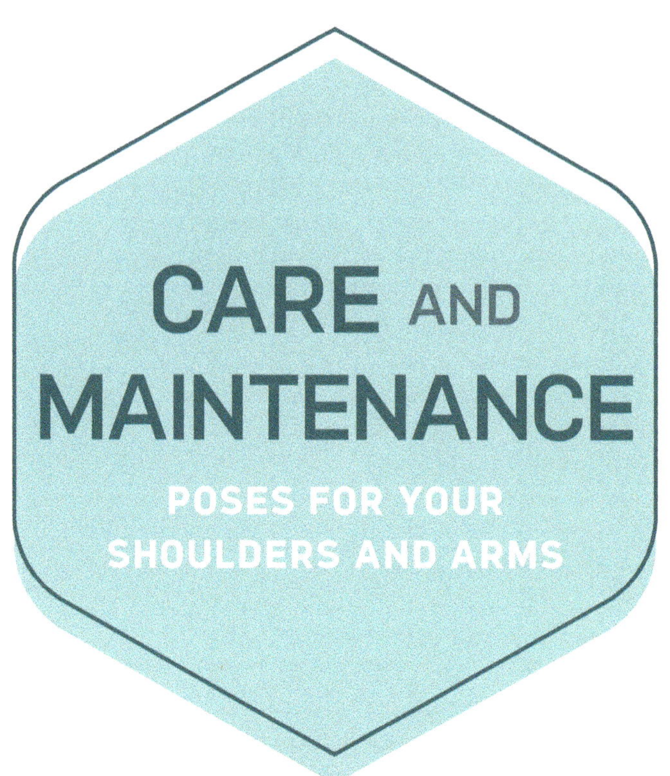

CARE AND MAINTENANCE

POSES FOR YOUR SHOULDERS AND ARMS

Your shoulder is already the most mobile joint in your body. Your focus in yoga should be to restore and maintain its normal full range of motion, by stretching tight muscles and strengthening weak ones. Your arms are in constant motion throughout a yoga practice, so your shoulder joint has plenty of opportunities to move through its full range of movement during class.

If you're struggling with the arm or shoulder position in a particular pose, stop pushing and steady your breath. Pause and explore where your arms or shoulders feel weak or tight. Investigate exactly what muscles seem to be limiting your arm and shoulder movement. Do not force your arms and shoulders into position. Remember, always approach your body with curiosity, not force.

Yoga poses are complex. Your shoulders are tied into your chest, your neck, and your upper back. Be curious, and change your position slowly and carefully; start scanning for central alignment, beginning with your feet and working your way up. By the time you get to your shoulders and arms, things may have rearranged themselves.

Observe. Breathe. Notice. Learn.

Locust Pose

ALSO CALLED: Salabhasana, Grasshopper Pose

WHAT IT DOES FOR YOUR SHOULDERS: This pose builds flexibility across the front of your chest and strength in your upper back. This is important because many of us have developed imbalances between the front and back of our shoulder girdle—tight chest muscles (pectorals) and weak upper back muscles—from sitting slouched over our phones, in front of our screens, or behind the wheel of a car.

TUNE IT UP: This pose can be done with a variety of arm positions, but the cues for correct alignment are the same. Start with your forehead and feet on the floor, to focus on drawing your shoulder blades together on your upper back (away from the floor) and stretching your chest muscles.

You can clasp your hands behind your back to help extend your chest muscles more. If your hands don't touch, either bend your elbows, or hold a strap across your backside with your palms facing the floor. Your elbows are straight when using a strap, pull it tight and roll your thumbs slightly outward and up toward the ceiling. Using a strap gives you an intense stretch in the front shoulder muscles and chest. Breathe deeply. Notice how the inhales intensify the stretching and strengthening benefits of this pose. Deepen your breath to work harder, and build more flexibility and strength in your muscles.

To make the pose more challenging, you can lift your head, chest, and legs up off the floor. Do not stick your chin forward as you lift; look slightly past the end of your mat, and keep the back of your neck lengthened. Draw your chin very slightly toward your throat.

The tendency to stick the chin forward in this pose is common, because it moves the muscle work out of your core abdominals, and into the back of your neck and shoulders (your trapezius muscles). Basically, if you stick your chin forward, what you're doing is shifting the weight of your head backwards, over your upper back and neck. Remember, your head is heavy, weighing eight to twelve pounds. Check it out for yourself: Get into Locust Pose and stick your chin forward. Notice how your ab muscles aren't working. Now pull your chin slowly in toward your throat, and feel how your core abdominals switch on.

As you work on this pose, don't forget about your legs. Pull your thighs together to protect your low back. Do not let your legs drift apart.

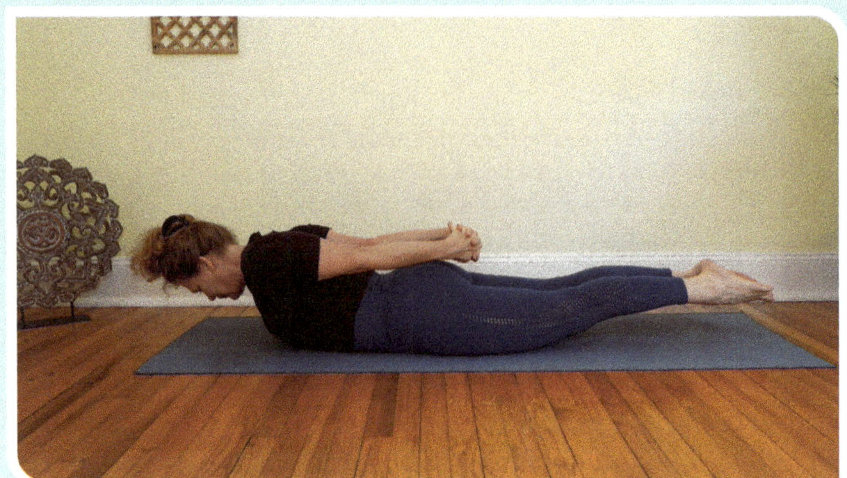

Locust Pose, variation with bound hands

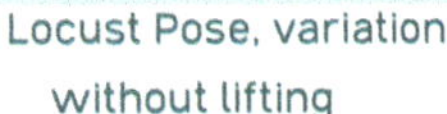

Locust Pose, variation without lifting

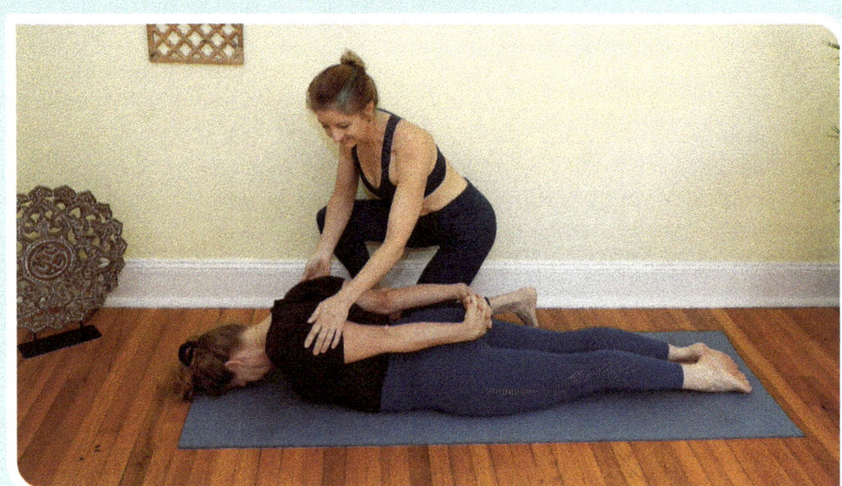

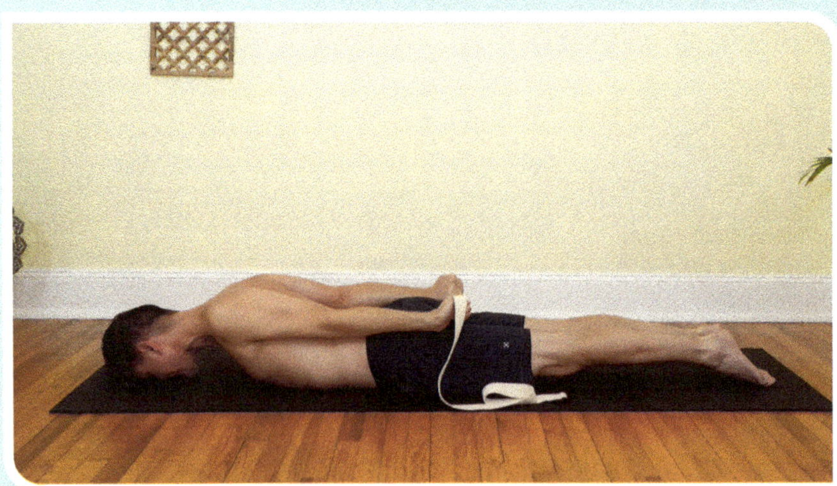

Locust Pose, variation with strap and without lifting

Intense Side Stretch Pose

ALSO CALLED: Parsvottanasana, Pyramid Pose

WHAT IT DOES FOR YOUR SHOULDERS: Although many people release their hands down toward the floor when doing this pose, the traditional variation requires clasping your forearms or hands behind your back. The purpose of using an arm bind here is to build more shoulder strength and flexibility and to challenge your balance.

TUNE IT UP: If you have limited shoulder mobility, start by touching the tips of your fingers together at your low back. Eventually you might hold opposite forearms or elbows, and one day you might press your palms together behind your back in Reverse Prayer (see photo, next page).

Whatever arm position you choose, focus on pulling your shoulder blades back and towards each other. In all standing poses where you bend forward, there's a tendency to round the shoulders and drop the elbows down toward the floor. Keep drawing your shoulder blades up onto your back.

If you have tight hamstrings, don't go so far forward that your back becomes rounded. Curving your back and bending over the front leg will pull your hands further apart. Instead, focus on extending your chest and ribs forward to your big toe, and lifting your elbows back.

Mechanic's Note: When you encounter a problem in your yoga practice, you must first stop fighting with your body, and learn to observe what's happening. Don't just start "fixing" your arms and shoulders. Scan your whole body's alignment to see what's out of whack. Although what you initially noticed may seem to be an upper body problem, it may well be caused by misalignment in your feet, legs, or hips.

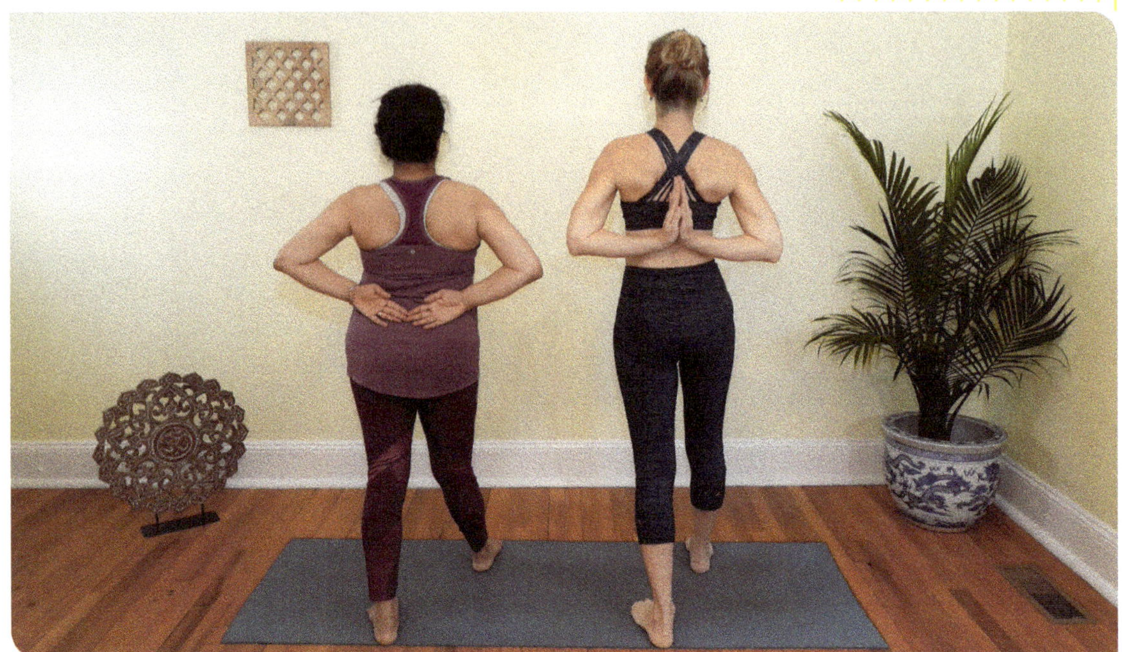

Intense Side Stretch Pose with arm variations

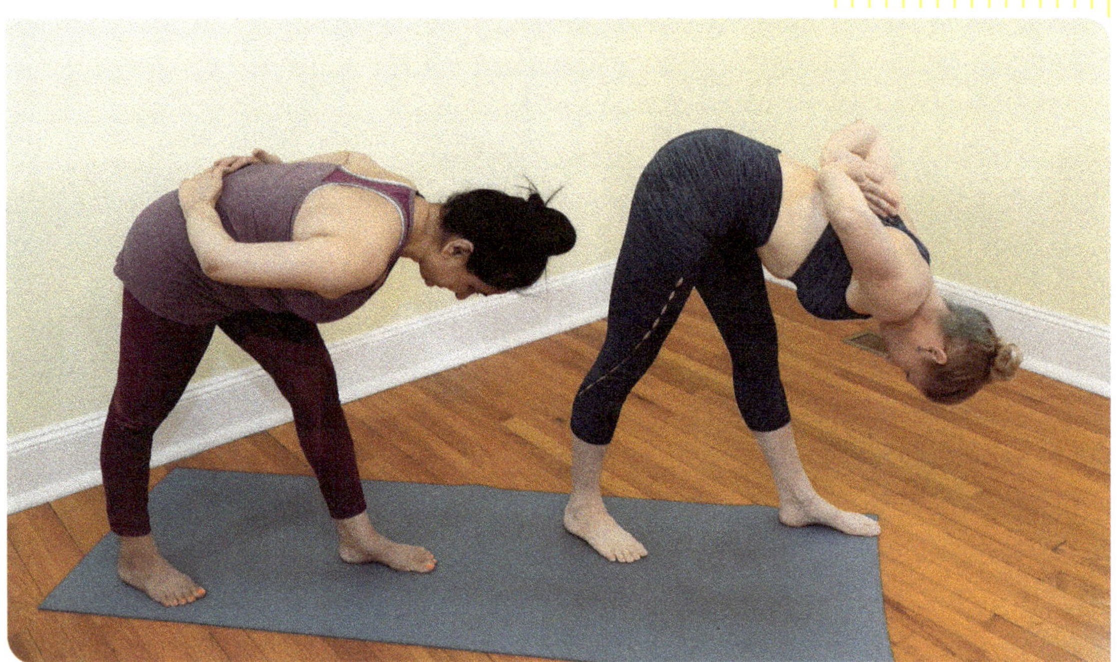

Intense Side Stretch Pose with arm variations

Wide-Legged Forward Fold, C

ALSO CALLED: Prasarita Padottanasana, C

WHAT IT DOES FOR YOUR SHOULDERS: This is another good stretch for the chest and front shoulders, while strengthening the upper back muscles.

TUNE IT UP: If you can't interlace your fingers behind your back with straight elbows, use a strap. Even if you can interlace your fingers, sometimes it just feels good to do this pose with your hands wider apart on a strap.

Do not force your hands overhead, or bounce to make your arms go further. Breathe. The muscular action that moves your arms further overhead is actually a shrugging motion of drawing your shoulder blades up toward the back of your neck.

Explore this shoulder motion when you're standing upright first. (It's never easier to figure things out when you're already upside down.) Stand up straight, feet wide apart, and hold your hands behind your back, either with your fingers interlaced or holding a strap with your palms facing forward. Pull the strap tight and roll your thumbs outward (toward the wall behind you) and then "shrug" your shoulders up toward your neck. Notice that your arms move *away* from your backside.

Relax your shoulders. Now, pull the strap tight and roll your thumbs outward while pushing your shoulder blades down your back toward your hips. Notice how your arms move *toward* your backside.

When you fold forward, you want your hands to move away from your backside—not toward it. So as you fold, shrug your shoulders up toward your neck. Don't force your arms overhead; let gravity slowly stretch your shoulders. This is a long-time pose. Don't hurry. It will come—little by little.

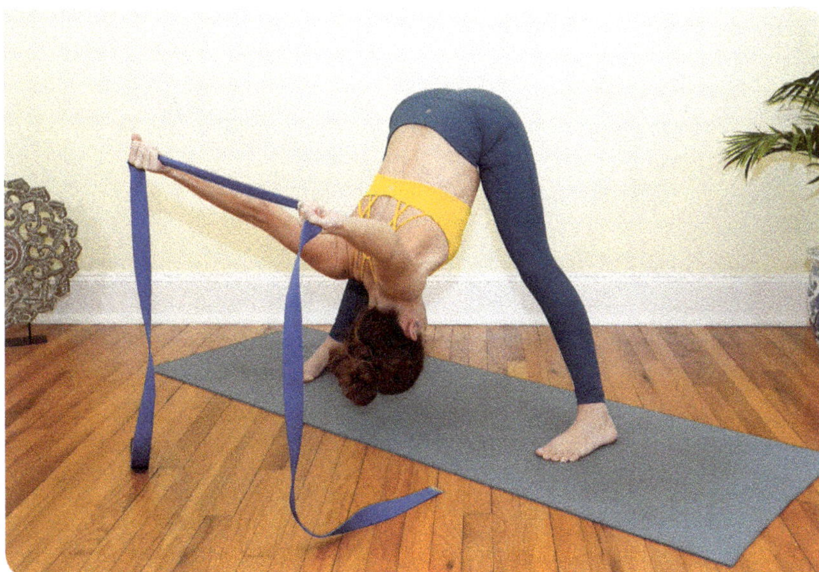

Wide Legged Forward Fold, C, variation with strap

Cow Face Pose

ALSO CALLED: Gomukhasana

WHAT IT DOES FOR YOUR SHOULDERS: This pose stretches the shoulder on each side differently. The raised side gets a big stretch in the muscles on the back and outer shoulder blade (triceps, serratus, teres, latissimus dorsi). The lowered arm gets a big stretch on the front of the shoulder (anterior deltoid) and the top of the shoulder up into the neck (trapezius).

TUNE IT UP: As with other poses, if you can't bring your fingers together behind your back, use a strap. Here's how: Put the strap over the shoulder on your top-arm side. Reach that arm up, bend your elbow, and grab the strap behind your neck. Reach your other arm out to the side, and turn that thumb down toward the floor. Bend your elbow and grab the strap behind your back. Now, wiggle your fingers along the strap to bring your hands a little bit closer. You'll know you've gone too far with your hands if your chin starts to stick forward, or your head drops down.

Keep sitting upright, and look forward (not down at the floor). Focus on pointing your top elbow up to the ceiling while lifting your chest and ribs up off your hips. Breathe. Do not force this pose; it's a mistake to stretch your shoulders aggressively. Remember, your rotator cuff is easy to injure and slow to repair. Take it easy. Stay calm, and cool, and collected. Make your yoga practice a therapeutic, healing experience.

If your shoulders are comfortable, you can try hinging slightly forward over your top thigh. Keep your back straight and keep lifting your top elbow. Don't round down toward the floor. Your leg and abdominal muscles must support the weight of your torso as you lean forward. Pull your thighs firmly toward each other and lift your low belly muscles. Pulling your arms away from each other will help activate your back and side waist muscles (your obliques). Your top hand pulls up and your bottom hand pulls down. Don't hold your breath. It's a lot, I know. Take it slow.

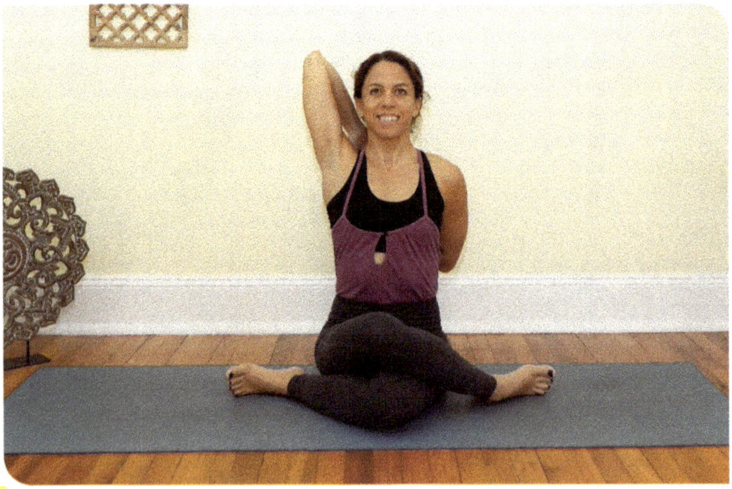

Cow Face Pose

One-Legged King Pigeon Pose

ALSO CALLED: Kapotasana, Eka Pada Rajakapotasana, Pigeon Pose

WHAT IT DOES FOR YOUR SHOULDERS: Stretches your shoulder and chest muscles while strengthening your upper back (rhomboids, rear deltoids, triceps, lats, and neck muscles). This is a big quad, glute, and hip flexor stretch as well.

TUNE IT UP: Start this pose by bending your back knee and turning your torso toward it to catch your foot. Turn forward again and place your other hand (on the bent knee side) on the floor, or a block for balance.

Once you're familiar with this one-handed variation, you can try holding the lifted foot behind you with both hands. As always, if you can't reach your foot, use a strap.

To use the strap, bring the back foot forward for a moment to make a little sandal with the strap to hold your foot when it goes back behind you. Start by running the middle of the strap behind the ankle on the leg that will be behind you. Then, bring both sides over the top of your foot and through the slot between your big and second toes (where your sandal thong goes). Take both sides of the strap underneath the sole of your foot, and hold them in one hand on the back leg side.

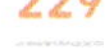

Now, swing that leg back behind you, holding the very ends of the strap as you get your leg into position. Facing forward, bend your back knee, and bring the hand that's holding the strap onto your shoulder. Pause here, resting your other hand on a block or the floor for balance.

If you feel balanced, bring the ends of the strap onto the top of your head, holding it with both hands. Pause here and breathe. Point your elbows forward (not out to the sides). If you're comfortable, lift your hands off your head and up towards the ceiling—as if trying to straighten your arms overhead. Breathe. Go slow. This is quite intense.

In all stages and all variations of Pigeon Pose, focus on lifting your chest and looking forward or slightly up. Don't look down. Take slow, full breaths.

There are a lot of sensations to explore in this complex pose. Pay attention. Notice what's going on in different parts of your body. Watch how your mind reacts to this intense physical challenge. Take these few moments in Pigeon Pose to learn something about yourself.

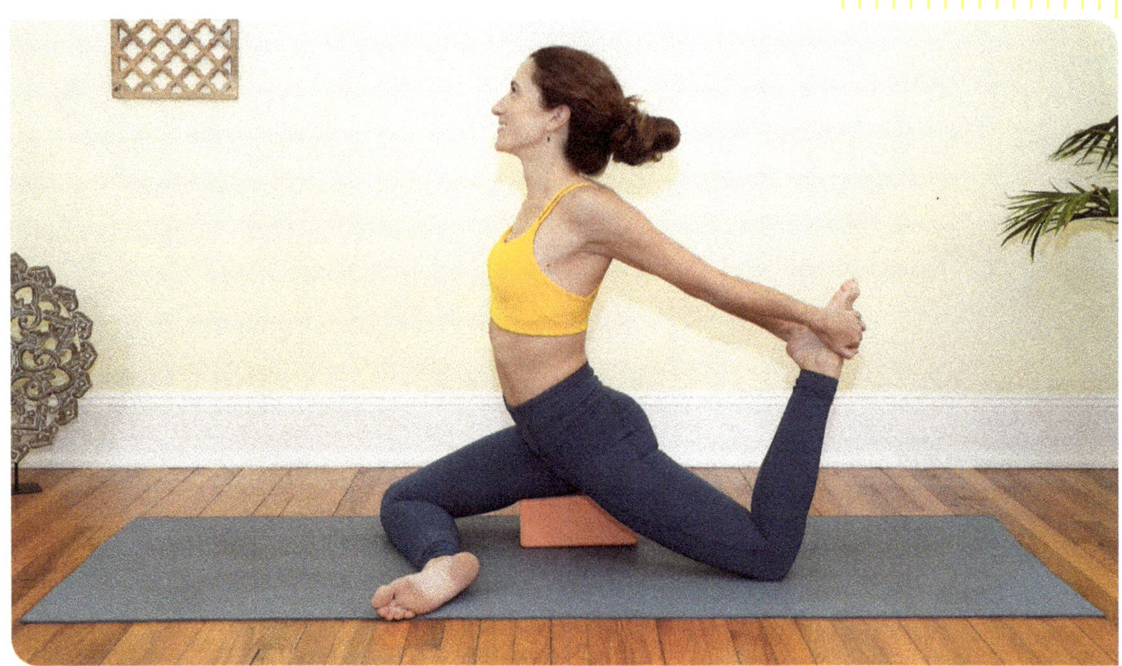

One-Legged King Pigeon Pose, variation with block

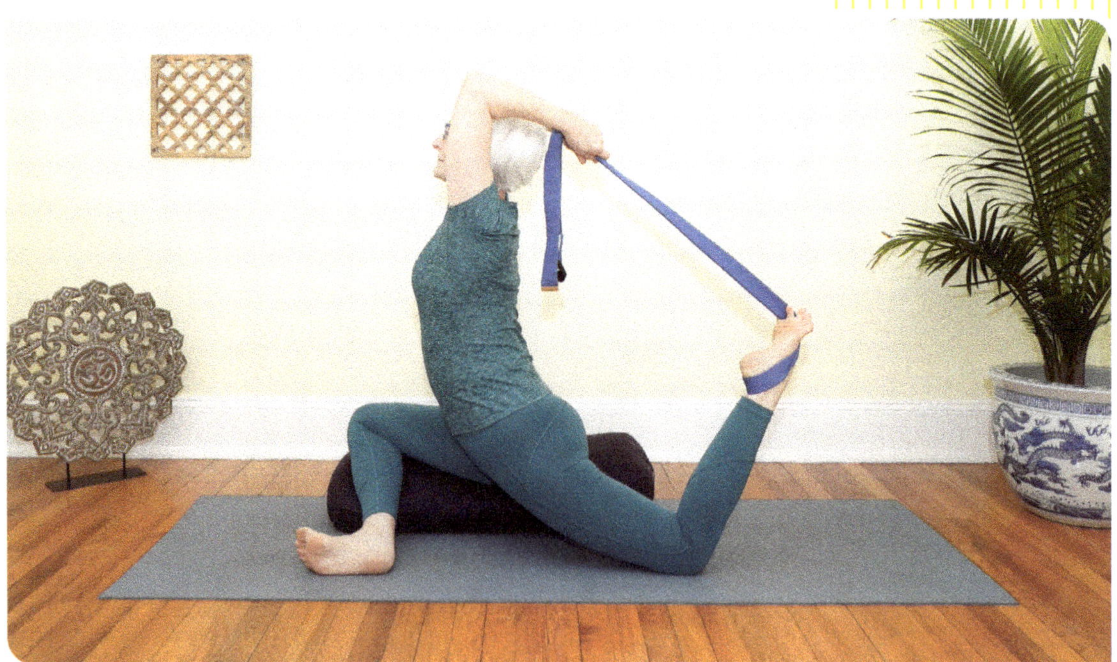

Variation with strap and bolster

Bridge Pose

ALSO CALLED: Setu Bandhasana

WHAT IT DOES FOR YOUR SHOULDERS: This pose builds a lot of chest and shoulder flexibility as well as shoulder strength. It's a preparatory pose for more challenging shoulder inversions, such as Plow Pose (Halasana) and Shoulder Stand Pose (Salamba Sarvangasana). Because these poses shift weight onto your upper back and shoulders, you need a lot of flexibility and strength in your upper back and chest to keep your shoulder blades together, and protect the spinal vertebrae in your neck from bearing too much weight.

TUNE IT UP: If you have limited shoulder mobility, use a strap in Bridge Pose. Hold it underneath you, with palms facing up. Externally rotate your upper arms by straightening your elbows and turning your thumbs outward (they'll roll down toward your mat). Press the backs of your upper arms and armpits firmly down into the floor, and pull your shoulder blades together. A gentle side-to-side rocking motion will help wiggle your shoulder blades further under your back.

There should be a very slight gap between the floor and your neck vertebrae (like someone could slide a thin pencil in there). Your neck should not be pressing flat down into the floor. As your chest and shoulder flexibility increases, you'll be able to interlace your fingers underneath. Keep your elbows straight, and press the backs of your armpits down.

Your legs provide the power to push your chest back, over your shoulders. The important action in Bridge Pose is to move more weight onto the tops of your shoulders—don't focus on shoving your hips up very high; that's not the point. Press the balls of your feet down and forward, and do not lift your heels or big toes off the floor (a common tendency). Keep your toes and heels on the floor. With your feet flat, push with your legs as if you're trying to stretch your yoga mat longer. Notice how this rolls your chest further back over your shoulders.

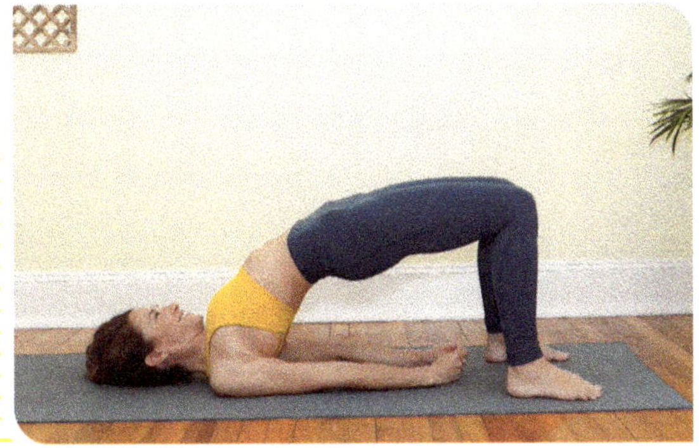

Bridge Pose

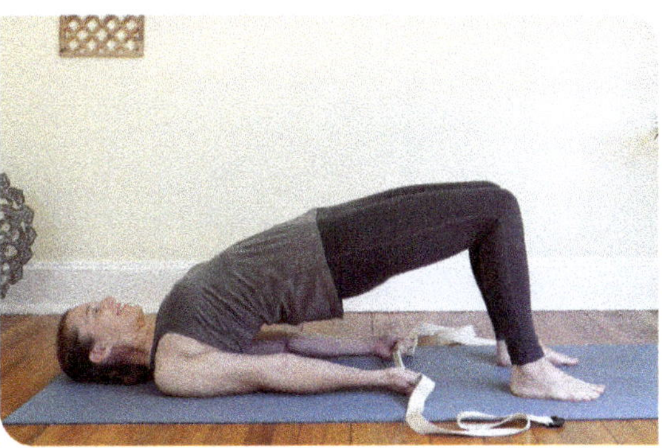

Variation with strap

Bow Pose

ALSO CALLED: Dhanurasana

WHAT IT DOES FOR YOUR SHOULDERS: Stretches your chest and shoulders, because you must reach back to hold your feet. Strengthens your upper back (rhomboids, lats, and trapezius) and upper arm muscles (triceps, teres, serratus).

TUNE IT UP: This variation uses a bolster to support your torso, and keeps your knees on the floor, so you can focus on the chest and shoulder stretch.

To do this, lie over the bolster with your elbows on the floor and your belly on the bolster. To test that you are in the right spot, lift your hands and elbows off the floor. If you do a face plant, pitching forward, you are too far forward. Shift back so that your mid-belly is on the bolster (not your hips). When you lift your elbows and hands up, your chest should stay up too. Bend your knees and rock from side-to-side to grab one foot behind you and then the other. Then lower your forehead to the floor. Wiggle your knees closer to each other, and pull your shoulder blades together on your upper back. Pause here and establish a deep, slow breathing pattern.

On an inhale, kick your feet backward, using the power of your legs and back to lift your chest and head. Do not lift your knees. Tilt your face slightly upward, but don't crimp the back of your neck. Look even further up with your eyes, but don't move your face—just move your eyes. Notice that taking deep inhales exponentially increases the stretch across your chest. Release your feet and rest your forehead on the back of your stacked hands. Rock your hips from side-to-side to release any low back tension, then try it again.

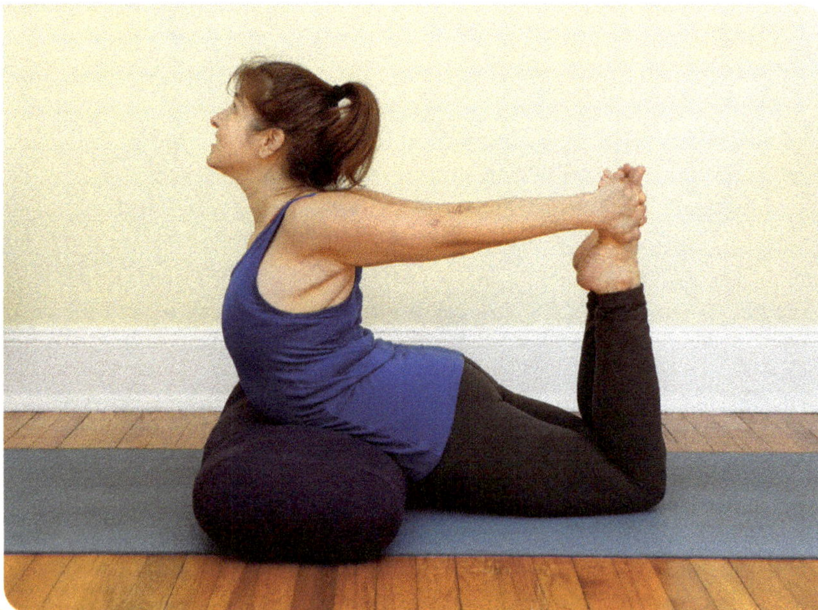

Bow Pose, variation with bolster

Camel Pose

ALSO CALLED: Ustrasana

WHAT IT DOES FOR YOUR SHOULDERS: Provides a deep stretch across your chest and shoulders.

TUNE IT UP: This variation using a two-block "speed-bump" is great for people who can't reach their heels. And even though I can reach my heels in Camel Pose, I like doing this variation on occasion to find some extra lift and opening in my chest and upper back.

For this variation, put two blocks end-to-end under your mat, and come onto all fours in front of your speed bump (all fours is called Table Top Pose, or Bharmanasana in yoga). Look backward, under your belly, and put your toes up on the front edge of the blocks. (See photo; don't put your toes on top of the speed bump, just hook them on the front edge.)

Come up to stand on your knees, which should be hip-distance or wider apart. Turn to one side and reach back, placing your fingertips inside your ankle or heel, with your palm facing outward to externally rotate your shoulder joint. Lift the opposite arm up to the ceiling with your elbow straight (palm in neutral facing the middle of your mat) and let it move back toward the wall behind you. Draw your knees slightly inward toward each other, to help engage your low belly muscles and protect your back. Take a few deep breaths and then come up and switch sides.

Eventually, you'll be able to put both hands on the insides of your ankles or heels at once. Push each heel or ankle outward with your hands, and squeeze your heels inward against that force. This push-and-resist action between your hands and your feet really helps to lift your chest.

Although Camel is a back bending pose, focus on lifting your chest. Don't think about going backwards or reaching down. Draw your knees slightly inward and press your thighs forward. This focus on lifting up your chest helps protect your low back.

In this pose, look up at the ceiling or slightly back, but don't drop the weight of your head back onto your neck. Use the muscles in the front of your neck and chest to support the weight of your head. Remember, your head weighs eight to twelve pounds, and your neck vertebrae are very small. These backward-looking poses in yoga help you develop strong muscles in the front of your throat to help protect your neck joints. Move your eyes back further than your face; move your eyeballs in their sockets like you're trying to look at your own eyebrows. Breathe deeply.

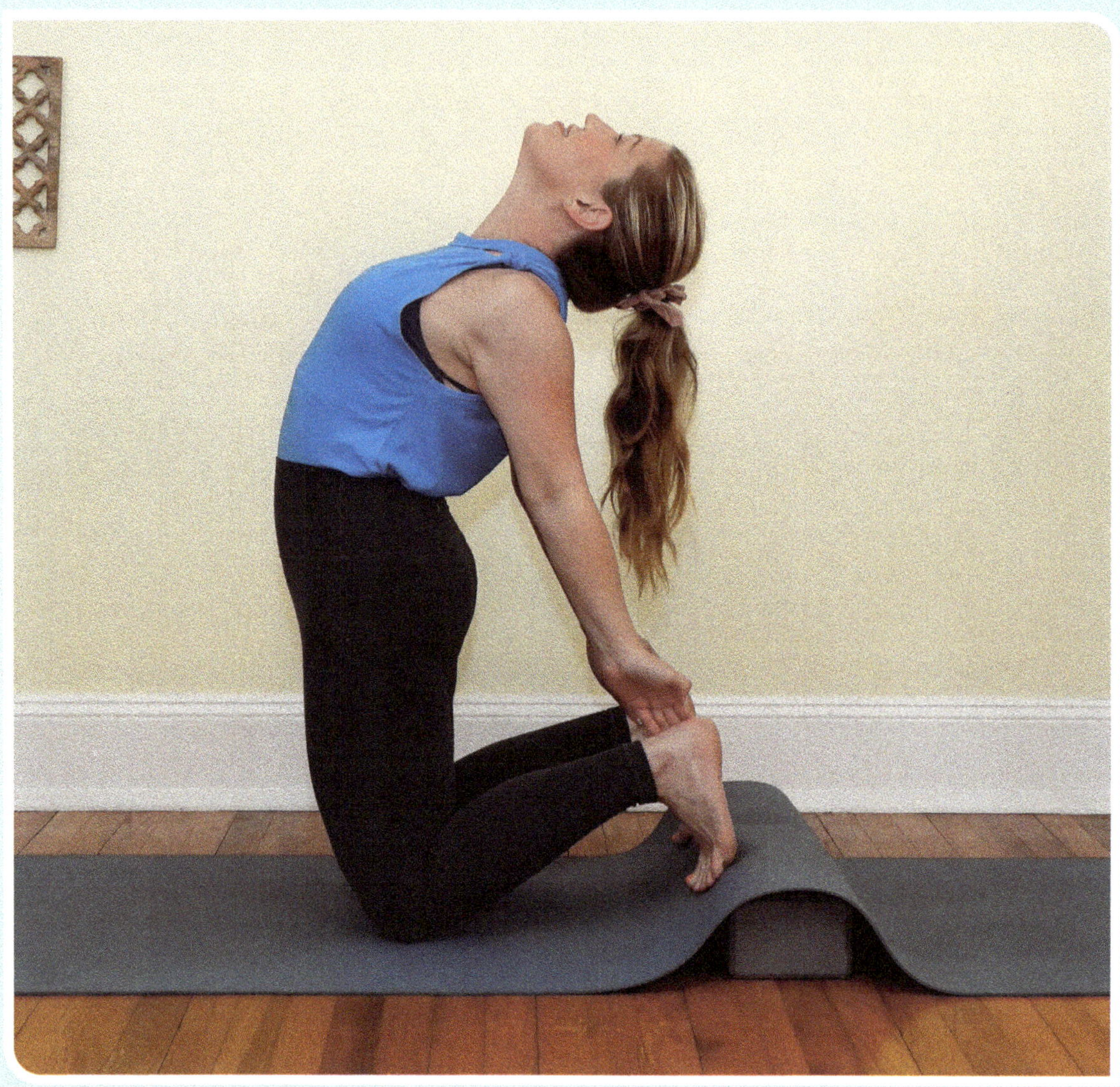

Camel Pose, variation with blocks

MECHANIC'S NOTE:
Why Straight Arms are Important

It's important to understand that to build shoulder strength in most yoga poses, your elbows must be straight. When your arms are fully extended, muscles on the back of your shoulders (your posterior deltoids) and upper back (serratus and teres) are activated. When your elbows are bent even slightly, they're not. Unless the instructor is teaching a special variation, or you have an injury, your elbows should be straight in most yoga poses.

Check it out for yourself. Stand in Mountain Pose (Tadasana), and raise your arms up overhead with straight elbows and your hands slightly wider than shoulder distance apart. If you can't get your elbows completely straight, move your hands further apart and forward of your body until they are straight-even if that means they are in a wide V-shape. Close your eyes and take a few deep breaths. Notice what muscles are turned on and working.

Now, keep your arms in place but bend your elbows. Notice how the muscles on the backs of your upper arms (your triceps), shoulders (your deltoids), and your upper back (serratus and teres) turn off as soon as your elbows bend.

Lifting your arms with straight elbows requires a lot of strength in the backs of your upper arms (your triceps), shoulders (your posterior deltoids), and upper back (serratus anterior and teres major and minor). Only raise your arms to the point that your elbows begin to bend. Don't practice with bent elbows. You'll miss most of the shoulder-strengthening benefits.

Extended Mountain Pose

ALSO CALLED: Utthita Tadasana

WHAT IT DOES FOR YOUR SHOULDERS: This is one of several basic yoga poses that are a lot harder than they look. It takes a tremendous amount of work to raise your arms, because all of the muscles that lift them are attached to your chest wall, front and back. It will take you quite a while to develop enough strength in the shoulders and chest to bring your palms together with straight elbows overhead.

TUNE IT UP: Start practicing Mountain Pose by raising your hands with your palms apart. Remember, the lifting action is always done on an inhale.

Once you develop enough strength and flexibility to raise your arms all the way overhead with straight elbows and your hands apart, begin bringing your palms closer together. There are two ways to practice this. One is to bring your palms together in front of your chest with straight elbows and gradually raise your arms from here. Go a few inches at a time, keeping your palms together and your elbows straight. You can cross one thumb over the other to help hold your palms together. As soon as your elbows bend, stop. Lower your arms to get them straight and work there. Little by little, your shoulders will get stronger, until you can keep your elbows straight and your palms together overhead. This will take many months. Give your body time to develop this strength across your upper back, chest, and shoulders.

The other way to build this strength is to raise your arms overhead with your palms apart and your elbows straight, and slowly draw them closer to each other. Go just an inch at a time, and stop as soon as your elbows bend. Move your palms apart until your elbows are straight, and work there. This method also takes many months to build the strength you need to have your palms together overhead with straight elbows.

Either version builds strength in your shoulders, upper back, chest, and core. Your "edge" in this pose is the limit of your strength and flexibility to hold your arms straight. As soon as your elbows bend, stop, back up, get them straight, and breathe there. If you practice with bent elbows, you'll never build this shoulder strength, because you can't fully engage these muscle groups when your elbows are bent. Be patient.

There's a very common tendency to hold your breath when you raise your arms, because the muscles that move your arms are attached to your chest wall. But holding your breath only makes it harder. Focus on taking deep inhales to fuel this work. It's surprisingly difficult.

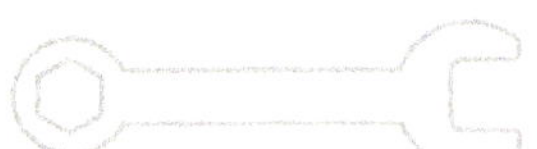

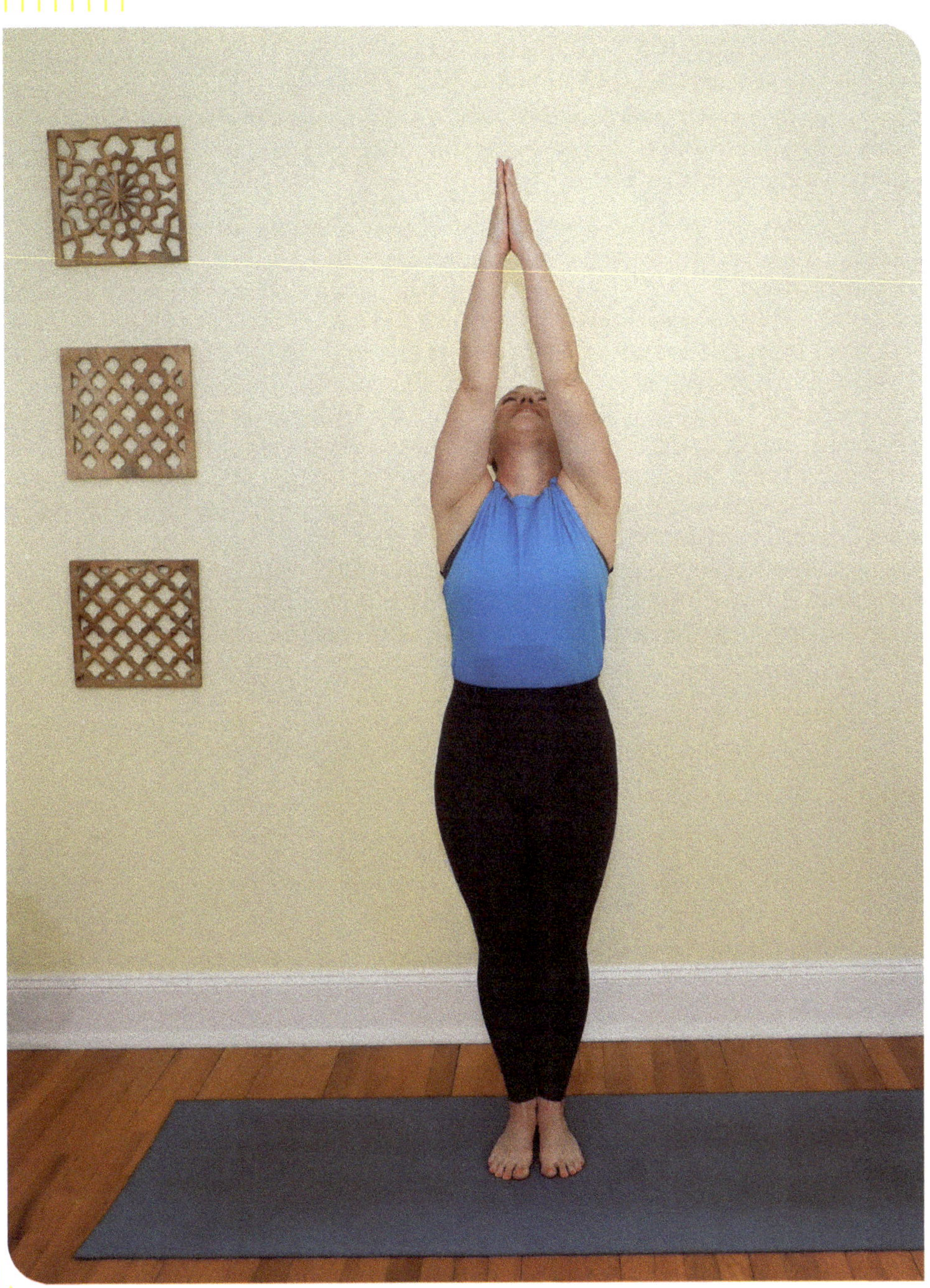

Extended Mountain Pose

High and Low Lunge Pose

ALSO CALLED: Anjaneyasana

WHAT THEY DO FOR YOUR SHOULDERS: These poses are a great for building shoulder and core strength because the leg position is relatively easy. That lets you concentrate on moving your arms from the shoulder blades on your back and building enough strength to start bringing your palms closer.

TUNE IT UP: Lowering your back knee helps steady your balance, so you can focus on keeping your elbows straight and breathing deeply.

In either low or high lunge, start with your hands in front of your chest and your arms together or apart and facing each other. Only raise your arms until your elbows start to bend; lower them a bit and get your elbows straight. Stay there and breathe.

If your palms are apart, as you build more strength try bringing them together with straight elbows. If your palms are close to each other, try crossing one thumb over the other to help hold the heels of your hands together. Eventually, you'll be able to uncross them and press flat palms together.

Expect it to take several months to develop enough strength to raise your arms all the way up with your palms together and your elbows straight. No matter where your hands are, your elbows must be straight. Remember, anatomically speaking, it's a different ball game when you work with straight elbows as opposed to bent elbows. You're using different muscle groups when your elbows are bent than when your elbows are straight.

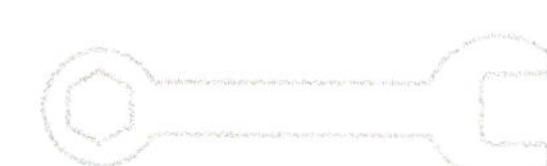

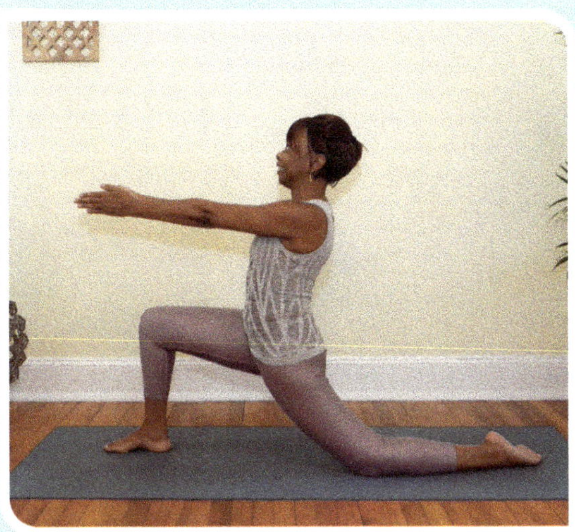

Low Lunge Pose, with arms forward

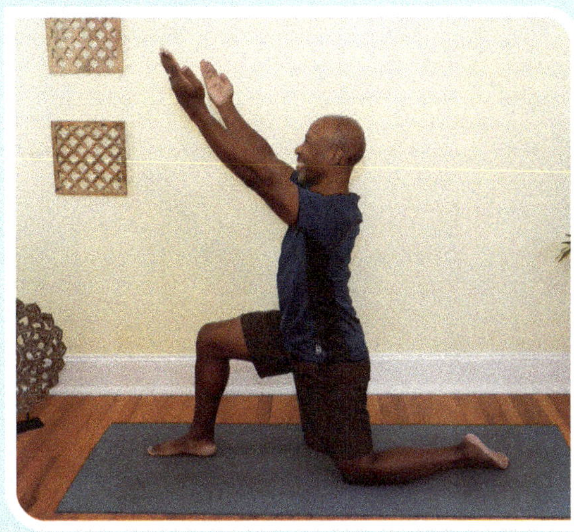

Low Lunge Pose, with hands apart

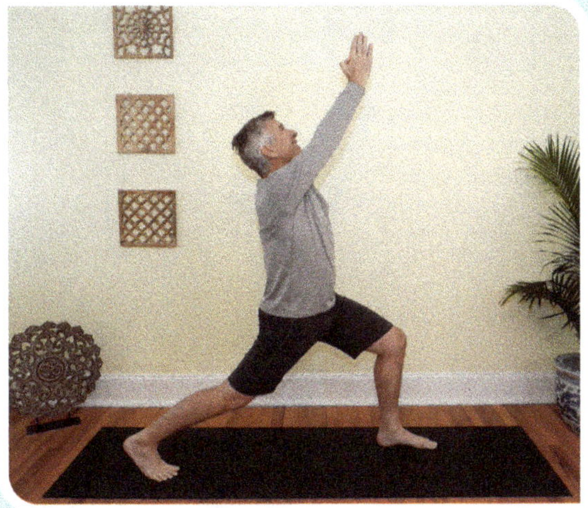

High Lunge Pose, with hands together thumbs crossed

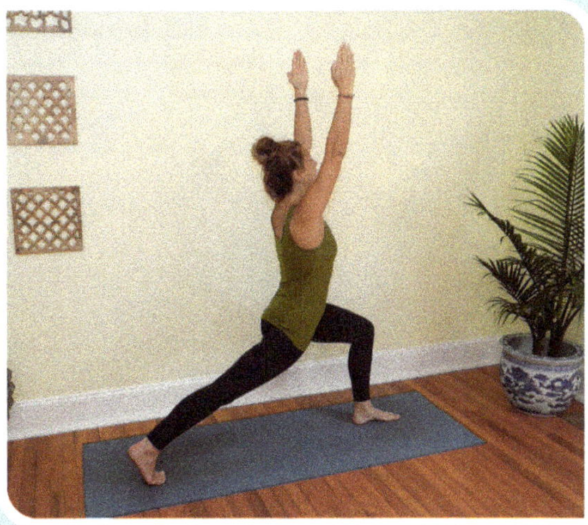

High Lunge Pose, with hands apart

Extended Triangle Pose

ALSO CALLED: Utthita Trikonasana

WHAT IT DOES FOR YOUR SHOULDERS: Holding your torso out over your front foot and drawing your shoulders back toward the wall behind you takes a lot of shoulder and upper back strength. Raising your top arm and pulling upward on your big toe with your lowered arm uses the muscles across your upper back and chest. This pose also builds a lot of core strength and hamstring length.

TUNE IT UP: Keep your back hand on your hip until it feels relatively easy to extend it upwards. Many people try to raise their arm before their legs, chest, and core are ready. Don't do that. It is not helpful. Focus first on building flexibility and strength in your core and legs to support correct alignment in your pelvis and spine. Moving your arm up is the *very last* thing you do in this pose. Don't get distracted from what's important by focusing on the wrong thing. Build a strong, flexible foundation first, and then work on the top arm position later.

To enter Triangle Pose, step your feet about 2 1/2 or 3 feet apart—about the length of one of your own legs from ankle to hip crease. Don't step your feet wider apart, doing so can injure your low back and hip joints. Keep your stance slightly narrower than you would for Warrior Two. This narrower stance ensures you can fully engage your leg muscles (especially your quads) to help lift the weight of your torso off of your low back and hip joints.

Make sure your back foot is turned at an angle so your heel points backward—more toward the short end of the mat behind you than to the long edge. This foot position turns your back hip inward, which is important as you lean out over your front leg for protecting your sacro-illiac (SI) joint (where your pelvis meets your sacrum at the base of your lumbar spine). Take a moment standing upright before you bend forward, to notice how the internal rotation of your back leg creates a nice stretch for that hip flexor.

Next, extended your arms out at shoulder height, and reach your front hand forward and down and bring your back hand to your hip. If your hamstrings are tight or your core

Extended Triangle Pose, variation with block and hand on hip

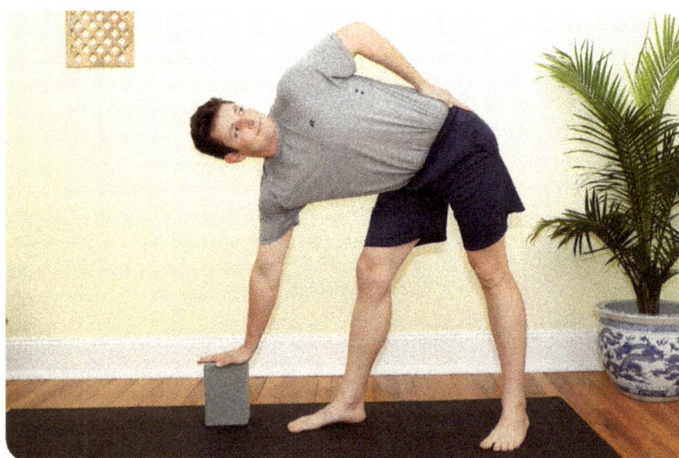

is weak (or both), don't put your front hand too low to the ground—rest it against your thigh or shin, or put it on a block.

A lot of people enter Triangle Pose with a big, dramatic, swoopy motion in their hips and chest. Please don't do that, because it flings your hips and legs out of alignment. Simply lean forward and bring your front hand to what it can reach—your thigh, your shin, a block, the front of your ankle, or your big toe.

Pause to take stock of your alignment, and fix it if needed. Your front sitting bone should be drawing in behind your front heel. If it's poking out behind, and you can't swing it in behind your heel, that means your bottom hand is too low. Lift up away from the floor until it comes behind your front heel. If your chest is turned toward the floor, your bottom hand is too low. Come up a little until your chest and shoulders turn to face the long edge of your mat.

There's a common tendency to shift your hips backward, over your back foot, when leaning forward into Triangle Pose. This brings too much weight into the back of your front knee joint. Make sure your pelvis is centered between your feet. If your front knee feels stressed, your hips are too far back. Don't bend your front knee to fix this discomfort. Instead, press down and backward with your back foot to shift your pelvis forward into the middle of your stance. If you can't shift your pelvis into central alignment, either your stance is too wide or your bottom hand is too low (or both). Narrow your stance and enter the pose again, keeping your bottom hand a bit higher off the floor.

When your hips are centered between your feet and your chest is turned toward the long edge of your mat, you can extend your top arm off your hip and look up toward your raised hand. Turning your head to look up is a balance challenge, so shift your eyes slowly.

Many people let the extended arm fall slightly behind their top shoulder or toward their back hip. Don't do that. Keep your extended arm directly above your shoulder, or slightly forward over your front ankle. You may be surprised that moving your top hand forward by only an inch creates much more work in your waist muscles (your obliques). Breathe.

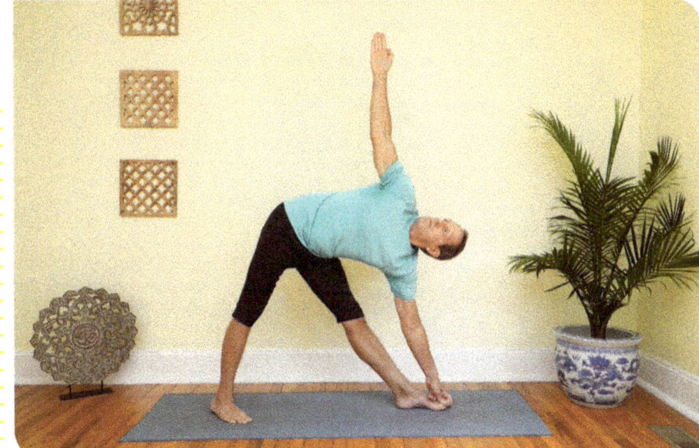

Extended Triangle Pose

Chair Pose

ALSO CALLED: Utkatasana, Fierce Pose

WHAT IT DOES FOR YOUR SHOULDERS: Even though it gets a lot of press for strengthening the quads, this is another good shoulder- and core-strengthening pose. Raising your arms forward or up, while sitting your hips low, asks the muscles in all sides of your shoulders and core to do a lot of work.

TUNE IT UP: As always, straight elbows are the key, regardless of whether you hold your arms out in front of your chest, or overhead. Work on gradually bringing your palms together while keeping your elbows straight.

To develop strength in your lower legs, press your knees together while pulling your ankles apart.

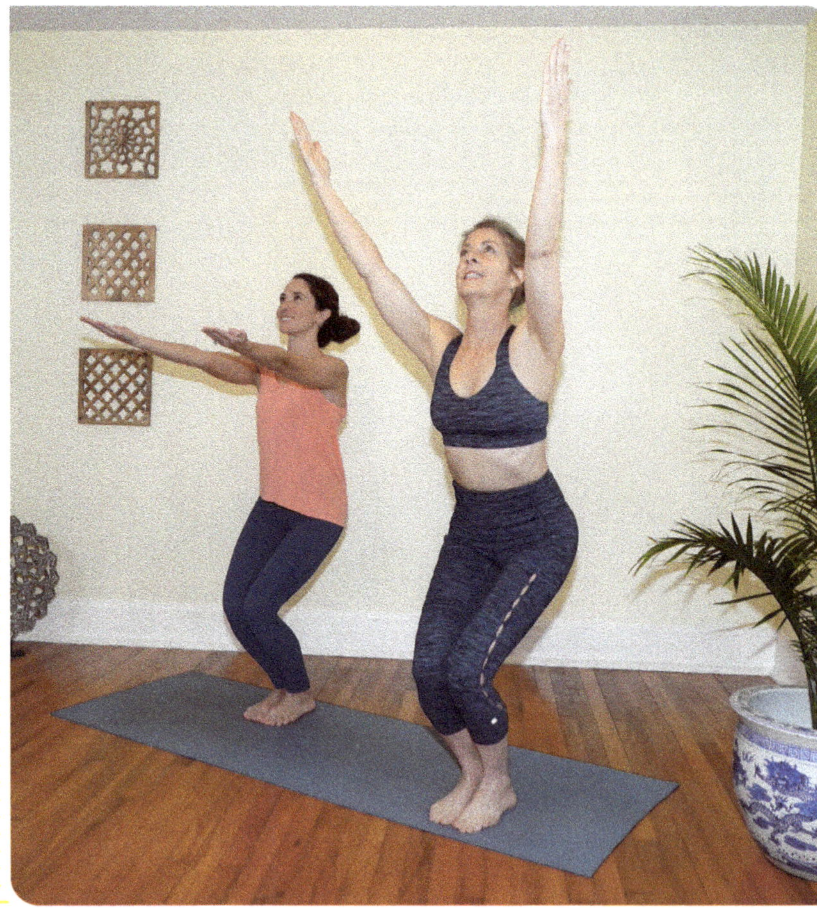

Chair Pose

Downward Facing Dog Pose

ALSO CALLED: Adho Mukha Svanasana

WHAT IT DOES FOR YOUR SHOULDERS: This is a foundational yoga pose that builds a lot of shoulder strength through the action of pressing your hips back, while extending your chest and ribs forward.

TUNE IT UP: Your hands should be placed slightly wider than your shoulders, so you can engage the muscles of your upper- and mid-back. Don't put your hands too close together in Downward Dog Pose. When your hands are directly in front of your shoulders, your trapezius muscles on the back of your neck are too active, and prevent rotating your upper arms fully outward (external rotation).

To experience how that works, try this: Get into Downward Dog Pose and move your hands wider apart than usual—maybe even put your pinky fingers off the outside edges of your mat. Then shift your shoulders forward by just an inch or two so you can wrap the back-edges of your armpits down toward the floor. This feels like drawing the outer shoulder muscles out and down. Hold this action in the shoulders and press your hips back into Dog Pose. With your hands wide apart, it's easier to find an outward rotation in your upper arms using your shoulder muscles (your posterior deltoids) and release tension in the back of your neck (your trapezius).

While in Downward Dog, imagine that you are reaching your rib cage slightly forward toward your thumbs, while pressing your legs firmly backward. These two opposing actions (chest and ribs going forward, while legs and hips press back) will activate your core abdominal muscles. Take slow deep breaths. Steady your eyes on one point behind you or up toward your thighs, and notice when they shift to look at something else. Bring them back to a single, soft focal point.

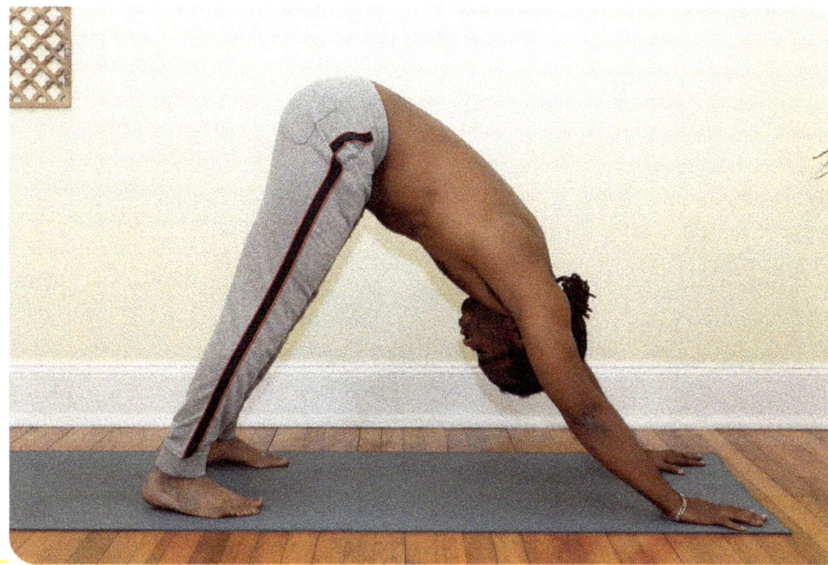

Downward Facing Dog Pose

Four-Limbed Staff Pose

ALSO CALLED: Chaturanga Dandasana, Plank Pose

WHAT IT DOES FOR YOUR SHOULDERS: This pose builds tremendous shoulder and core strength, because you have to stabilize your entire shoulder girdle in central alignment by pitting one muscle group against another. Muscles in your chest, outer shoulders, and upper back have to balance out their efforts to keep your weight evenly distributed. It's really hard to resist sagging down into the shoulder joints or rounding up into your mid-back. Your collarbones should be a straight line between the tops of your upper arm bones.

TUNE IT UP: This one's another basic yoga pose that's surprisingly difficult. Fortunately, there's a Plank Pose variation for everyone, no matter your strength level.

When first learning this pose, start with both knees, or just one knee, on the floor. Focus on keeping your elbows and any lifted knees straight. Keep your leg and core abdominal muscles very firm.

Once you're strong enough to lift both knees off the floor, you can try raising one foot a few inches to increase the challenge for your shoulder and abdominal muscles.

Next, try lowering your body a few inches by bending your elbows straight back toward the back of your mat. Be careful. Many people mistakenly lower too far in this pose. When you first start lowering, only bend your elbows one or two inches. Bending your elbows too far will risk injuring your shoulders, elbows, and wrists. Many people lower themselves too far because they're not strong enough to stop when they're only a few inches down. It's much harder, but also much safer for your joints to just lower a little bit. In this pose, less is more. Take time to build your strength, don't waste the time you spend on your mat. Work hard until the end of practice—then rest hard.

I strongly suggest using two medium-height blocks to support some of your body weight while you explore the muscles you need to lower safely (see photo). Put one block under your lower ribs and another under your upper thighs. Get the blocks in the right spots, and then press into Downward Facing Dog Pose. Inhale and move forward into Plank Pose over your blocks. Exhale and bend your elbows to lower your body onto the blocks. Pause to explore. Pull your elbows in against your ribs, and keep your toes tucked under. Firm up your leg muscles. Then press back into Downward Dog Pose.

Eventually, you'll be strong enough to lower yourself without the blocks until your elbows touch your sides (your rib cage). Never lower further than that; keep your elbows alongside your ribs. Some people mistakenly think they should touch their nose to the floor. This is incorrect and dangerous. You can damage your shoulder and elbow joints by lowering too far. Your elbows should never rise higher than your sides.

Your leg muscles (quads) and abs should be kept very firm to help protect your low back in this pose. If your low back sags down like in Cow Pose, put one or both knees on the floor, and work on building more core strength. There is also a tendency to stick your chin forward in Plank Pose. Keep it tucked very slightly toward your throat. The back of your neck should be elongated, not crimped.

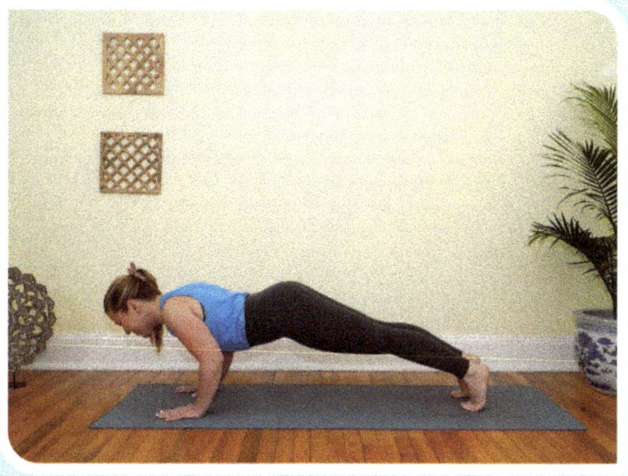

Four-Limbed Staff Pose with bent elbows

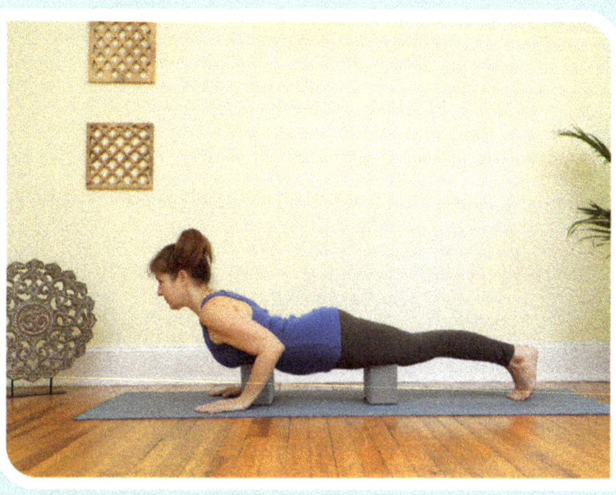

Four-Limbed Staff Pose, variation with blocks

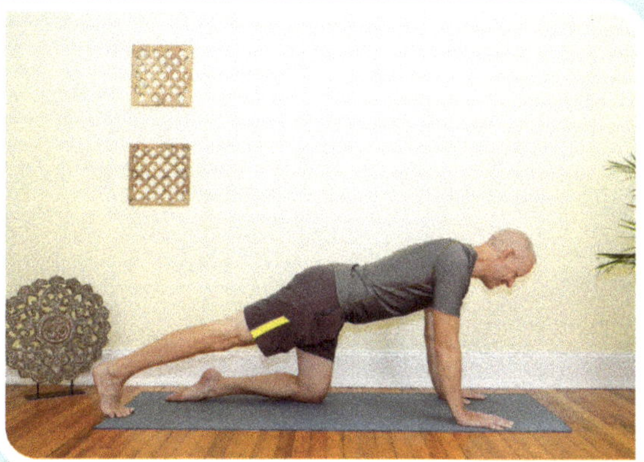

Variation with one knee down

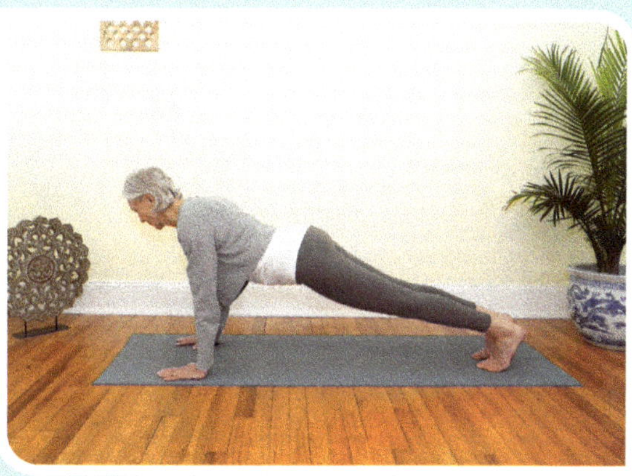

Four-Limbed Staff Pose with straight elbows

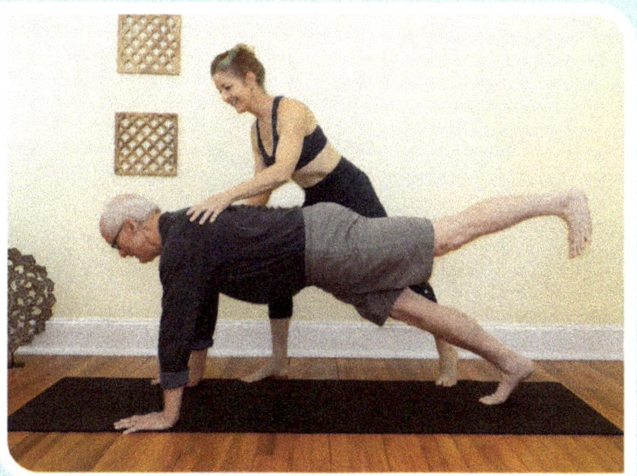

Variation with one foot lifted

Side Plank Pose

ALSO CALLED: Vasisthasana

WHAT IT DOES FOR YOUR SHOULDERS: This pose builds a lot of shoulder and core strength because those muscle groups must both stabilize your torso and lift it up off the floor. Your lower shoulder must press firmly down, while your upper shoulder, chest, and abdominal muscles lift the weight of your raised hips and arm.

TUNE IT UP: Lowering one knee to the floor will reduce the weight you have to lift. Traditionally this pose is done on the palm of the lower hand, but if your wrists are irritated or balancing is difficult, you can do this pose on your forearm instead of your palm.

There's a natural tendency when you first start doing this pose to wrap your top foot over the bottom one (see photo). Try not to do that—although it will be hard to avoid for a while. Eventually your feet will be stacked side-by-side and flexed, as if you're standing on the floor.

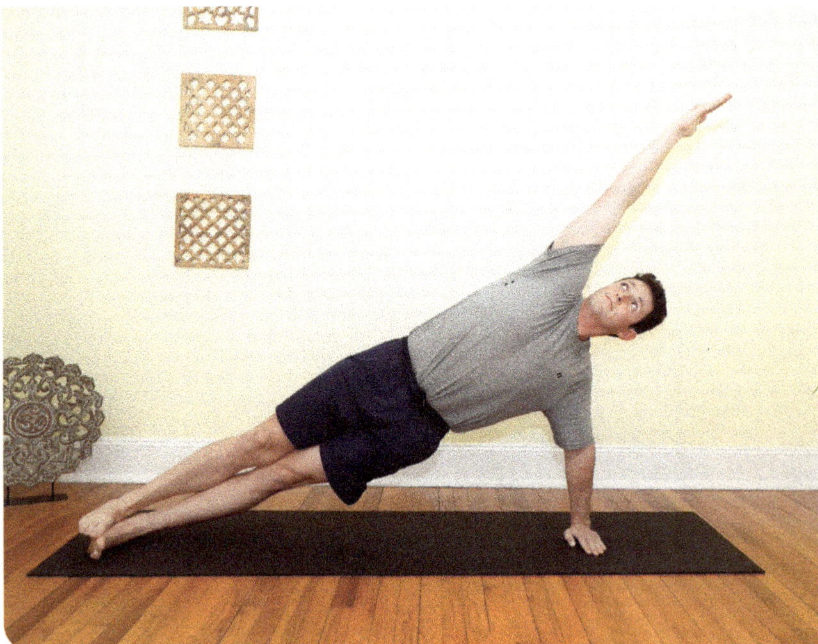

Side Plank Pose

Upward Facing Dog Pose

ALSO CALLED: Urdhva Mukha Svanasana

WHAT IT DOES FOR YOUR SHOULDERS: Like all back bends, this is another great way to strengthen your shoulders. In Upward Dog, you have to support the weight of your body while simultaneously drawing your shoulder blades back and together on your upper back.

TUNE IT UP: Push firmly down with your hands and lift up through your chest to prevent too much weight from dropping down into your low back joints. It's helpful to put a medium-height block under your thighs to support some of your body weight until your shoulders and arms are strong enough to lift your torso. When using a block, keep your toes tucked under and firm up your leg muscles (your quads, glutes, and hamstrings).

The muscular action is to pull your shoulder blades together on your back, which presses the center of your chest forward. Imagine you are pulling your chest through your upper arms. Tilt your face slightly up, but don't crimp the back of your neck, or throw the weight of your head back onto your neck joints. Look further up with your eyes than with your face by moving your eyeballs in their sockets.

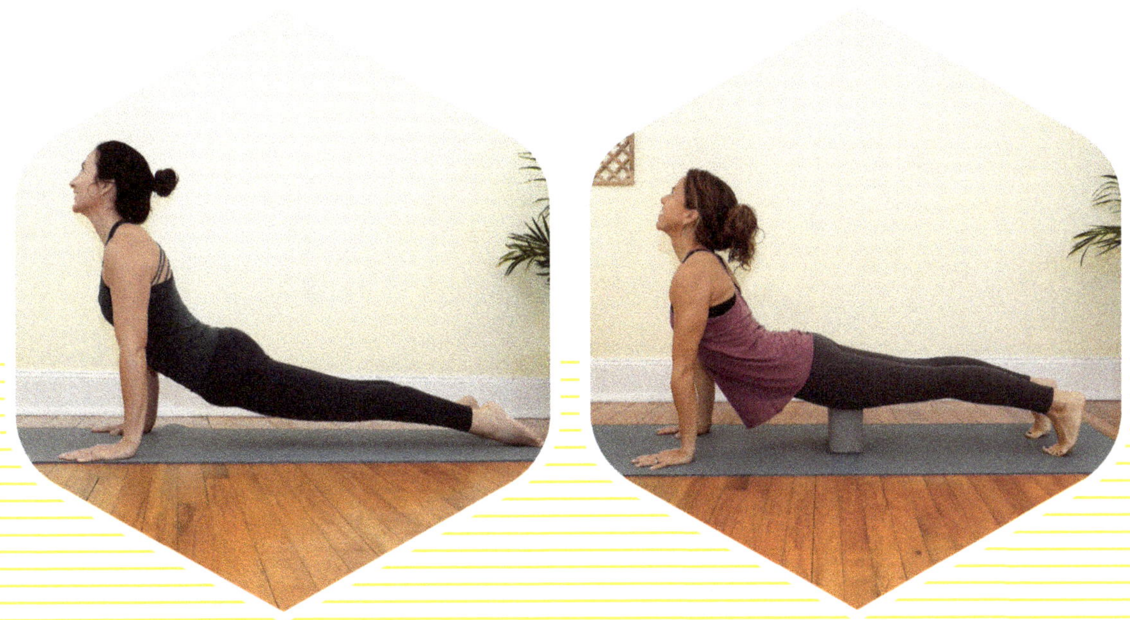

Upward Facing Dog Pose

Upward Facing Dog Pose, variation with block

Bridge Pose

ALSO CALLED: Setu Badhasana

WHAT IT DOES FOR YOUR SHOULDERS: A very good pose for building shoulder strength while creating flexibility in your abs, hip flexors (psoas major and minor), and thighs (quads).

TUNE IT UP: Try approaching this pose by first lying on your back with your knees bent and a block in each hand. Lift your hips and slide the blocks under the back of your pelvis at your sacrum. Adjust the height to provide a stretch to your hip flexors but don't force yourself into a deeper backbend than your body is ready for today. Put your feet hips-distance apart (or slightly wider), and a bit forward of your knees.

Take a moment to lift your hips an inch or two, and lengthen your low back by tilting your sitting bones toward your heels. Then, lower your hips back to the floor or blocks. Feel how your chest is popped up but your low back is long and flat underneath you. Hold the outside edges of your mat to help engage your shoulder muscles to lift your chest from the back and press your feet down and forward. Notice what is easy or difficult about being in this position.

Take time in Bridge Pose to explore your strengths and weaknesses and to calm down your mental chit-chat. Work here to focus on building more stength across your chest, arms, and shoulders. Remain calm and positive. Don't let your thighs fall outward.

If you are using blocks, the higher you're able to set the blocks under your pelvis, the easier it will be to feel your shoulder and back muscles lifting your chest up and back toward the alignment of your shoulders. Breathe.

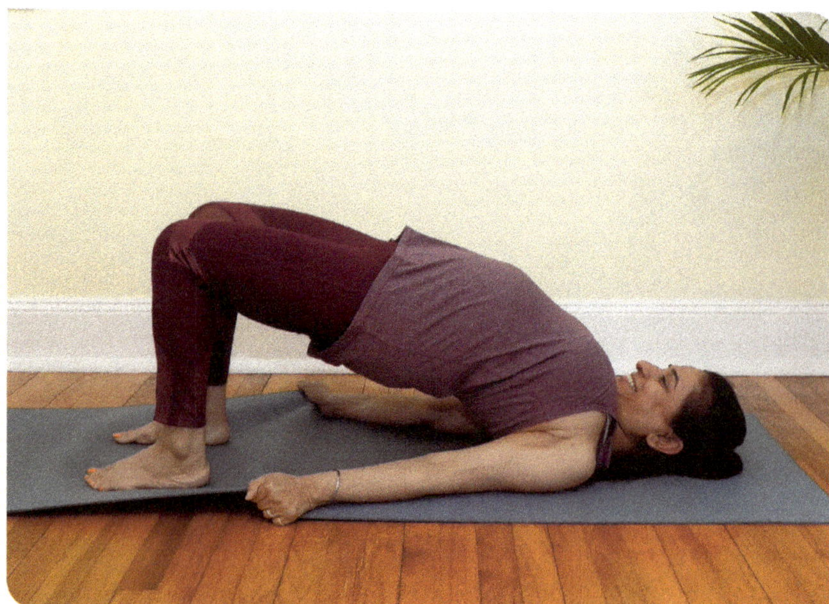

Bridge Pose, holding sides of mat

Locust Pose

ALSO CALLED: Salabhasana

WHAT THEY DO FOR YOUR SHOULDERS: This pose is a prone backward bend that builds more or less shoulder and core strength, based on the position of your arms and how much of your body you lift up.

TUNE IT UP: You can reach your arms forward, lifting one at a time along with the opposite leg. You can also lift both arms and both legs at the same time. You can keep your hands down while lifting only your head and chest and/or your legs. You can leave your forehead down on the floor or lift your head. Remember, it weighs eight to twelve pounds. If you lift your head, keep your nose pointed down—there's a common tendency to stick your chin forward. Don't create tension in your neck by looking forward. That's just your abdominal muscles trying to shift the work into your back. Make them work. Tuck your chin very slightly toward your throat.

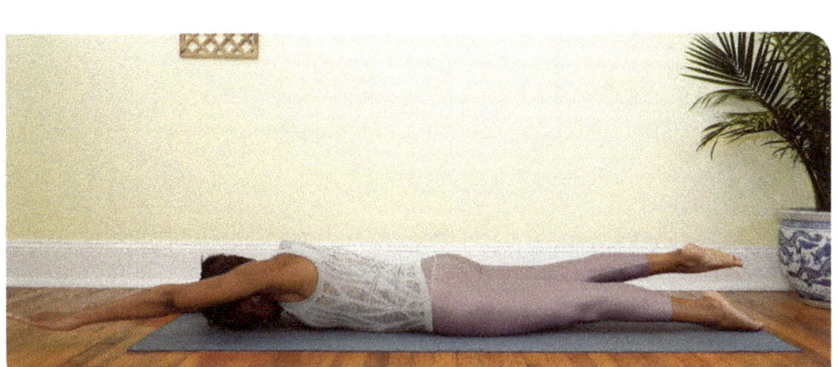

Locust Pose, variation with head down and one arm and leg lifted

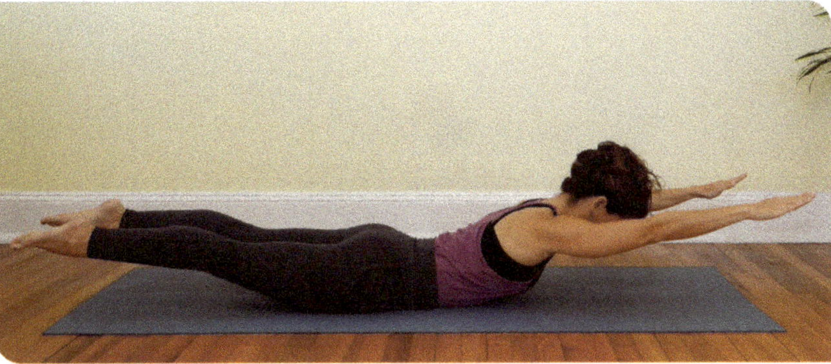

Locust Pose, variation with head raised and both arms and legs lifted

Half-Bound Lotus Intense West Stretch Pose

ALSO CALLED: Ardha Baddha Padma Paschimottanasana

Head of Knee Forward Fold, A

ALSO CALLED: Janu Sirsasana, A

WHAT THEY DO FOR YOUR SHOULDERS: Like all seated forward folds, these poses are a good way to build strength across the back of your shoulder girdle.

TUNE IT UP: When you fold forward in these poses, you must draw your shoulder blades strongly toward the center of your back. Many people misunderstand forward folds, and let their shoulders round down as they lean over. In fact, your shoulders must move up and away from the floor as you hinge forward. This is one of the most important actions to figure out in your yoga practice—how to pull your shoulder blades up when you're bending down. I promise, learning to lift your shoulders away from the floor in forward folding poses will change your yoga practice and save your low back from strain.

This muscular action not only generates great shoulder strength, it also turns on your abdominal muscles to support your low back. To protect your low back, learn to distribute the weight of your torso into the most muscle groups possible including your legs, feet, shoulders, sides, and waist muscles. For example, gently draw the bent knee forward in both of these poses; it won't visibly move much, but this action will activate muscles in your legs and low belly for support. It can take a while to figure out how to do some of these actions—so be patient.

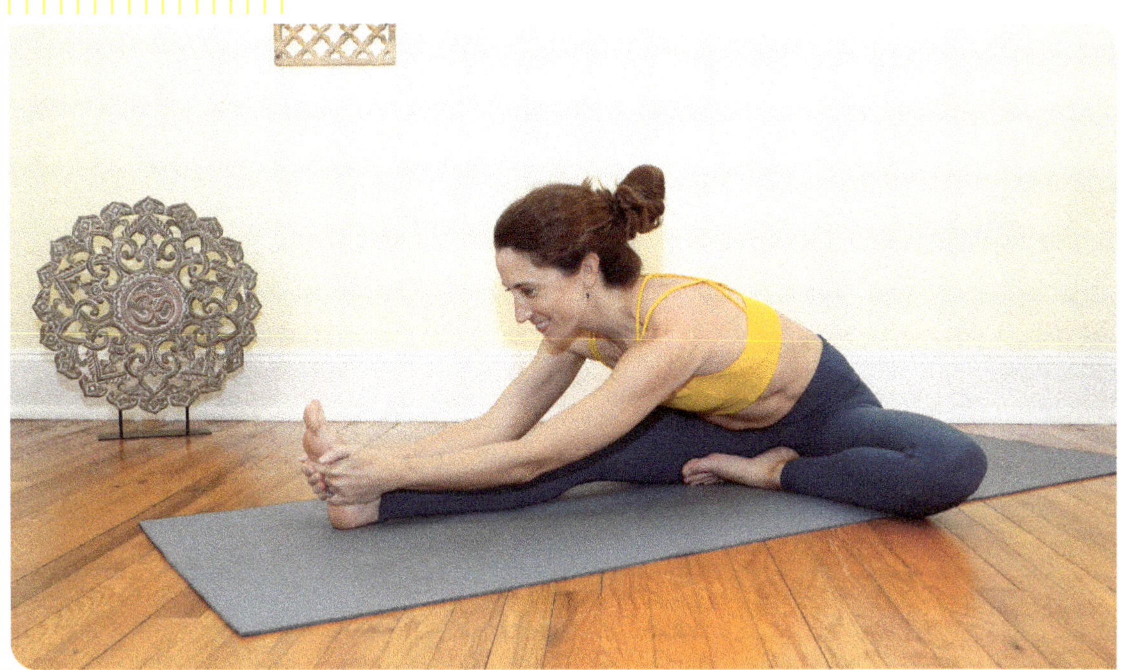

Head of Knee Pose, A

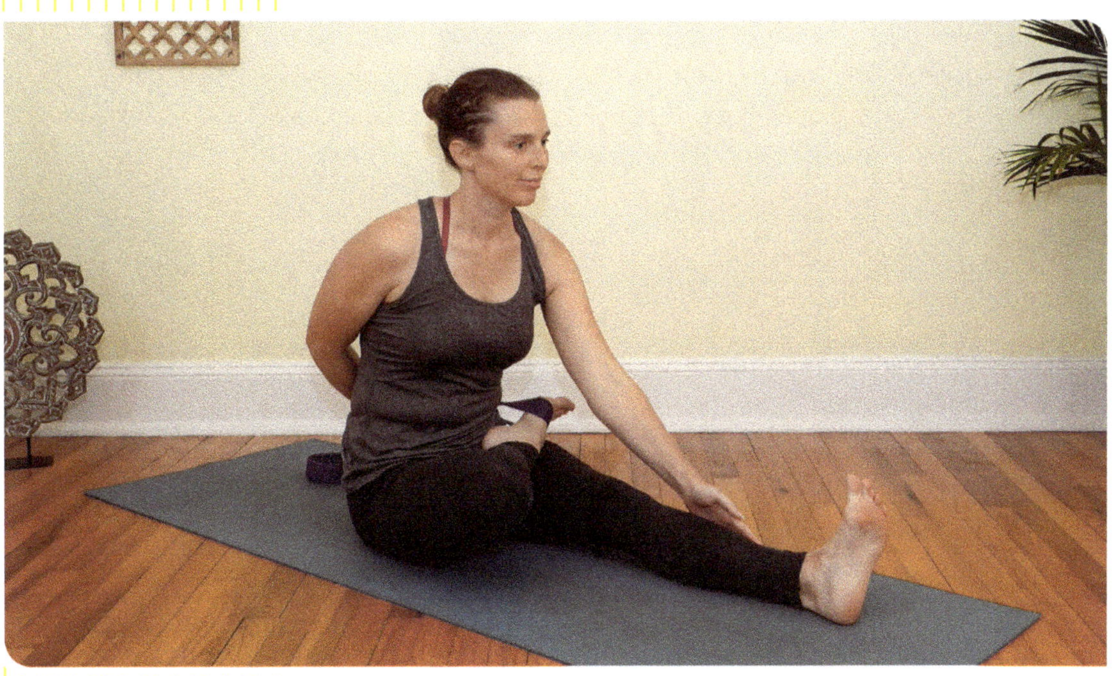

Half-Bound Lotus Intense West Stretch Pose, variation with strap

MECHANIC'S NOTE:
Move Your Shoulders to Lift Your Chest

When you draw your shoulder blades together on your back, your chest moves forward. By contrast, when you round your shoulders forward, your chest retreats backward. Try it: Sit comfortably and draw your spine up straight. Focus on your breast bone (your sternum) at the center of your chest, and then round your shoulders forward. Feel how your breast bone (your sternum) sinks back? Sit up straight again and draw your shoulder blades back toward your spine. Feel how your breast bone (your sternum) moves forward? That's what you want to do in all forward folds.

Be careful not to squeeze your shoulder blades back with too much intensity. This is a subtle motion that moves your shoulder blades back and down just one or two inches. Many people have a hard time figuring out how to move their shoulder blades without letting their shoulders lift up into their necks. This subtle action of shifting the shoulder blades happens on the back, not in the neck. It should not increase tension around your neck. Maybe practice while looking in a mirror to see what's going on. Don't worry, you can learn to change that "neck clenching" pattern and eventually move your shoulder blades by themselves. Little by little, you'll notice your upper back, shoulders, and abs getting stronger. It's really important to break the habit of rounding your back in forward folds. Don't be a downer.

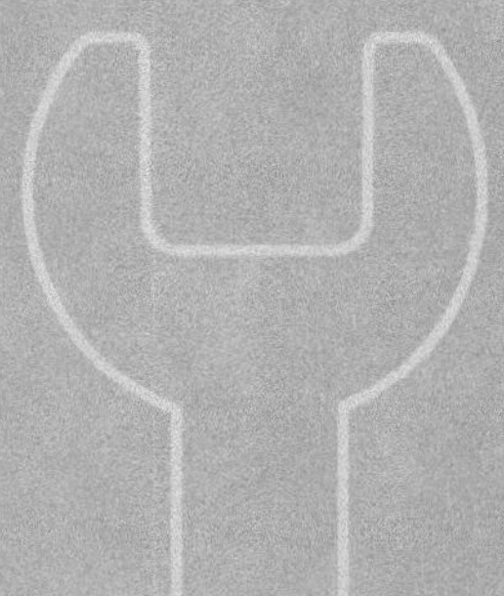

Both Big Toes Pose

ALSO CALLED: Ubhaya Padangusthasana

Wide Angle Seated Pose, B

ALSO CALLED: Upavistha Konasana, B

WHAT THEY DO FOR YOUR SHOULDERS: These are also good shoulder strengthening poses. Technically speaking, these are forward folding poses because they close the angle between your torso and your legs. So, they require the same chest-lifting action as seated forward folds, with an additional level of mental focus to balance on your backside. Although these poses do stretch your hamstrings and groins, I recommend doing other poses when that's your focus. I prefer to use these poses to focus on building shoulder, back, and core strength and developing mental clarity for balance.

TUNE IT UP: Although you can use a strap in Both Big Toes Pose to help reach your feet, I recommend simply bending your knees as needed to reach your big toes or the outside edges of your feet. In both poses, start with your heels on the floor and your knees bent. Hold your feet (big toes or outer edges) and rock back to lift your heels a few inches off the floor to balance just behind your sitting bones. Gaze upward (tilt your face a little, and look further up with your eyeballs).

Very slowly, straighten your knees, stopping when you can't straighten them anymore. Shift your focus to lifting your chest. Push your feet out and pull back with your shoulders on your back (not with your biceps). Keep your elbows as straight as possible.

In both poses, you have to figure out how much to push and how much to pull back. It's a subtle push-me-pull-you game. Lift your chest and rib cage up away from your hips. Breathe.

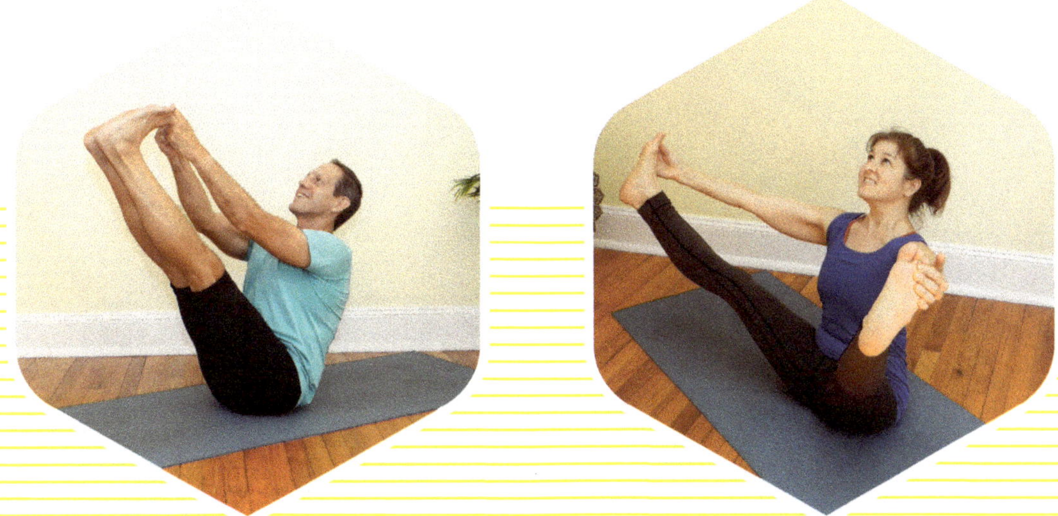

Both Big Toes Pose

Wide-Angle Seated Pose, B

Plow Pose

ALSO CALLED: Halasana

WHAT IT DOES FOR YOUR SHOULDERS: This pose builds shoulder strength, but also requires a lot of flexibility in your neck and upper back muscles. Your hands press firmly into your back while your shoulder blades draw together toward your spine. This is the next step after you're comfortable doing Bridge Pose. Be sure you're ready by taking the time to build up your shoulder strength and chest flexibility in Bridge Pose. Plow Pose is a more intense shoulder and chest stretch, and requires more strength because it stacks the weight of your legs and hips over your shoulders.

TUNE IT UP: Approach this pose with clear mental focus, and do not attempt Plow Pose unless your elbows can point to the front of your mat with your palms flat against your back. If your elbows point out to the sides, or only your fingertips touch your back, work in preparatory poses such as Bridge Pose (Setu Bandhasana), Camel Pose (Ustrasana), and Wide-Legged Forward Bend, B and C (Prasarita Padottanasana, B and C), to build the strength and flexibility you need to do Plow Pose safely and effectively.

When you are ready to start trying it, raise your shoulders on several (one to three) folded blankets to make the stretch on the back of your neck less intense. If your toes do not touch the floor, put them on the wall, a block, or a bolster. Don't let your legs float in the air. Your feet must have contact with something so you can use your leg muscles (your glutes, quads, and hamstrings) to help lift the weight of your hips up off of your neck.

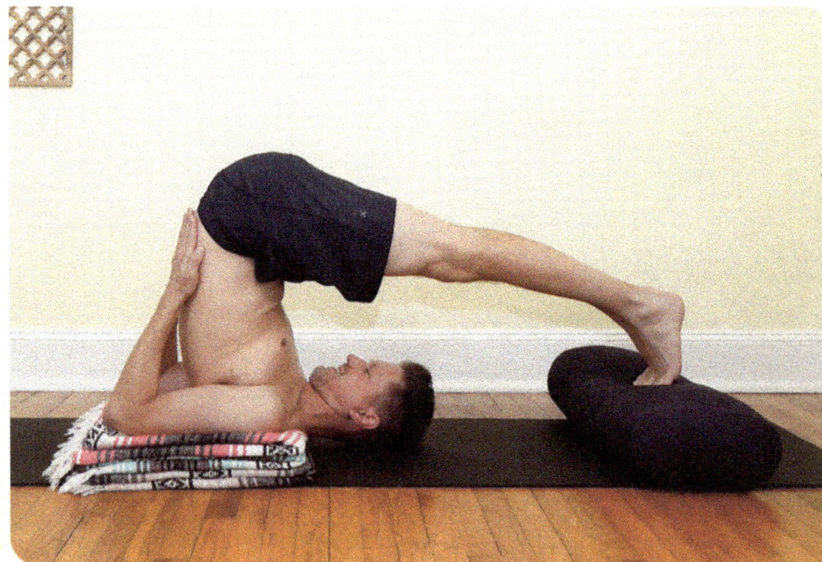

Plow Pose, variation with blankets and bolster

In all variations of Plow Pose, focus on squeezing your shoulder blades together and lifting your hips up by pressing the backs of your arms down. It's important to use your arm muscles, by pressing your palms firmly into your back to help shift your hips back and over your shoulders. Your arms should be working hard, not just resting on your back.

If you get tired, come out of it and do Bridge Pose, which strengthens and stretches many of the same muscle groups. Know how to get the benefits without overdoing it. Tomorrow is another day when you can try again.

When you develop enough strength and flexibility to keep your neck vertebrae off the floor (by squeezing your shoulder blades and lifting your hips), you can straighten your elbows and clasp your hands on the floor behind you. Again, your arms don't just lie on the floor. Press your arms firmly down.

In Plow Pose, try to maintain a gap between your neck vertebrae and the floor by pulling your shoulder blades close together, and using your leg strength to lift your hips upward.

Your neck vertebrae are quite small, so it's crucial to protect them in this pose by using your leg and shoulder strength. Do not release your arms unless you have a good gap between your neck vertebrae and the floor. This takes time. Be patient. Do not rush into this (or any) pose with incorrect alignment.

Many people mistakenly think that Plow Pose is just the entrance for Shoulder Stand Pose. This is incorrect. Until you can do Plow Pose safely and effectively, do not lift your legs into Shoulder Stand Pose. It makes no sense to move even more weight above your shoulders and neck, when you do not have the strength and flexibility to lift just some of that weight in Plow Pose.

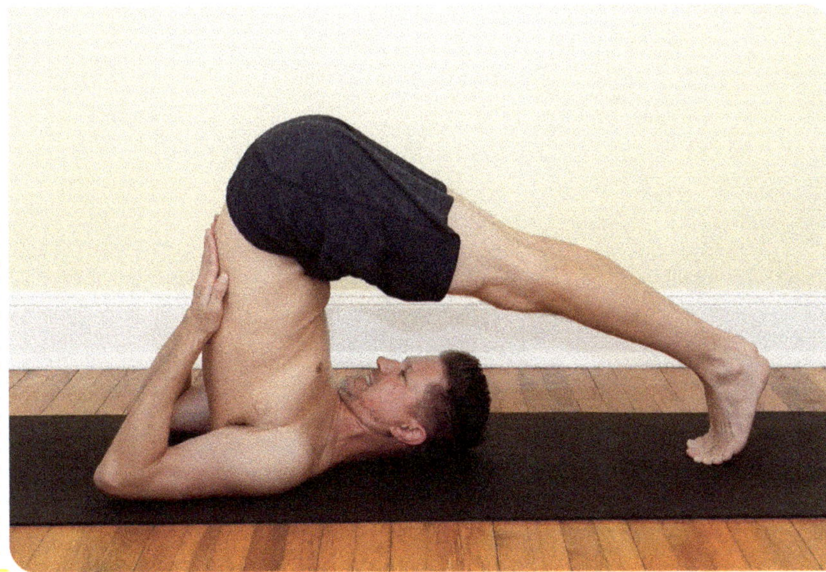

Plow Pose with hands supporting the back

If you're not yet able to use your leg and shoulder muscles to protect your neck, it simply makes no sense to continue stacking more and more weight above it. Don't let your ego injure your neck. Develop the strength and flexibility you'll need for Shoulder Stand Pose by first working on your alignment, flexibility, and strength in Plow Pose.

Your patience will be rewarded. You'll be amazed at how easy Shoulder Stand can be after you develop a strong practice in Plow Pose. Yoga is not a race. There's no finish line. Relax. Work on one pose at a time. Only move on to the next challenge when the initial pose is quite comfortable for you.

Once your feet can reach the floor with your toes tucked under, the final stage (krama) of Plow Pose is to un-tuck your toes and press your toenails down on the mat. This will come with time and practice. Be content to notice your body becoming stronger and more flexible in each stage. Your body is miraculous. Treat it kindly. Give it time.

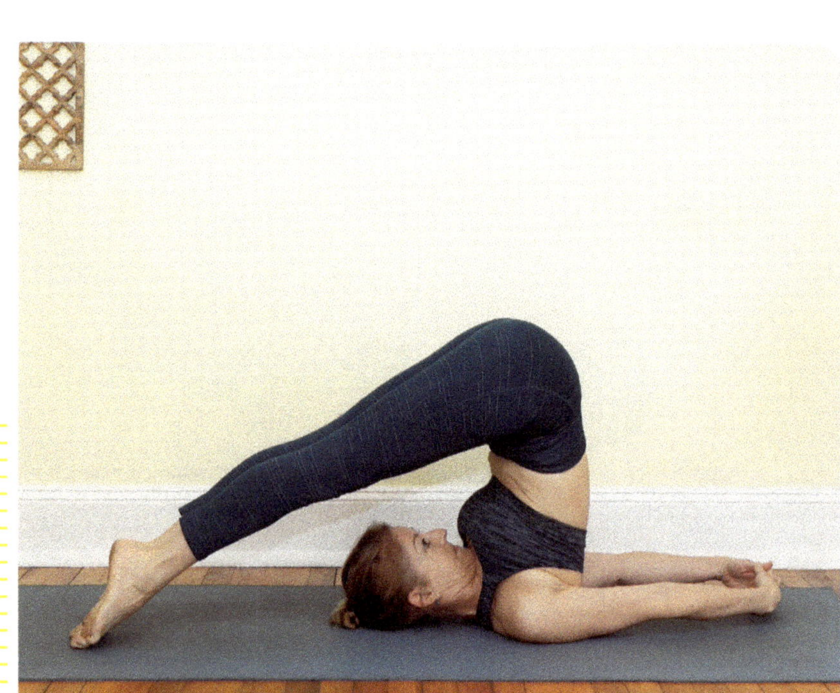

Plow Pose

Shoulder Stand Pose

ALSO CALLED: Salamba Sarvangasana

WHAT IT DOES FOR YOUR SHOULDERS: The very name, Shoulder Stand, lets you know that this pose takes a lot of strength, because you've got to stand on your shoulders. The pose also takes a lot of flexibility across your chest and upper back, because your shoulder blades have to move into the center of your back to keep weight off your neck vertebrae. So be sure you've taken the time to build up all the strength and flexibility this pose asks for before you go upside-down with no additional support, like from the wall or some blankets.

TUNE IT UP: This is another pose that should be approached slowly and in stages (kramas). You may spend several months, or even many years, building the strength and flexibility needed to do this pose safely and effectively. Work on it step by step. Notice your body changing and adapting. Do not let your ego injure your wonderful body.

Please understand that each stage working up to this pose has tremendous benefits of its own. You never have to do the full Shoulder Stand Pose to build a lot of strength and flexibility while you're working in the most appropriate karma for your body. Learning to breathe while you're upside down is, in itself, a big accomplishment. Inversions like this one, and all the stages leading up to it, strengthen the muscles of breathing and increase your lung capacity.

When you're just starting out, try Shoulder Stand near a wall. Sit very close to it and swing your legs up, as you roll down on your back. Bend your knees and put your feet flat on the wall. (Don't be up on your tip-toes.) Walk your feet up the wall a little bit, and press into it to lift your hips.

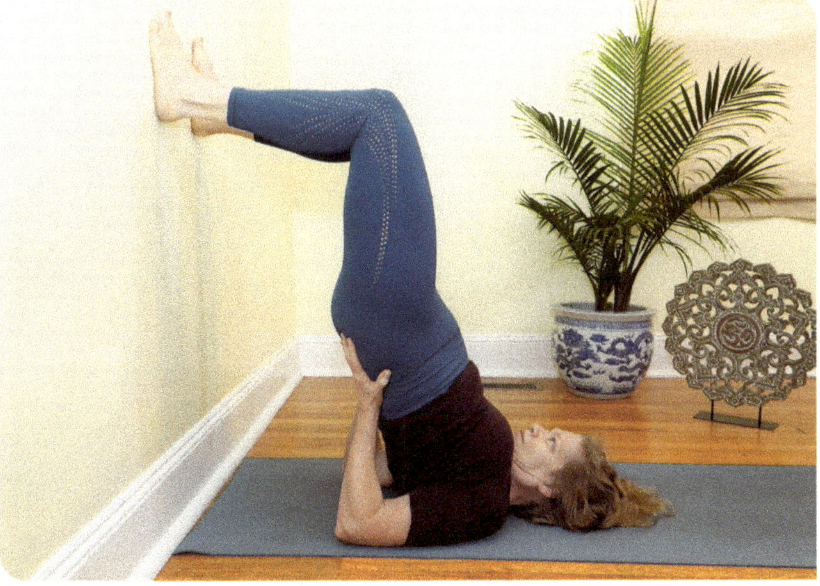

Shoulder Stand Pose, beginning variation with feet on wall

Now, with your hips lifted, bend your elbows and put your hands on your back. Keep using your legs to lift your hips toward your shoulders. Rock gently side-to-side to get your elbows further underneath you. As you build strength and flexibility, your elbows will point straight back at the wall, not out to the side.

Squeeze your shoulder blades together and try to create a small gap between the floor and your neck vertebrae. Breathe.

Try to equalize the effort into both feet evenly. There's a common tendency to press into the heels more than the forefeet, and into the outside edges (pinky-toes sides) more than the inner edges (big toe sides).

Do not sit your hips down onto your hands. Keep using your powerful leg muscles (your quads, hamstrings, and glutes) to press your hips back over your chest and shoulders. Most people work here—with both feet on the wall—for several months to build the shoulder and core strength, and the chest and shoulder flexibility, needed to lift their feet off the wall. Be patient. Rushing will not help, and you might injure yourself. Breathe.

Once your elbows can point at the wall (not out to the side), your hips are nearly over your chest and shoulders, and your neck vertebrae don't feel like they are being mashed into the floor, raise one foot toward the ceiling, keeping the other foot on the wall. Do not let the raised foot drop back past your face. The raised foot should not pass your hips. This is a difficult step.

Press with the foot that's still on the wall to keep lifting your hips. If you rush to do this step before you're ready, your hips will drop onto your hands and the lifted foot will fall back over your head. This is a sign that you may need to work with both feet on the wall for a little longer.

If you don't yet have the strength and flexibility to put more weight over your shoulders, don't kid yourself. It will only risk an injury.

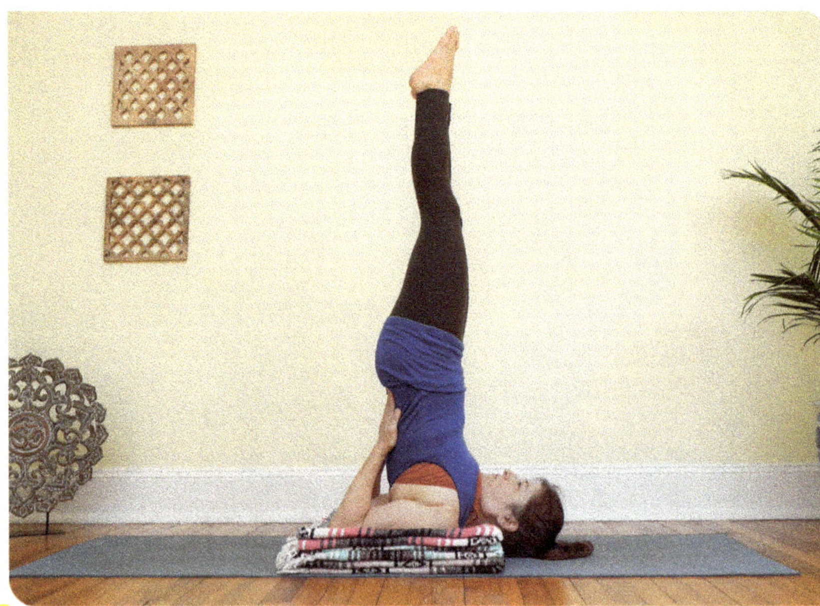

Variation with blankets

Mechanic's Note: Patience and self-honesty are two of the hardest and most valuable lessons in yoga. Be honest with yourself. Work step by step to develop a safe, effective practice. Don't skip steps. You're not a special exception to the laws of anatomy, gravity, and alignment. Set up correct alignment, and breathe while your body builds up the strength and flexibility you're asking of it.

If one foot is lifted, keep it directly above the hip. Notice that the lifted leg actually feels a little lighter when it's aligned correctly over the hip. Hold this position for a few breaths and then switch sides to lift the other foot off the wall.

When your hips are stacked almost directly above your chest and shoulders, and there's tiny gap under your neck keeping your neck vertebrae off the floor, you've developed enough strength and flexibility to safely lift both feet off the wall.

As in Plow Pose (Halasana), you can stack a few folded blankets under your shoulders to reduce the stretch in your neck muscles. However, beware, the balance can be a bit trickier when you're lifted on blankets. Move slowly.

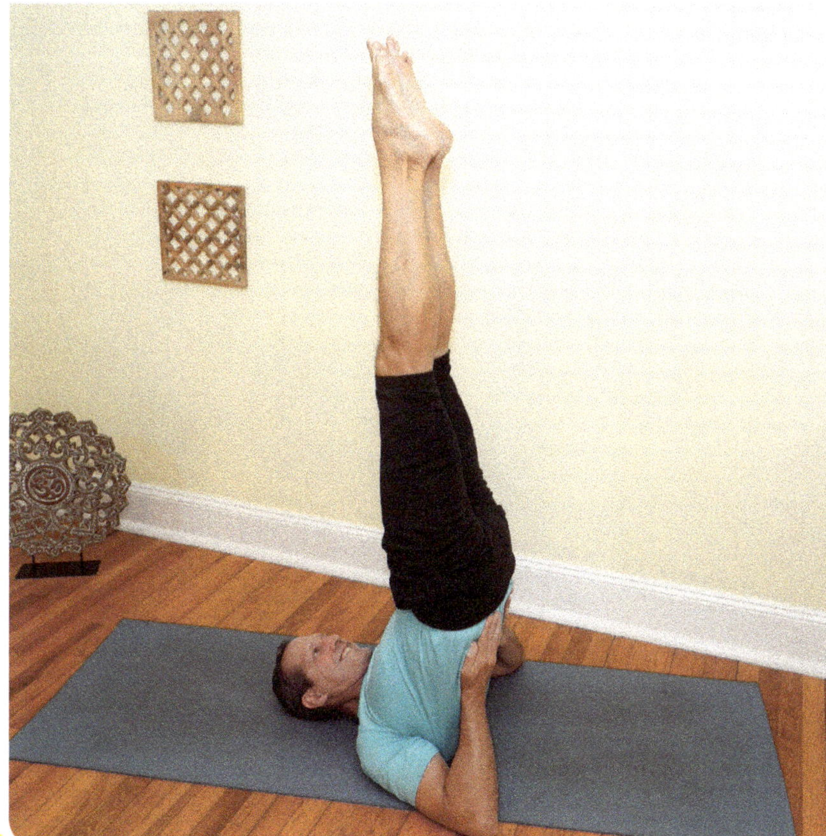

Shoulder Stand Pose

Head Stand Pose

ALSO CALLED: Sirsasana

WHAT IT DOES FOR YOUR SHOULDERS: This pose develops a great deal of shoulder and core strength, even if you work on the preparatory poses and never take your feet off the floor. Some folks are surprised to learn that Head Stand requires a lot of hamstring flexibility, because to enter the pose, your hips have to come over your shoulders while your feet are still on the floor. That's why so many folks end up trying to hop or kick up into headstand. They have not taken the time to build the hamstring length needed to walk their feet close enough so they can lift their legs calmly. Don't use momentum—it's dangerous to kick up. Use your strength and flexibility.

TUNE IT UP: Like Shoulder Stand Pose, many people rush into Head Stand without first taking time to build the strength and flexibility they need to do it safely and effectively. Remember, your neck vertebrae are very small, and not designed to bear the weight of your body. It helps to think of Head Stand as more of a forearm balance than a head balance. You must use your forearms, wrists, and the sides of your hands to distribute weight in this pose.

I like to break complex, long-time poses like Head Stand into multiple steps so you can see the progress you're making from week to week. Everyone starts with Steps One and Two (see photos).

Head Stand Pose, Steps One and Two

Step One: I recommend starting to explore the strength and flexibility needed in headstand by lying on your back with your hands interlaced behind your head (not behind your neck). Grip your fingertips to hold onto your head, point your elbows up (not out to the side), and press out through your heels. Draw your low back slightly down into the floor to turn on your core muscles. Imagine that you're in Head Stand Pose. Take several deep, slow breaths. This step is harder than it looks.

Step Two: Next, try doing all those actions while standing upright. Point your elbows forward (not outward), draw your low back gently toward the wall behind you, and make your leg muscles very firm. When standing, you can slide your hands an inch or two up the back of your head to help lift your forearms. Eventually, your forearms are level with the top of your head or higher. This requires a great deal of strength in your upper and outer back muscles (your lats). Remember, when you do this upside-down, most of the weight is on your forearms, wrists, and the sides of your hands. Your body weight does not rest on the top of your head in Head Stand, because your neck vertebrae are not designed to bear so much weight.

In both of these steps (kramas), you're practicing the muscular action and alignment of Head Stand Pose without putting any weight on your upper body. These preparatory steps help you build the strength and awareness needed to hold your body in correct alignment as you begin stacking more weight over your shoulders. If your elbows fall out to the sides when lying down or standing, or if you can't breathe smoothly—keep practicing these steps until it seems quite comfortable and easy.

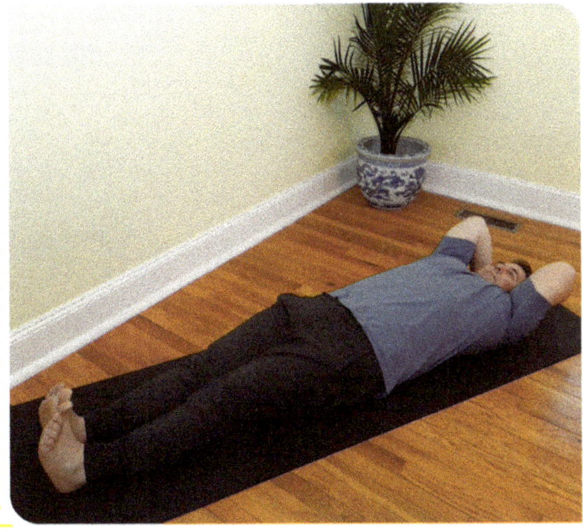

Head Stand Pose, step one

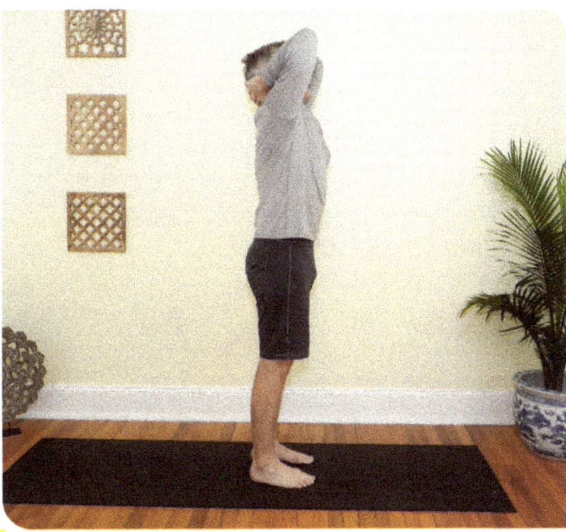

Head Stand Pose, step two

Head Stand Pose, Steps Three and Four

In the next stages of Head Stand Pose, you begin building more strength and flexibility by bringing a little more weight onto your arms.

Step Three: Start in Table Top Pose (Bharmanasana, or All Fours) and put your elbows on the floor. Now, grasp opposite elbows with your palms. Be sure to wrap your hands all the way around your elbows—don't simply touch your elbows with your fingertips. Your elbows should be directly in line with your shoulders.

To see what I mean, touch your elbows with your fingertips and notice that they're still wider than your shoulders. Now, wrap your hands further around your elbows. See? They're all lined up. Now, let go of your elbows, and pivot your forearms forward so you can join your hands by interlacing your fingers. Keep your elbows exactly where you set them down; don't move them. When you interlace your fingers, your thumbs should stick up to the ceiling.

Put the very top of your head on the floor inside your hands, and grip your head with your fingers. Don't let your hands be limp—use your fingers to grip your skull. This helps turn on the bicep muscles in your arms.

Tuck your toes and lift your hips into Downward Facing Dog Pose (Adho Mukha Svanasana). Firm your thigh muscles to make your knees completely straight. Breathe here, and get your bearings. You may be able to tip-toe your feet a few inches toward your face. Notice if your knees start to bend and stop there. This step (krama) is testing whether your hamstrings are flexible enough to get your hips stacked up over your shoulders.

Step four: If you have tight hamstrings, it can be helpful to put a block under your feet to help get your hips up over your shoulders.

Pause here. Focus on making a solid foundation with your forearms, wrists, and the sides of your hands. Grip your skull. Lift up onto your tip-toes and lower your heels a few times. Notice how your weight shifts forward and back when you do this.

Press down strongly with your forearms, and flatten your shoulder blades onto your upper back. Focus on lifting your hips and using your shoulder strength to take weight off of your head and neck. Work on this step until your hamstrings get long enough for you to line up your hips over your shoulders.

Do not rush into Head Stand Pose. It takes a long time to develop the strength and flexibility you need to do it safely and effectively. You'll be ready when you're ready. Never try to kick, hop, or jump up into a Head Stand. You'll injure yourself. Be patient. Prepare your body for the poses you want to do. Don't force your way through your yoga practice; learning to prepare patiently and thoroughly is a valuable life lesson. Listen to what each step tells you. Your yoga practice is full of good advice. Try taking some of it.

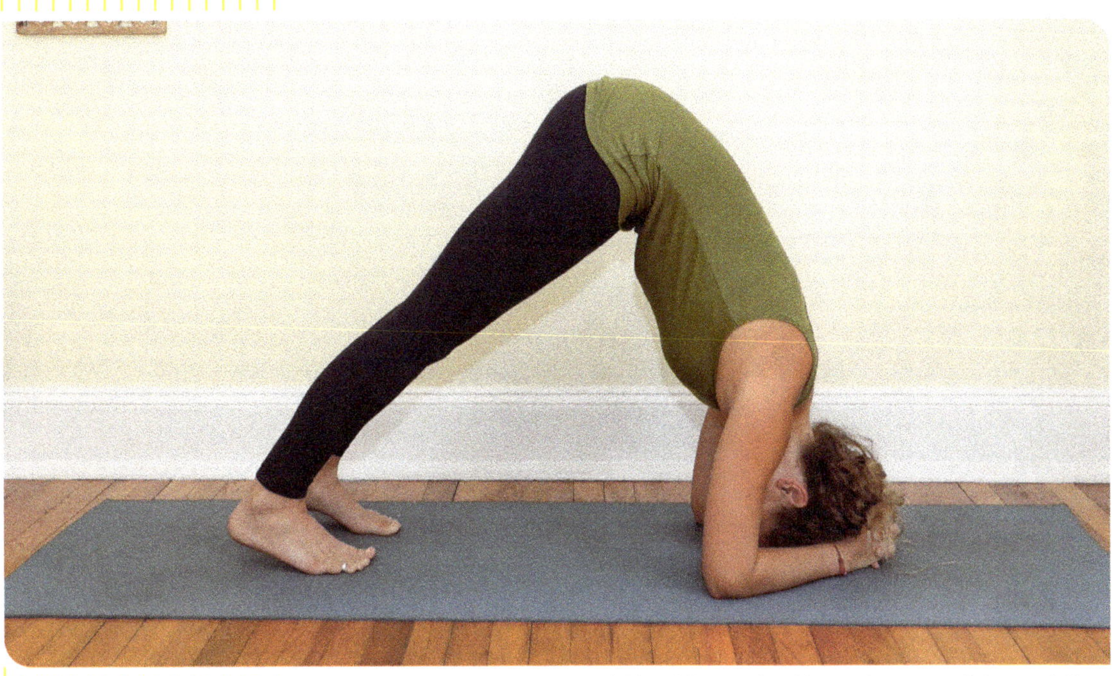

Head Stand Pose, step three, downward dog variation

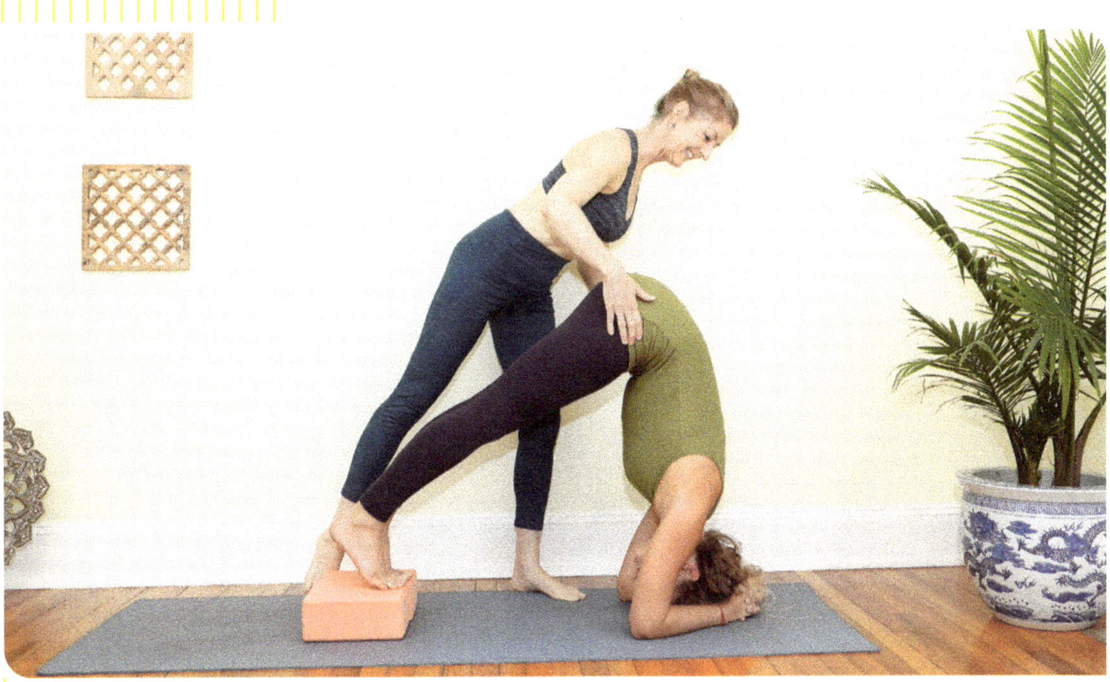

Step four, variation with block

Head Stand Pose, Step Five

The next steps (kramas) of Head Stand Pose (Sirsasana) use the wall to develop even more strength and steadiness. Remember, your hamstrings need to be long enough to shift your hips (your center of gravity) over your shoulders.

Step Five: Sit with your backside against the baseboard and your legs extended in front. Put something (a block, a strap, your water bottle) beside your heels to mark that place. Now, lean forward and get into Table Pose (on all fours) with your feet back toward the wall (where your butt just was).

Wrap your hands all the way around your elbows and place your elbows on your mat, *closer than your marker* object. Once your forearms are on the floor, release your hands and pivot on your elbows to interlace your fingers, so that your hands are now level with your marker (the block, strap, or water bottle). Do not move your elbows, and don't let them point far out to the side.

Put the top of your head down into your hands and grip your skull with your fingers. You'll feel like you're almost "too close" to the wall behind you or a little "crunched up". Don't worry. You're in the right spot, believe it or not.

Slowly straighten your legs so that your heels are on the baseboard, and your toes are on your mat, with your head still in your hands. If you can't completely straighten your knees, stop and go back to Step Three and Step Four. Your hamstrings need to become more flexible before you move on. Breathe here. Don't hurry. Work on lengthening your hamstrings and strengthening your shoulders and core in a prior step before trying this one again.

Many people with tight hamstrings mistakenly try to kick or hop up to get their hips up over their shoulders. Don't do that. You'll risk injuring your neck and you won't build the strength, flexibility, and mental focus to do this pose safely. Take your time and show respect for your body by preparing it. Don't put your entire body weight on top of your neck and shoulders until your muscles can handle those loads. It's silly to rush into this pose. Remember, your yoga practice should be therapeutic and healing—not stressful and damaging.

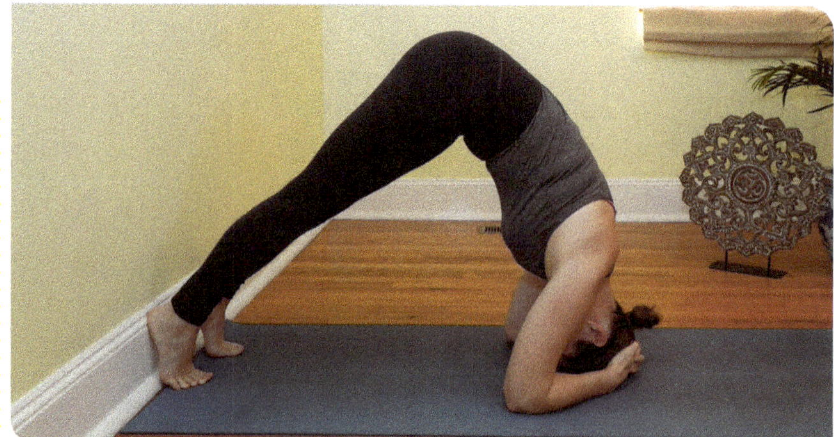

Head Stand Pose, step five with wall

Head Stand Pose, Step Six

When you can get your legs completely straight with your toes on the floor, you're ready to start lifting your legs in step six. Put one foot at a time on the wall at hip height. It's common for people to put their feet high up the wall above their hips; don't do that. Your feet should be exactly at hip height, so your body is in a 90-degree angle.

Many people get so excited and distracted when they first try going upside-down, that they forget they can see their feet. You're facing the wall. Look at your feet. Put your feet in line with your hips. Don't put your feet far up the wall into a sort of plank position. This is incorrect. Your legs should be at a 90-degree angle with your knees completely straight. If your knees are bent, come down and work in the previous step for a while longer.

This step adds even more weight over your neck and shoulders. Press down with your forearms and focus on flattening your shoulder blades onto your upper back. Use your shoulder strength to lift some weight off your head. If your shoulders feel very strong and your mind is calm, come up onto your tip-toes on the wall (see photo). This shifts your center of gravity (your hips) further over your shoulders. Breathe. Raise and lower your heels a few times, to get used to the feeling of your hips stacking up over your shoulders.

Spend several weeks or months practicing this step until you can breathe fully and deeply while using your shoulder strength to lift some weight off your head and neck. Focus on building mental focus and a calm attitude in Head Stand Pose.

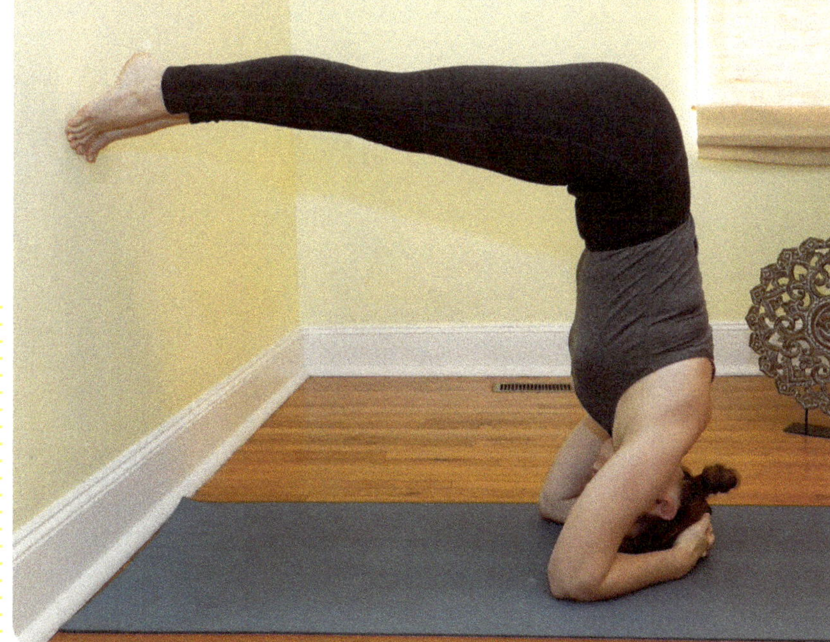

Head Stand Pose, step six, feet at hip height

Head Stand Pose, Step Seven

Once you feel very strong and steady in the previous steps, and you can breathe deeply and calmly with both feet on the wall, both feet on the wall, you're ready for step seven. Lift one leg. Only one. Don't lift both feet yet. Stretch the lifted toes to the ceiling and keep your lifted foot directly over your shoulders. There's a common tendency to let the lifted leg drift overhead, back toward the front of the mat behind you. This is incorrect. The lifted foot should stop moving when it is stacked directly over your hips.

There is also an unhelpful tendency for your thighs to move out, away from each other. Pull your inner thighs slightly toward each other—do not let your legs drift apart. This inward action of the thighs helps engage your core to steady your balance. Press down with your forearms.

The next movements in this krama build more strength and flexibility to prepare you to do Head Stand Pose without the wall. While at the wall with one leg lifted, flex the lifted foot and slowly draw it down, passing the wall and hovering it just off the mat in front of your face. Don't let your knees bend. Don't touch the floor with the moving foot. Then slowly draw that foot back overhead. Put it back on the wall and release the pose, stepping down and taking a rest in Child's Pose (Balasana). When you're focused and calm, repeat all of Step Seven with the other leg lifted. Practice this "leg-sweeping" stage of Head Stand for several months.

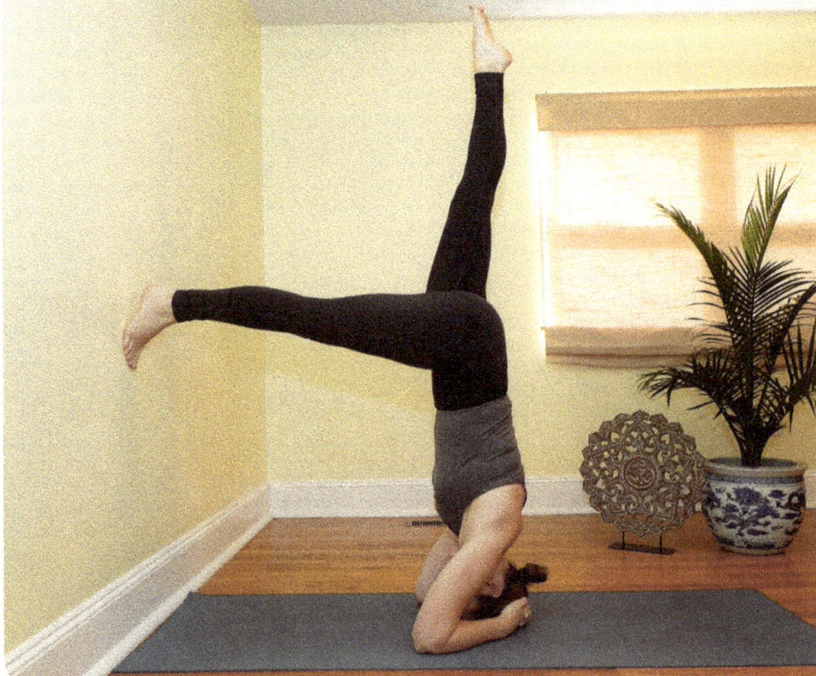

Head Stand Pose, step seven with one leg lifted

Head Stand Pose, Steps Eight and Nine

Practice the preparatory steps (kramas) of Head Stand Pose until you develop enough core and shoulder strength and hamstring flexibility to calmly and easily do all of these early stages. Your shoulders should feel very stable, your hips (your center of gravity) should stack easily over your shoulders, and your neck should not be bearing the majority of your body weight. Then—and only then—move away from the wall and try the pose without support. Remember, there's no kicking, jumping, or hopping into Head Stand Pose!

Step Eight: Set up your arms and hands as described in the prior stages. With your head in your hands in Table Pose (on all fours), wrap your palms around your elbows, pivot your forearms forward to interlace your fingers, and put the crown of your head inside your hands. Then, straighten your legs and lift your hips into Downward Facing Dog Pose. Slowly walk your feet toward your face to bring your hips over your shoulders.

Lift one foot to the ceiling and bend the other knee into your chest. Do not extend the second leg. Keep it bent into your torso in a sort of "stag leap" position (see photo). This ensures that if you drop out of the pose quickly, you'll come down the way you went up. Your body will not topple over your head toward the front of your mat, which is very dangerous for your neck and shoulders. Keeping one knee bent keeps more weight on the "entry and exit" side of the pose. Stay in this "stag leap" position and explore your breath. Is it steady, full, and calm?

Focus on pressing your forearms down and flattening your shoulder blades onto your upper back. Keep pulling your inner thighs toward each other so your core is activated. Do not let your legs drift apart. Practice for several weeks or months with your legs in this stag-leap position. Take slow, deep, calm breaths.

It's normal for lifting one leg or the other to be significantly easier. Don't worry about trying to do this step on both sides at first. Get comfortable and secure on one side, before you try the other. Also know that it's not a crime to always enter and exit Head Stand Pose with the same leg (i.e., on the same side). The yoga police will not write you a ticket. Don't worry. You'll have many years to work on the other side. Get comfortable on one side first. Breathe.

Step Nine: After many months, or years, doing this stag leap position, you can extend the bent knee to bring both feet together overhead. Keep pulling your thighs together, and press up through the balls of your feet. Calmly and quietly congratulate yourself. Good job!

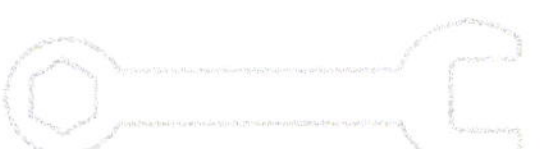

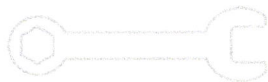

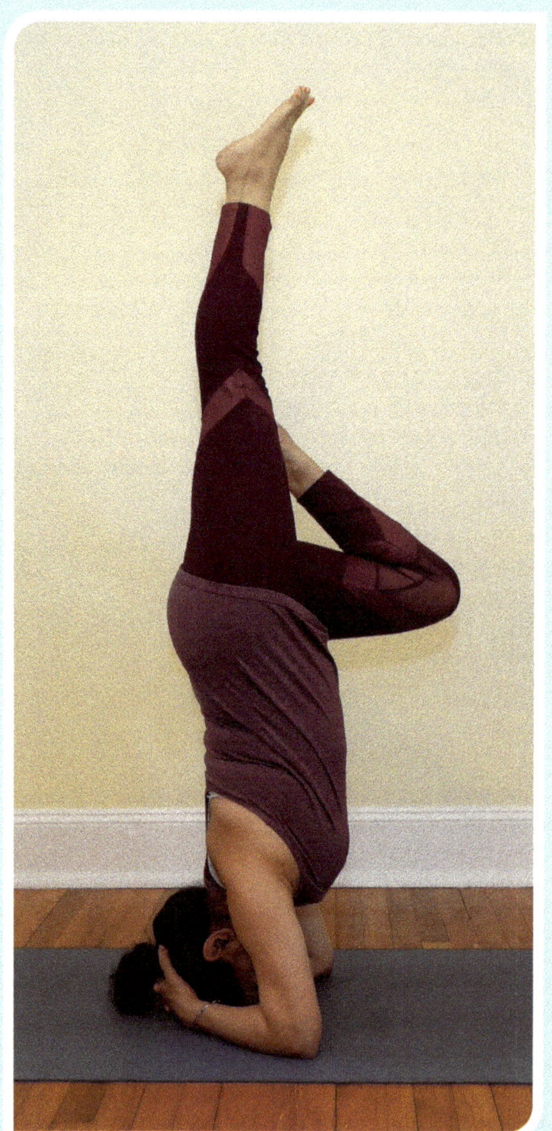

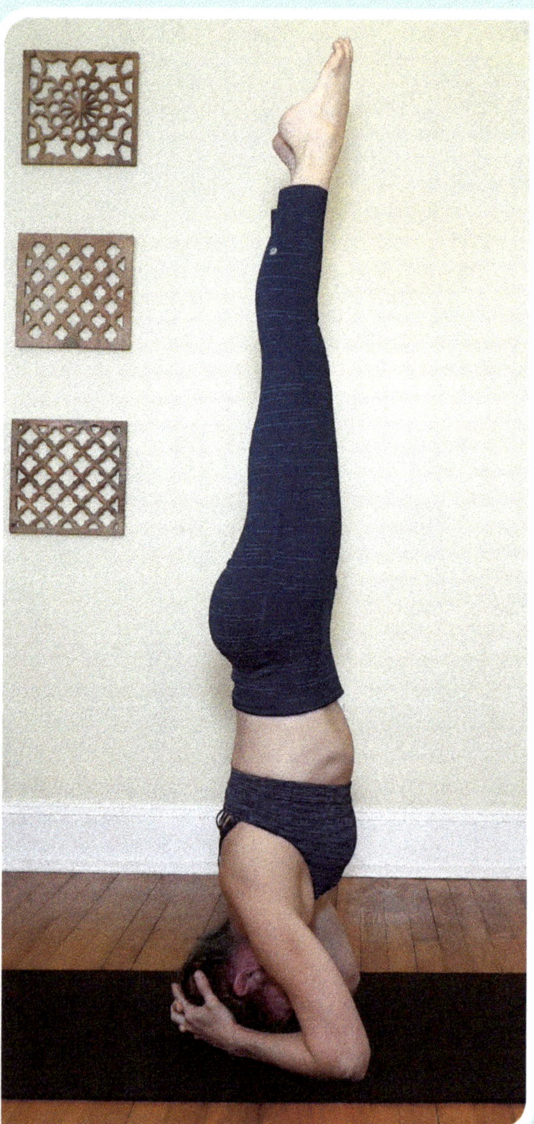

Head Stand Pose, steps eight (stag leap position) and nine

Hand Stand Pose

ALSO CALLED: Adho Mukha Vrksasana

WHAT IT DOES: Like Shoulder Stand, just the name Hand Stand tells you that this pose will require a lot of arm, back, core, and shoulder strength, because you'll be supporting your entire body weight on your hands. Again, it's important to work on each preparatory step, until each krama feels relatively comfortable and easy, so you'll avoid injury when you finally put your entire body weight up over your hands (or don't; Remember, the preparatory positions have many benefits). There are a lot of muscular actions to become familiar with, which will help you step calmy, safely, and effectively into Hand Stand. Take your time to learn them. Try not to fixate on kicking your feet up overhead. That moment may or may not come in the future. There are a lot of steps to practice before you get to that point. Stay present. Do what's right for your body today.

TUNE IT UP: The steps (kramas) for Hand Stand Pose are similar to those used to prepare for Head Stand.

Hand Stand Pose, Steps One and Two

Step One: Start by lying on your back and reaching your arms overhead to touch the floor behind your head. Move your hands apart until your elbows are completely straight, and your fingertips touch the floor when you flex your palms toward the wall behind you. Note, your arms may need to be in a very wide V-shape to get your elbows straight. That's fine. Don't work on this pose with bent elbows because you'll never build the strength you need in the back of your shoulders if your elbows are bent.

Flex your feet and firm up your leg muscles while pressing your low back down toward the mat. Look slightly up and back by moving your head a little, but moving your eyeballs in their sockets more. Don't crimp the back of your neck or hold your breath. Do not let your elbows bend. This is much harder than it looks.

Step Two: Once your breath is smooth and full in krama one, try it while standing up. Stand with your feet together and raise your arms overhead. Bring your hands apart until your elbows are completely straight. Do not allow any bend in your elbows; just keep moving your hands further and further apart until your elbows straighten. Flex your fingertips back and press your palms up toward the ceiling. Draw your low back slightly toward the wall behind you and make your leg muscles very firm. Look slightly up toward your hands (moving your eyes more than your face) and breathe.

There's a common tendency to hold your breath in this pose, because the muscles that move your arms are attached to your chest wall. With your arms overhead, it becomes more challenging to breathe deeply. You may be surprised at how hard this is to do. Stay calm. Observe your body and your thoughts.

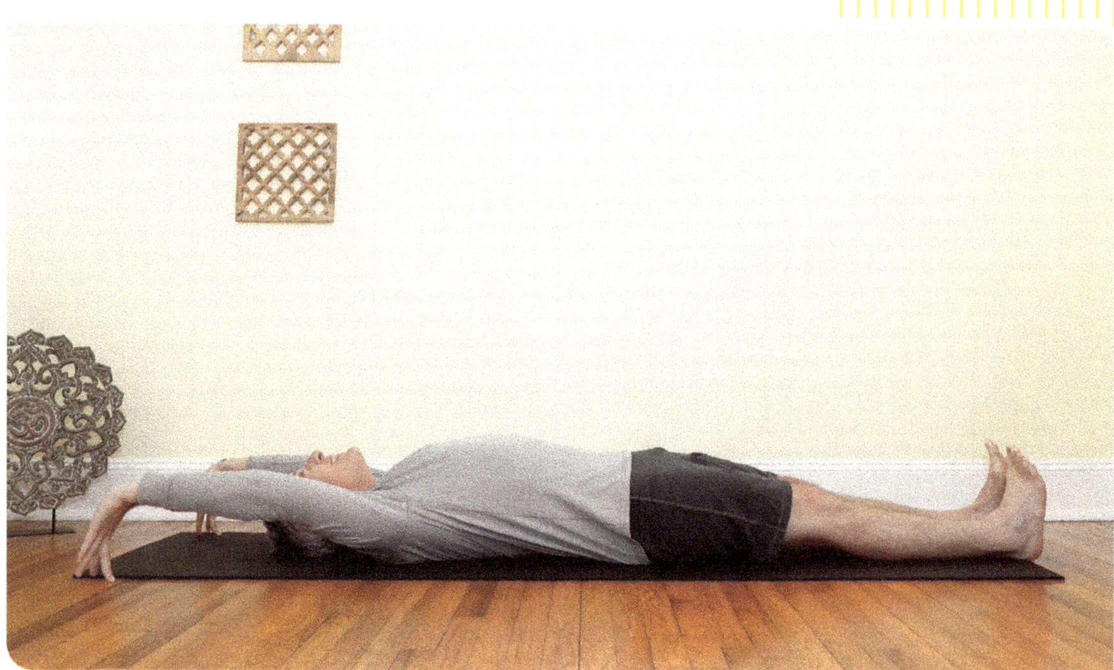

Hand Stand Pose, step one

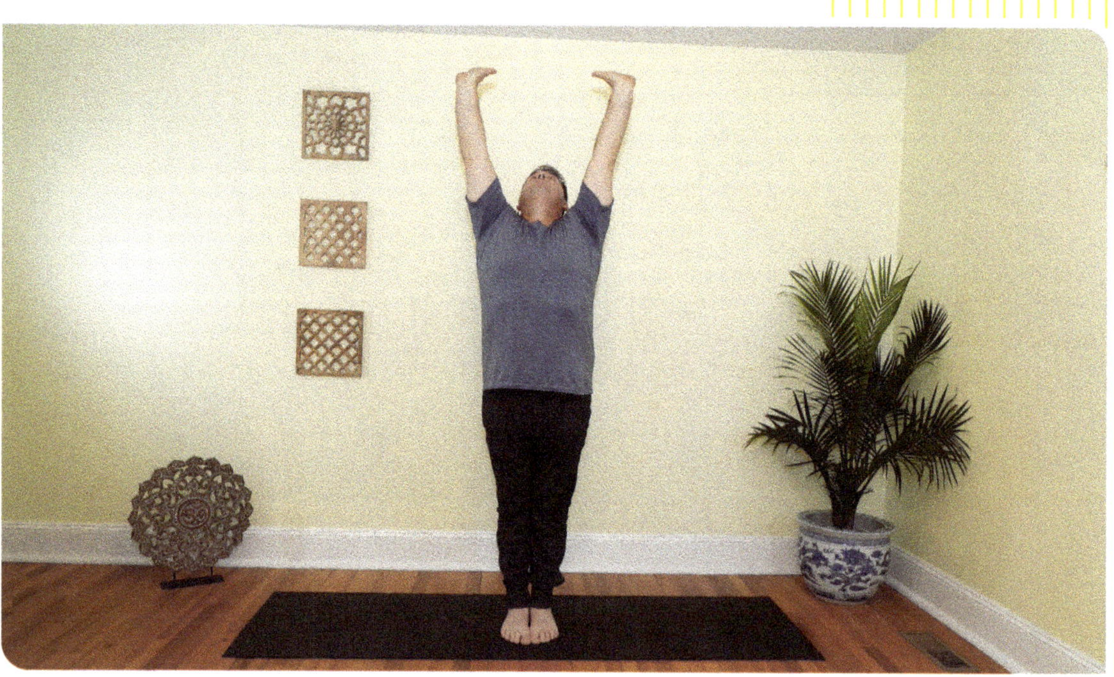

Hand Stand Pose, step two

Hand Stand Pose, Steps Three and Four

In these steps, you build more strength and flexibility for Hand Stand Pose by working from Downward Facing Dog Pose (Adho Mukha Svanasana).

Step Three: As in the steps toward Head Stand, start in Table Top Pose (Bharmanasana, or all fours) with your knees close together or touching, and put a block behind each foot. Place your hands flat and slightly wider than shoulder distance apart. Don't put your hands too close together. (I put my pinky fingertips on the outside edges of my mat.) Placing your hands wider than shoulder distance makes it much easier to access the strength of your upper back, shoulder, and chest muscles. With your hands wide apart, you can feel your latissimus dorsi muscles, which connect your mid-back to your arms, engaging to stabilize your shoulders. Eventually your hands will be closer, but for this step keeping them a bit wide helps you feel what's going on in your shoulders and upper back.

Look at the mat between your thumbs, lift your hips into Downward Facing Dog Pose, and step up onto the blocks behind you. Get your legs as straight as possible, and maybe walk your hands back a few inches toward your feet. This step tests whether your hamstrings are long enough to get your center of gravity (your hips) stacked up over your shoulders. Having your feet raised on blocks makes it easier to move your hips over your shoulders. Try lifting up onto your tip-toes and lowering your heels a few times, and notice the feeling of shifting your hips forward and back over your shoulders. If your hamstrings are tight and your hips are still far behind your shoulders, work on this step until your hamstrings get longer.

Step Four: Keep looking at the mat between your thumbs. Your gazing point (your drishti) is very important in Hand Stand Pose. Keep your eyes steady and still. Breathe. Press down strongly from your shoulder blades and focus on lifting your hips. If your knees are straight and your shoulders feel strong and stable, you can raise one leg at a time to build more core strength and mental focus.

Don't hurry to kick up into Hand Stand Pose. That's not an effective way to learn this pose—you'll kick, and kick, and kick forever without making much progress. Take your time to build the strength and flexibility needed to do this pose safely and effectively. Be patient. Learn not to automatically hold your breath when you go upside down—that's a big task in itself.

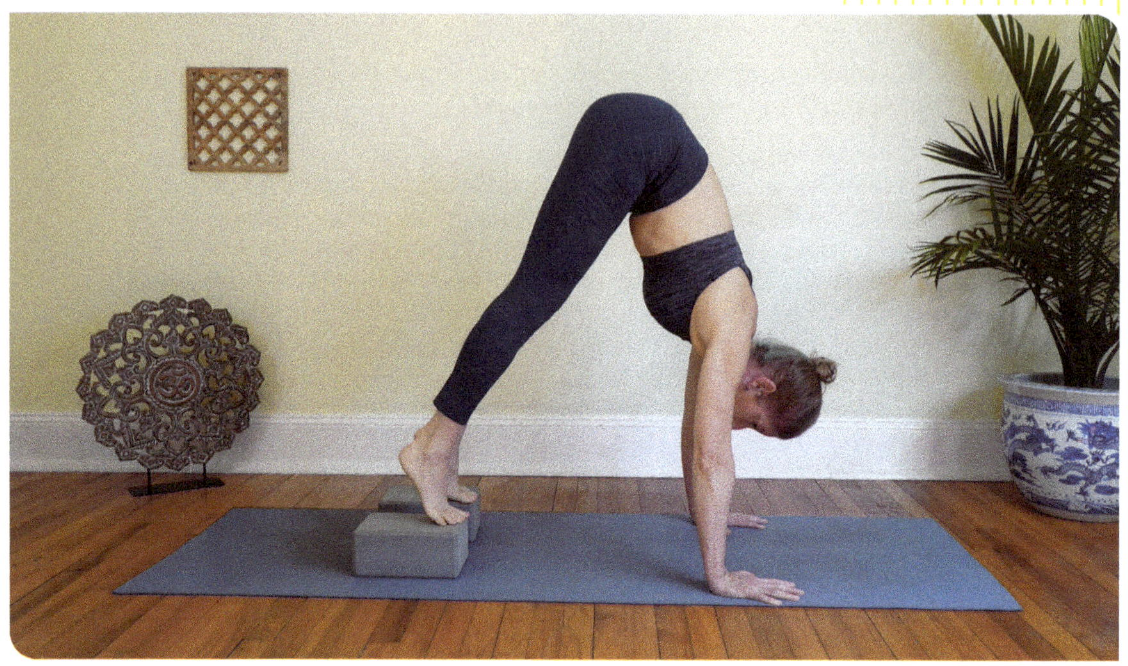

Hand Stand Pose, step three, Downward Dog variation

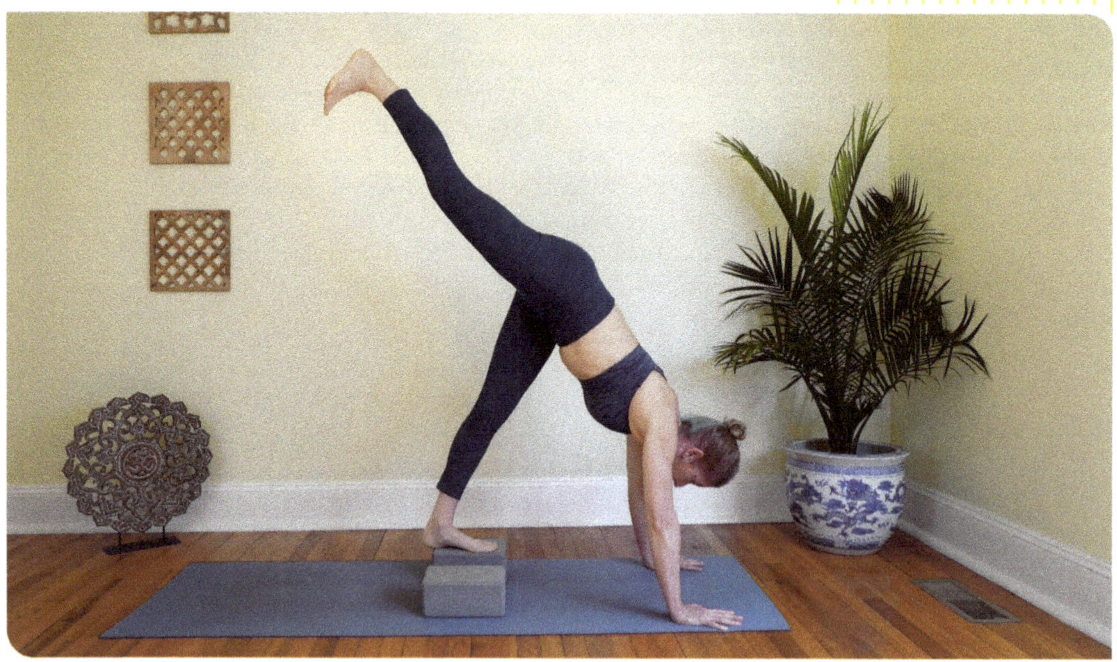

Hand Stand Pose, step four

Hand Stand Pose, Steps Five and Six

Just as in Head Stand Pose (Sirsasana), the next steps into Hand Stand Pose use the wall to build more strength.

Step Five: Sit with your back and hips against the wall and extend your legs forward. Place a marker off the side of your mat even with your heels (a block, a strap, or your water bottle). Come forward into Table Top Pose (all fours) and line your palms up with your marker, placing them slightly wider than your shoulders. Your feet are now back at the baseboard.

It's normal to feel like you're too close to the wall, or a little "scrunched up" at this point. You're not. Don't move your hands forward. Begin to straighten your legs into Downward Dog with your heels on the baseboard and your toes on the floor. If you can't get your legs completely straight, pause and work here or in a previous step. Your hamstrings need to become longer before you move on to the next step.

Set your gazing point (your drishti) on the mat between your thumbs. Hold your eyes steady and focus on stretching your hamstrings and building shoulder and core strength. If you try kicking up into Hand Stand Pose before your hamstrings are long enough, you'll have to kick too hard, and will lose your alignment. It's impossible to catch your balance on your hands from a misaligned, wonky, reckless kick-up. Not to mention it's dangerous for both you and your neighbors. Correct alignment and a calm, focused mind give you the control you need to try moving your legs up safely and effectively. Be patient. Prepare by building the strength and flexibility this pose requires. Throwing your body weight up over your wrists and shoulders is not a productive use of your energy or your time on the mat.

Step Six: You should be able to almost stack your hips over your shoulders with your feet on the ground before you start lifting your feet. This ensures that you have enough flexibility to enter Hand Stand using strength and mental focus. Do not rely on momentum to fling yourself into this pose. Learn to enter Hand Stand with the grace and lightness that comes with strength and mental clarity.

When you can keep your legs straight with your feet on the baseboard and your breath steady, you can bring one foot at a time flat onto the wall. Look back at the wall and step one foot then the other up to hip height. There's a common tendency to put your foot high up the wall so that you're in a plank-type position. Don't do that. Keep your feet at hip height so your legs and torso are at about a 90-degree angle. Notice how it feels to shift your hips, your center of gravity, directly over your shoulders. Breathe. Look at the mat between your thumbs with a steady gaze.

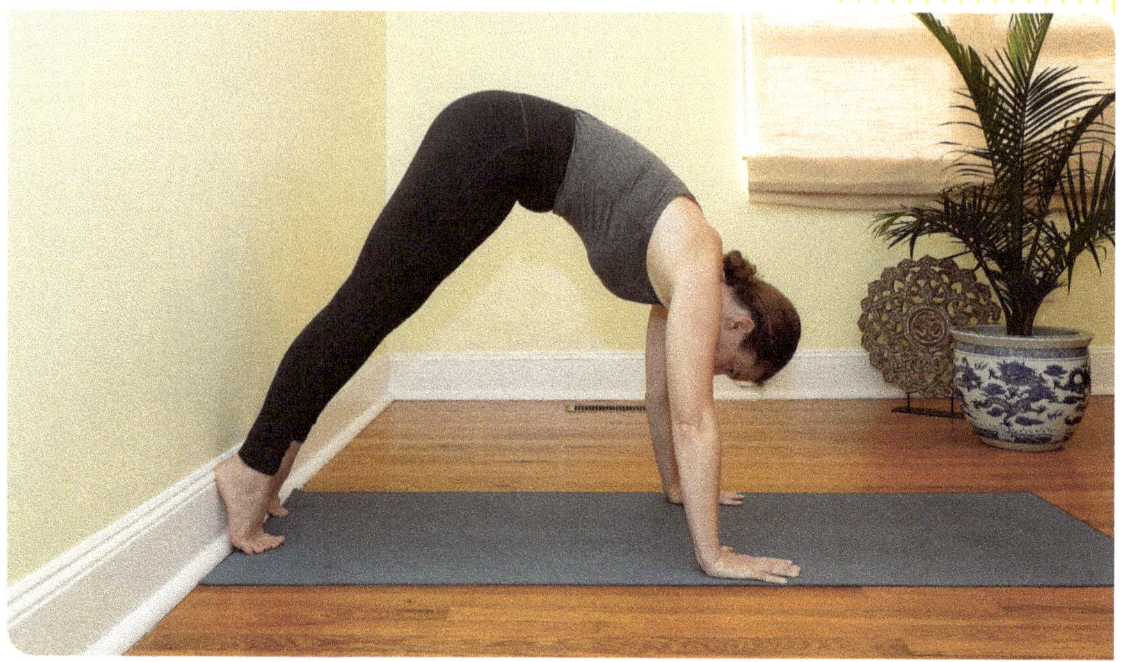

Handstand Pose, step 5

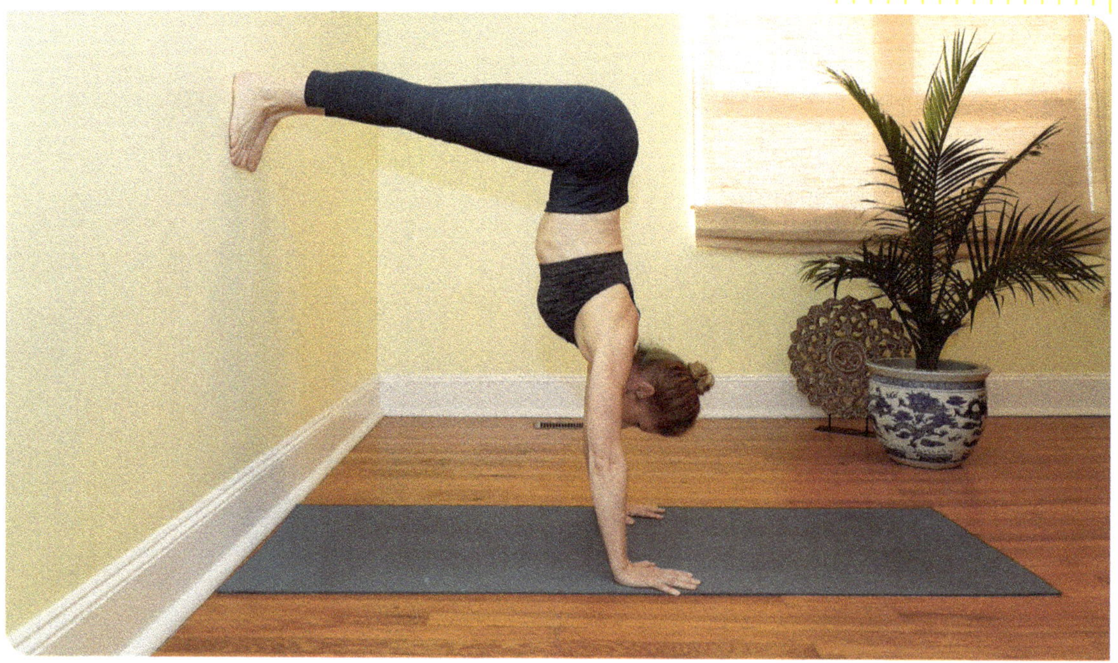

Handstand Pose, step 6

Hand Stand Pose, Step Seven

Eventually you'll feel strong and steady enough to lift one foot at a time toward the ceiling. Do not let the lifted leg drift overhead, back past your shoulders. The lifted foot stays over your hip. Also, do not let your legs drift apart. Pull your inner thighs toward each other to keep your core muscles activated. Keep your eyes (your drishti) on your mat between your thumbs.

Press down with your shoulder blades and grip your mat with your fingertips—imagine you have talons and dig them into your mat.

When the pose feels controlled, flex the lifted foot, and slowly draw that leg down towards the floor, until that foot hovers above the floor in front of your chest. Do not bend either knee, or let the lowered foot touch the floor. Use your core, shoulder, and back strength. Inhale and slowly draw the moving leg back up overhead. Place the foot back on the wall and come down for a rest in Child's Pose (Balasana), before repeating Step Seven with the opposite leg raised. Practice this step for several weeks or months.

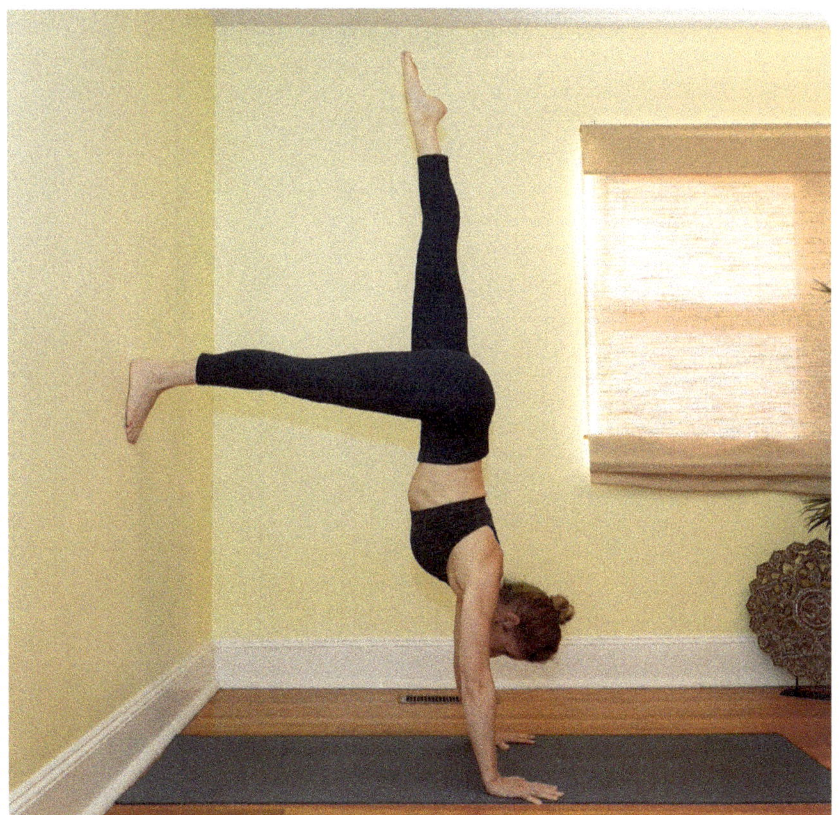

Hand Stand Pose, step seven

Hand Stand Pose, Steps Eight and Nine

When you've built enough shoulder strength and hamstring length, and can breathe slowly and calmly in the preparatory steps (kramas) of Hand Stand Pose, you're ready to try lifting into it.

Step Eight: Turn around to face the wall. Place your hands on the floor slightly wider than shoulder distance apart with your fingertips quite close to the baseboard. If you put your hands too far from the wall, you'll end up with a big arch in your back, which is incorrect, and makes it much more difficult to eventually get your heels off the wall. Start with your hands close to the wall.

Get into Downward Facing Dog Pose (Adho Mukha Svanasana) and step one foot about six to eight inches forward. Bend that knee and extend the other leg straight back behind you. The forward knee is bent, but your back knee should be firm and as straight as an arrow.

Next, gently sweep your back (straight) leg up, and give a very tiny hop with your bottom (bent) leg. Keep gently swinging the straight leg and hopping with the bent one. Do not get overly excited. These are very slow, gentle pulses, like you would give to a small child on the swing set. Do not hop and swing with gusto. Don't scare the children! Eventually the sweeping heel will land softly on the wall like a butterfly landing on a flower.

Focus on your straight leg—not on your hopping leg. Keep it completely straight. It's harder than you think. Swing and hop. Swing and hop. Nice and easy. Keep your eyes focused on the mat between your thumbs throughout. Many people make the mistake of trying to bring the lower (hopping or pushing) leg up. Don't even think about getting both feet on the wall. Just focus on the first heel. One thing at a time.

Eventually, one day, when your heels naturally land one at-a-time on the wall, you'll pull your inner thighs together and firm up your leg and shoulder muscles. With both feet up, draw your low back toward the wall and look at the mat between your thumbs. Take a few breaths. Come down and rest in Child's pose (Balasana). Try again. Practice this for several weeks or months, until it's easy. Your feet should hardly make a sound when they land on the wall—no CLUNK CLUNK. Remember, float up like a butterfly.

Step Nine: You'll be relieved to learn that—if you've approached this pose slowly and built your strength and flexibility over time—getting your heels off the wall is not really very difficult. It's a matter of focus and concentration. With both heels on the wall, draw your inner thighs toward each other and make your leg muscles very firm. Squeeze your heels together, press the balls of your feet up to the ceiling, then pull your low back slightly back toward the wall to activate your core. Look at the mat between your thumbs and, *very slowly*, dig your fingertips into your mat like talons. This action in your fingertips will float your heels off the wall. If you dig your talons into the mat too hard and too fast, your heels will pop off the wall and you'll drop down from the pose. The hand action is very subtle. Try to see how gently and slowly you can grip your fingertips, while noticing your heels getting lighter and then lifting away from the wall. I promise, the first time you do this you'll be amazed at how little effort it takes to make this subtle shift.

After your heels leave the wall, your task is to practice balancing, which is a matter of learning to alternate between either pressing your fingertips or your palms into the mat. A little softness in your elbows helps with balancing. You'll learn to use your hands and arm strength to catch your body weight as it shifts forward and back. We actually do this same thing to balance on our feet, but it's so automatic that we don't realize what we're doing. Standing up, we instinctively sway slightly back-and-forth between the balls of our feet and our heels, all the time. When you're upside down, you have to learn how to do this with your hands by catching and shifting weight from your finger tips to the heels of your hands to stay vertical.

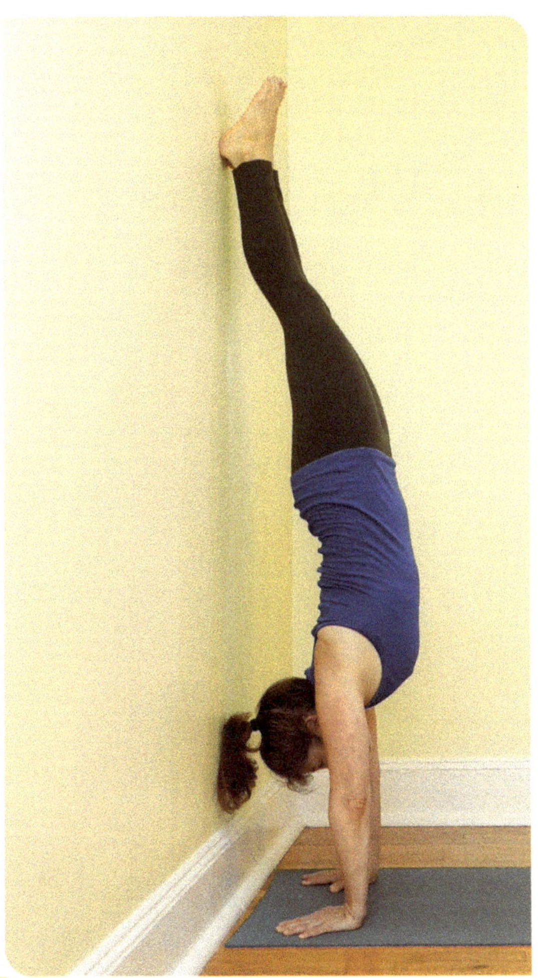

Hand Stand Pose, Step Eight, heels against wall

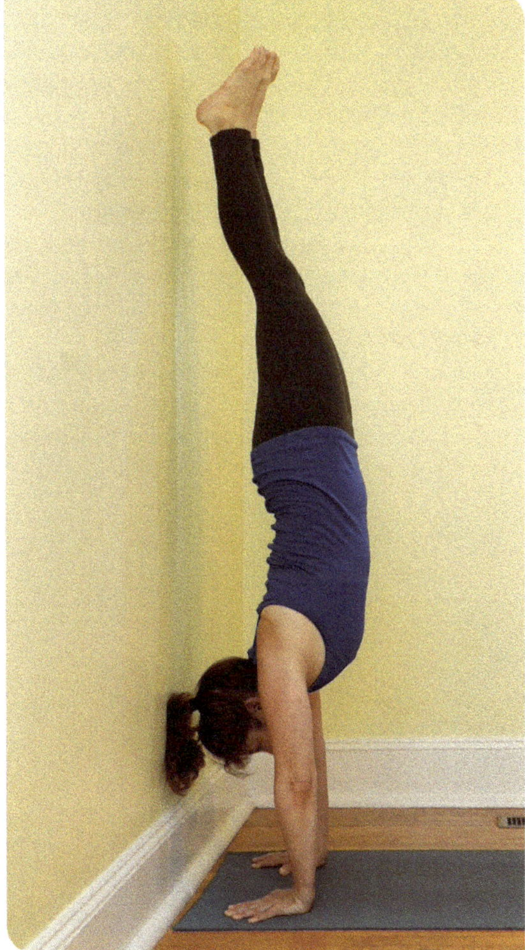

Hand Stand Pose, Step Nine, heels off wall

Crow Pose

ALSO CALLED: Bakasana, Crane Pose

WHAT IT DOES FOR YOUR SHOULDERS: Another great shoulder strengthening pose. This pose also requires a great deal of core and leg strength, especially in the groin muscles (your adductors).

TUNE IT UP: As in all arm balances and inversions, you need to spend some time building the strength and flexibility needed to do this pose safely and effectively. I recommend preparing for this pose by first practicing it lying on your back (see chapter 3, page 151).

When you feel strong and flexible in the pose while lying on the floor, and your breath is deep and steady, try it upright. Squat down with your knees and toes pointing outward and your heels turned in toward each other. Put a block in front of you, so your forehead can eventually rest on it.

Place your hands flat on the mat, slightly wider than shoulder distance apart. Remember, placing your hands wider than your shoulders makes it easier to activate your shoulder and back muscles. Bend your elbows deeply, lean forward and wiggle your knees as high as possible onto your upper-arms. Look slightly forward, and begin shifting your shoulders toward your hands to eventually rest your forehead on the block in front of you. Your toes can stay on the floor, or try lifting one foot at a time toward your backside. Come out of the pose and take a rest in Child's Pose (Balasana). Give your wrists some rotations. Then try it again.

Eventually, you'll be strong and flexible enough to remove the block from under your forehead. Your focus is on shifting your chest and shoulders forward (not down), and drawing your big toes together to pull your feet up toward your backside. Gradually work on straightening your elbows.

Eventually, this pose will feel more and more like you are lifting your body forward and upward. Take your time. Crow Pose builds a tremendous amount of core and shoulder strength, as well as mental focus. But that takes time. Try. Rest. Then try again.

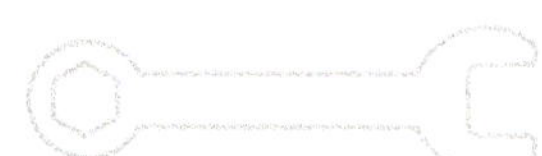

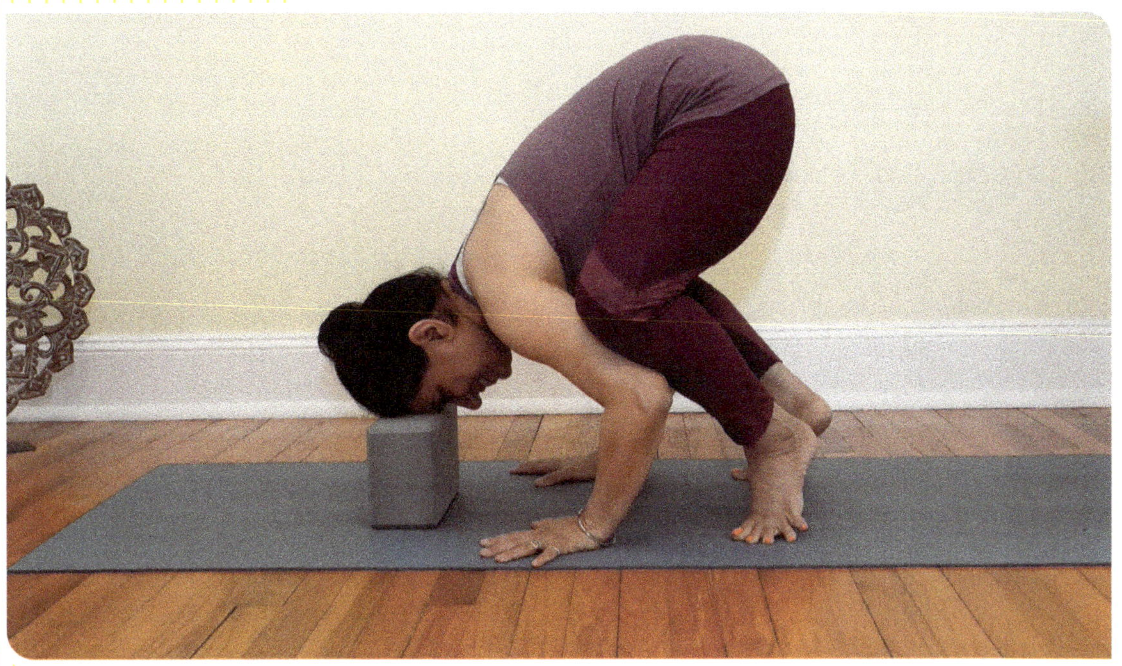

Crow Pose, variation with block

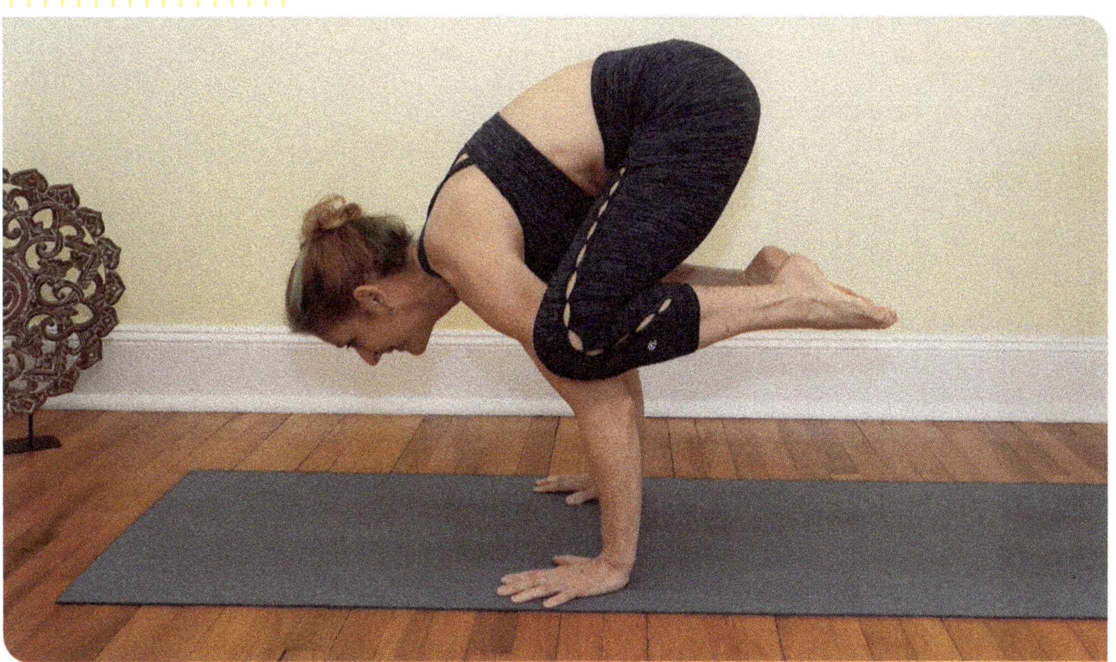

Crow Pose

Side Crow Pose

ALSO CALLED: Parsva Bakasana

WHAT IT DOES FOR YOUR SHOULDERS: Here's a fun variation that many people prefer to plain, old traditional Crow Pose. Side Crow builds shoulder, core, and back strength while helping you grow a lot of self-confidence.

TUNE IT UP: You can start finding the muscular actions and flexibility needed for this pose by using blocks to support most of your body weight, keeping it off of your wrists and hands.

Stack two blocks across the center of your mat. Squat down behind the blocks on your tip-toes, and turn to face one side with your knees pointing toward the long edge of your mat. Lean over the blocks and put your hands flat on the floor in front. At the same time, sit your hip on top of the blocks.

Look forward toward the end of your mat, and bend your elbows *very* deeply. Lean *very* far forward and bend your elbows as much as you can. Your face should be almost touching the floor. As your shoulders go down, your feet will automatically lift off the floor behind you. Pause here with your knees bent and drawn in together so that you are curled up in a ball. Take a breath in this curled position. Make sure that your palms are absolutely flat on the floor. Many people unconsciously lift the heels of their hands, bending their palms in half backwards. Don't do that—it's bad news for your hand tendons. Keep your palms flat and your elbows bent deeply. Breathe.

Now, flex your feet to activate your leg muscles, and stretch your top leg back and your bottom leg forward. Lift your chest toward the front of your mat. Don't drop your shoulders. Firm all of your leg muscles down to your toes as you press your feet in two different directions. Smile. Have fun! Enjoy your flight.

To exit this pose, bend your knees and curl yourself back up over your hip on the blocks. Press your hands down to tip yourself upright and bring your toes back down behind the blocks. Turn around and try the other side.

Eventually, you'll be strong and flexible enough to do the pose without blocks. The set-up is the same as above, except that you'll sit the side of your hip and thigh on your elbow(s) instead of on the blocks. Now, your arms will be supporting your entire body weight.

To enter Side Crow Pose without blocks, you have to bend your elbows even deeper and lean much further forward than you do when using blocks. When you first try this pose without blocks, you'll use both elbows to support your weight—with your hip on one elbow and your outer knee or thigh on the other.

Once you're comfortable using both elbows, you may be able to twist far enough past your thighs to only rest your mid-thigh on only one elbow, leaving your other elbow free. This takes a lot of practice and a tremendous amount of strength. Don't force your way into this pose. It will only lead to injury. Remember, the patience and humility you learn on your yoga mat are valuable tools for life. Try. Rest. Try again.

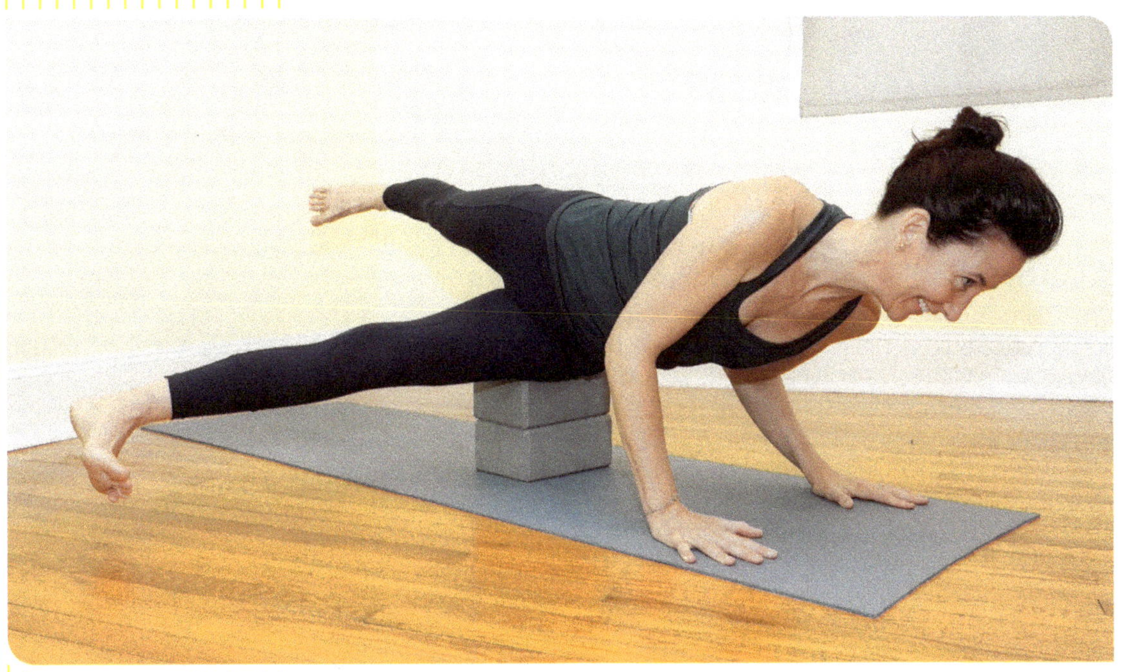

Side Crow Pose, variation with blocks

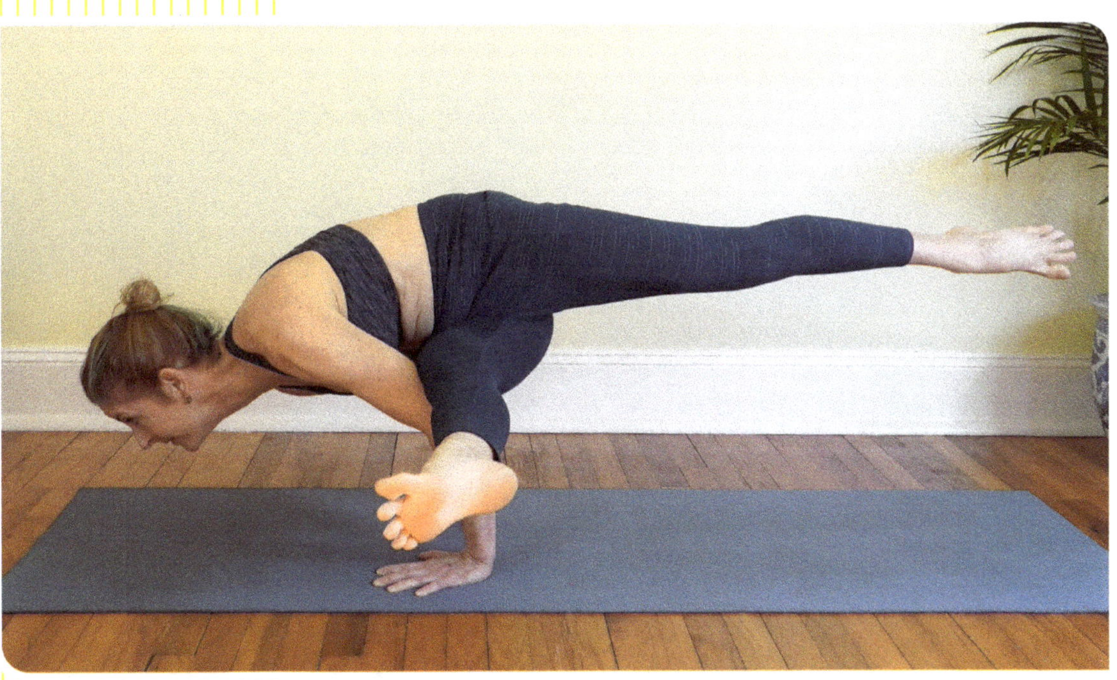

Side Crow Pose

Scale Pose

ALSO CALLED: Tolasana

WHAT IT DOES FOR YOUR SHOULDERS: Another great shoulder strengthening pose that takes a lot of patience, preparation, and mental focus. It also builds strength in your core and adductors.

TUNE IT UP: If your hips are tight and your legs will not fold into Lotus Pose (Padmasana), sit in Comfortable Seated Pose (Sukhasana) with your shins crossed.

To start, put a block beside and slightly in front of each hip, with your palms flat on top. This pose requires you to do two different muscular actions at the same time—push down from your shoulder blades and draw your knees in and up toward your belly.

Don't grip the blocks with claw-like fingers. It won't help. Keep your hands calm and flat. Focus on pushing down from your shoulders and pulling your thighs and knees up and inward. If your shins are crossed, don't worry about getting your feet off the floor. Push and squeeze inward. Lift on an inhale and hold for a few breaths. Lower. Take a rest for a moment and try it again.

When your hips are flexible enough to fold your legs into Lotus Pose, Scale Pose actually becomes a lot easier, because your legs are now bound into one unit. It's much easier to lift your lower body off the floor when it's all tied up into a single, tidy package.

Again, focus on pressing down from your shoulders and pulling your thighs up and in. Look forward. There's a common tendency to drop your head and look down at the floor. Don't do that. Shift your gaze slightly forward even if you do this by mostly moving your eyes.

If you can smile in this pose, you'll know you've developed an advanced yoga practice! One day you'll be strong and flexible enough to lift your lower body off the floor without using the blocks. Put your palms flat on the mat slightly in front of your hips. Gradually build up to holding Tolasana for ten deep breaths. No hurry. No worry. Just breathe.

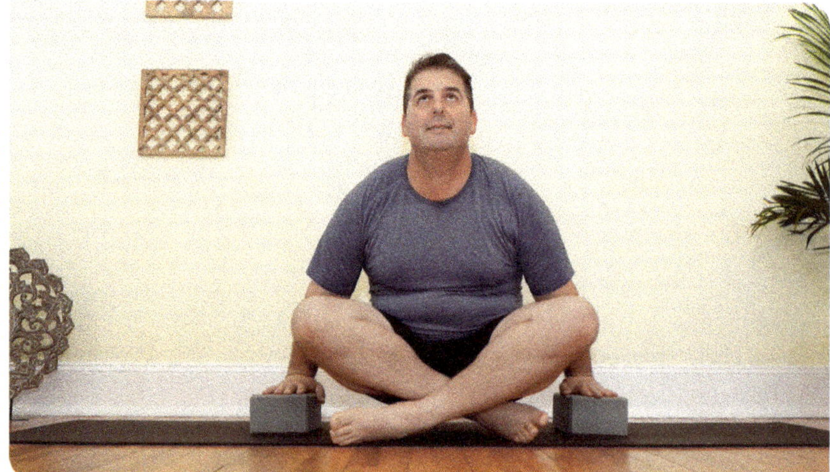

Scale Pose, variation with blocks and shins crossed

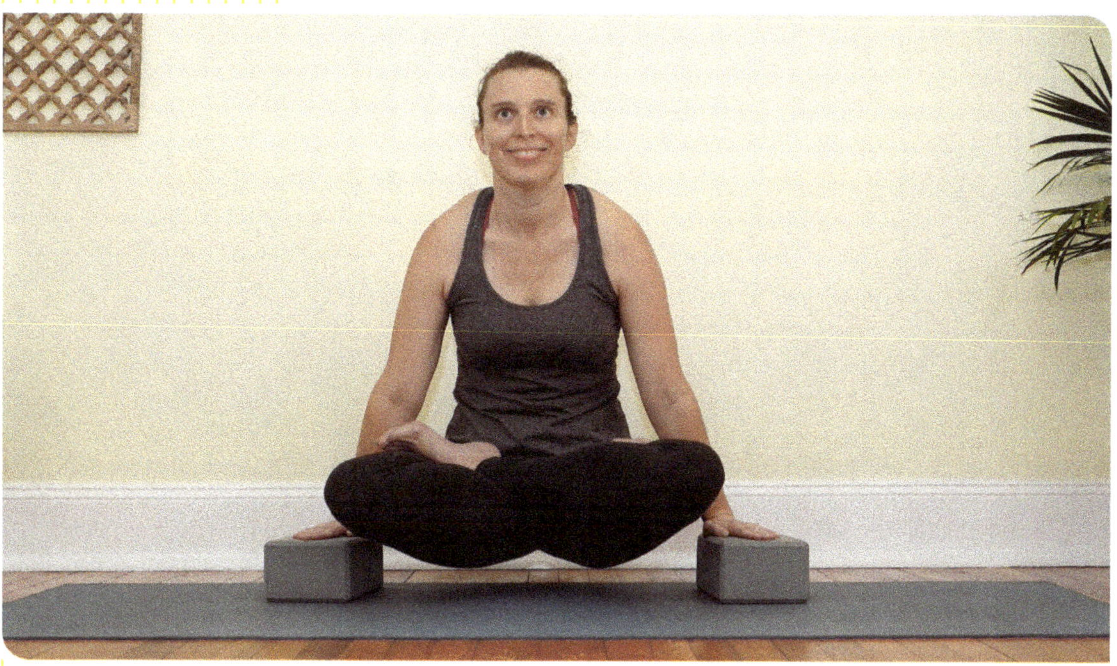

Variation with blocks and Lotus Pose legs

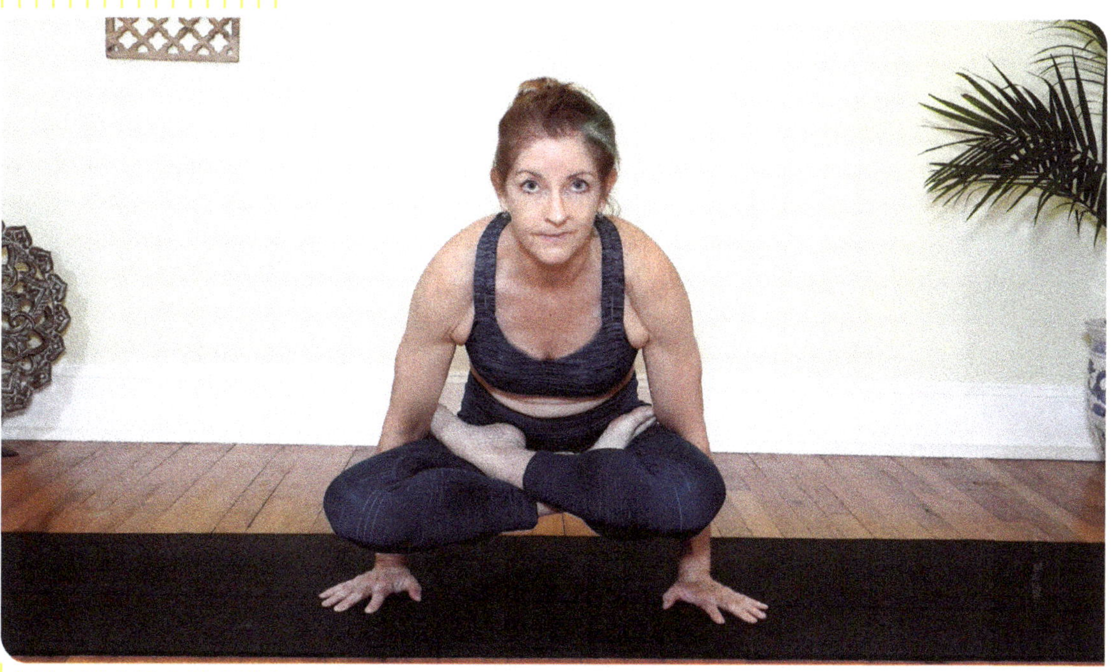

Scale Pose

CHAPTER 6

NOTES FOR STUDENTS AND TEACHERS

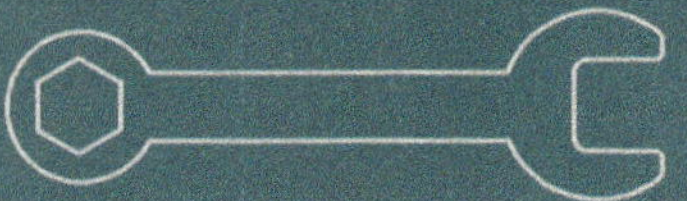

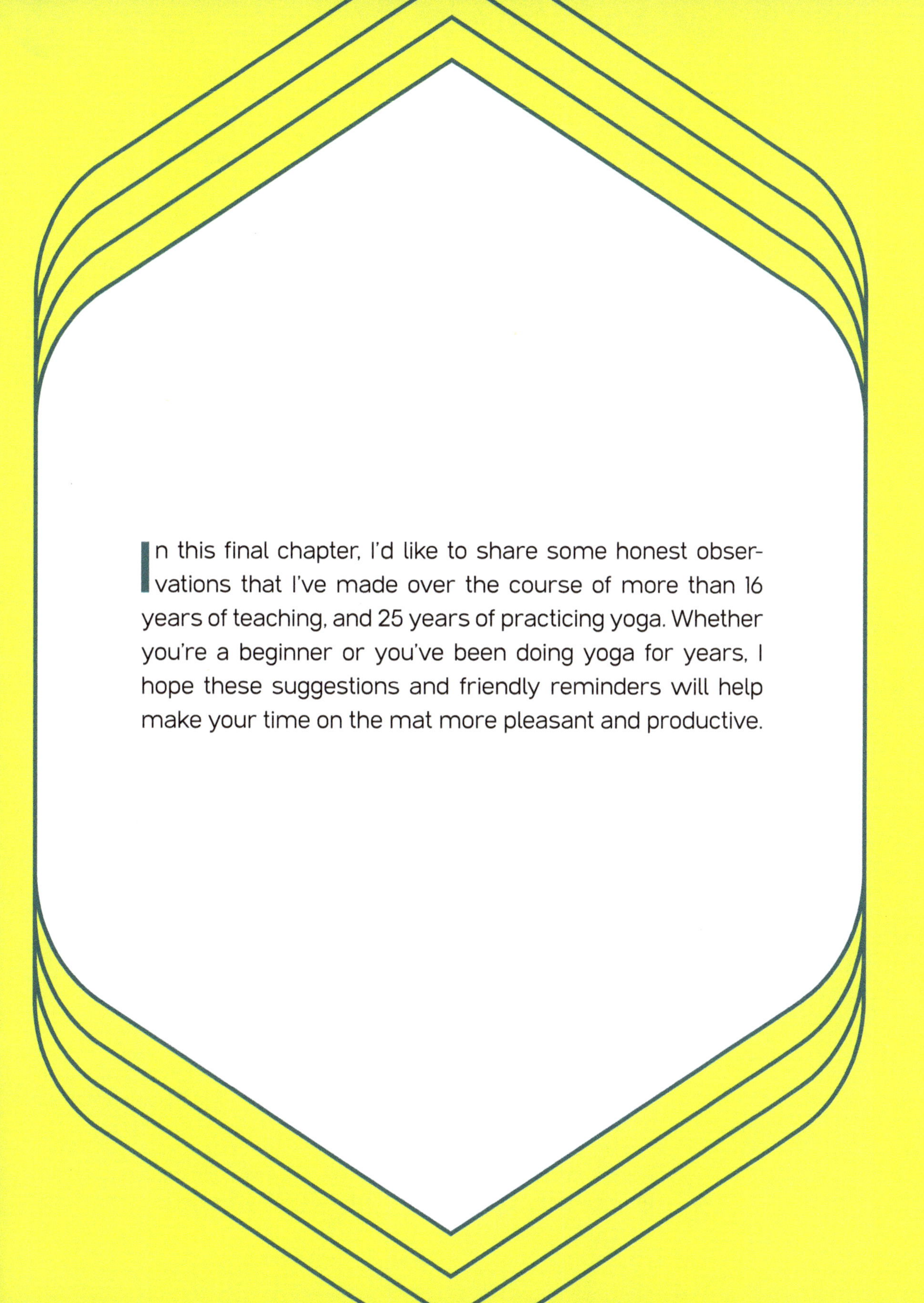

In this final chapter, I'd like to share some honest observations that I've made over the course of more than 16 years of teaching, and 25 years of practicing yoga. Whether you're a beginner or you've been doing yoga for years, I hope these suggestions and friendly reminders will help make your time on the mat more pleasant and productive.

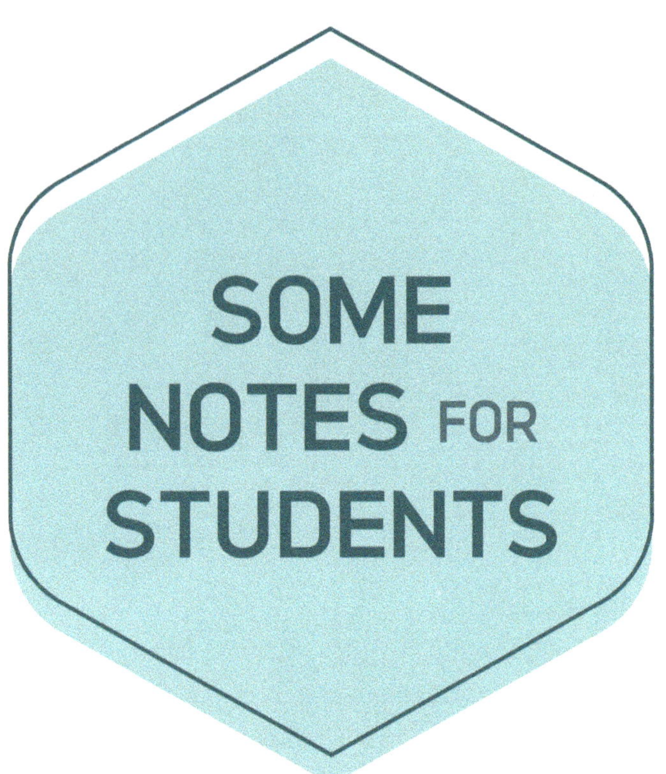

SOME NOTES FOR STUDENTS

When you practice on your own at home, taking an online class or following your own sequence, you're free to suit yourself. Everything from the temperature of the room, to the music, to the poses you do are under your control. You can do what you want when you want. But getting the most out of a group class requires a slightly different mindset. So here are some important rules of the road.

Respect the Group

Always remember, a yoga class is a community experience, and that comes with certain expectations and responsibilities. To ensure that everyone feels comfortable, welcome, and respected, you should:

Have reasonable expectations. Your instructor can only provide so much individual attention to each student. If you'd like more instruction, consider scheduling a private lesson or asking in-depth questions before or after class.

Accept the environment. Think about how you can adjust yourself to the environment, instead of asking for the lighting, music, or temperature to be adjusted just to suit you. If you get easily overheated, don't push so hard; wear breathable clothing, and bring a bottle of cold water to sip during class. If you tend to get cold at the end of class, bring a long-sleeved tee or hoodie to pull on. One of my students wears sunglasses so the lights don't make his migraines flare up.

Mute or turn off your phone and other devices before class begins. Even if you leave your phone outside the room, it can still be audible inside—especially if several people's devices go off at the same time. And don't forget to mute your wrist device, too.

Share the space. You may have a certain place in the room that you prefer, but it's not "your spot." Don't be annoyed if someone else puts their mat there. Instead, think of it as an opportunity to expand your horizons.

Be on time. Entering class late is a distraction for the instructor, and for other students who may have to stop practicing to move their mats and make room for you.

Stay until the end. Leaving class early is also a distraction. Yoga classes always end with a few minutes of quiet relaxation. Rolling up your mat and rustling around to get out the door keeps your classmates from enjoying what is, for many, the best part of class. Chill out for the last few minutes.

When we start noticing our own behavior, we put ourselves squarely on the path of positive personal growth. This is the true purpose of practicing yoga—to become more like the person you want to be, by noticing how you actually behave. Only when you notice what you're really like (without judgment, if possible) can you begin taking small steps toward being a more optimal version of yourself—someone you'll be happier living with, someone others will be happier to meet on their own journeys.

Follow the Instruction

It's a mystery to me why some students will pay an instructor their hard-earned money, yet refuse to accept any instruction. Years ago, I took class from a very experienced, knowledgeable instructor; there was one student who simply would not follow along. Throughout class, this person insisted on doing her own thing—jumping back into plank when everyone else stepped forward, doing Shoulder Stand while the instructor taught Plow Pose. At the end of class, when everyone else was sitting quietly for a few minutes of meditation, this student recited a lengthy prayer in a whispered but audible voice. As we gathered our belongings afterward, I overheard the teacher say, "You have such a lovely home practice. There's really no need for you to come to a studio."

It was an awkward conversation-starter, but I admired the teacher for her compassion and courage to bring the subject up. They went on to have a longer conversation about the benefits of practicing in a group. Students who "freelance" during class are a distraction, or worse, a hazard to themselves and others. Consistently refusing to follow the instruction being provided is disrespectful—both to the instructor and to the other students. Of course, if you know that a variation other than the one being taught is safer or more effective for your body, you should do it. But make sure it's a variation of the pose being taught, not a completely different pose altogether. Then, do it without fanfare or making a commotion. If you have an injury or health condition, tell the instructor before class that you'll be adjusting your practice to accommodate it. Doing that allows the instructor to give you helpful cues, too.

One of the beautiful things about a yoga class is that it's a shared journey each person takes alongside their fellow students. Rest assured, skilled instructors constantly assess the levels of ability and energy in the room, which informs their choice of poses and variations. Go off on your own, and you miss all the benefits of preparing your mind and your muscles more gradually and arriving together as a group. There's a collective, unspoken agreement that we're all in this together. Enjoy it. If you still crave a particular pose after class, take a moment and do it on your own.

Take a Break When You Need to Rest

If you feel exhausted and can't breathe steadily through your nose, pause for a moment in Downward Dog or Child's Pose to collect yourself. Taking a break when you need one is much more productive than forging ahead when you're overwhelmed. Remember, learning to listen to your own body is part of yoga.

Say 'Hi' to the People Next to You

After all, you're going to spend the next hour beside each other–smiling and struggling, balancing and tipping over. It's a nice gesture to briefly greet those who are nearby either at the beginning or end of class. It doesn't need to be a big deal, just a simple 'hi' might brighten your day and theirs.

Put Your Scent in Neutral

In a small space where you're in close proximity to other people, it's polite to take responsibility for your own scent. Try to minimize the amount of perfume, essential oils, body spray, cigarette smoke, vape flavors, and plain old b.o. that ride into the room on your skin and hair. Even smells you think are pleasant may be unpleasant to someone else. That said, going 'nose-blind' is real, and we can't always be aware of our own funk. So regularly clean your mat with warm water and dish soap, then let it air dry before rolling it back up. If you notice a petri-dish thing going on, wipe your mat down with a 10% vinegar and water solution to kill any bacteria that might be growing on it. Keep a packet of unscented hand-wipes in your bag to swipe your neck, pits, and wrists before class, and use it to knock down your perfume, any vape or smoke scents, and the day's grit and grime. You'll enjoy class more if you start off feeling a little bit refreshed.

Think Beyond Physical Poses

People who are new to yoga often get hung up on accomplishing the physical positions, because they view yoga as just another fitness endeavor. But the asanas, the physical yoga poses, are only one part of practicing yoga. They're just positions that build strength and flexibility in particular muscle groups of your body.

Throughout this book, we've touched on the importance of breath, of focus, of how yoga can help you build concentration, and other matters besides strengthening and stretching your body. Even though this book focuses mostly on anatomy, I want to be clear: Avoid the common misperception that practicing yoga is just like going to the gym, or putting in your miles running or cycling, or some other exercise regimen. That perception raises your risk of injury. Thinking of yoga as just another fitness routine creates an unhealthy attachment to "mastering" the poses, and attempting only the most challenging variations—whether you're ready or not.

I've practiced yoga for over twenty-five years, and I don't consider myself to have "mastered" many poses at all. Every time I step onto my mat, at least a few poses really poke a stick in my ego's eye, and it's almost never the same ones. Those reality-check moments during practice, when I have to stop struggling, slow down, and breathe, are what keep me interested, grounded, and humble. Those are the moments that keep me coming back.

Mastery isn't the point. The attitude that you're on your mat to accomplish physical feats will suck all the joy out of your practice by fostering a competitive, striving attitude. You'll tend to push your body too far, too hard, and too fast. Worse, this attitude creates feelings of failure and frustration instead of steadiness and contentment. When you can't do a certain pose, you'll feel dejected instead of curious. These are exactly the negative self-judgments that a patient, steady yoga practice can free you from. Focusing on pose accomplishment, instead of on your alignment, breath, and mental steadiness, builds a wall between you and the contentment your practice can bring.

I've seen it happen. Some folks become what I call "pose hoarders." They relentlessly pursue certain poses to check them off their list of accomplishments. They mistakenly believe that making progress down a list of poses is the same thing as making progress in their practice. They're like bird watchers who focus mainly on making a list of all the different species they've seen, so they can impress other bird watchers. That's fine, but it doesn't do anything to actually protect, feed, or support the birds.

Being primarily attached to the physical aspects of your practice is like jogging up and down the same path. Week after week, you jog from here to there and back again—liking the poses you can do easily, and disliking the ones you find difficult. It's hard to ever arrive somewhere new by going over the same old ground. Remember, you have to do something new to get something new. Instead of trying to "master" a difficult pose, try shifting your focus to your breath, and to your gazing point (your drishti). Move your effort onto those things while holding your body steady in correct central alignment. See what happens.

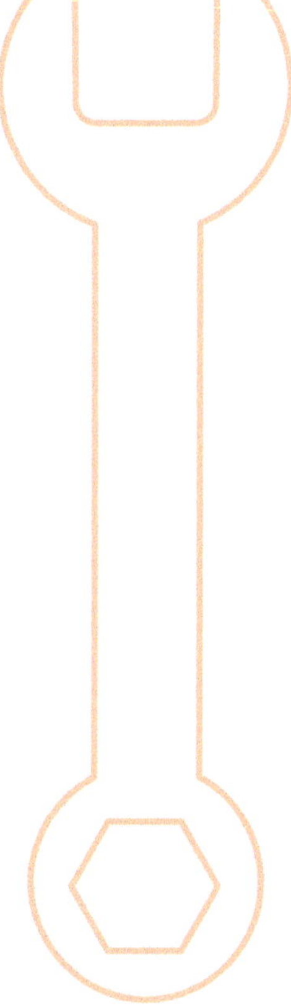

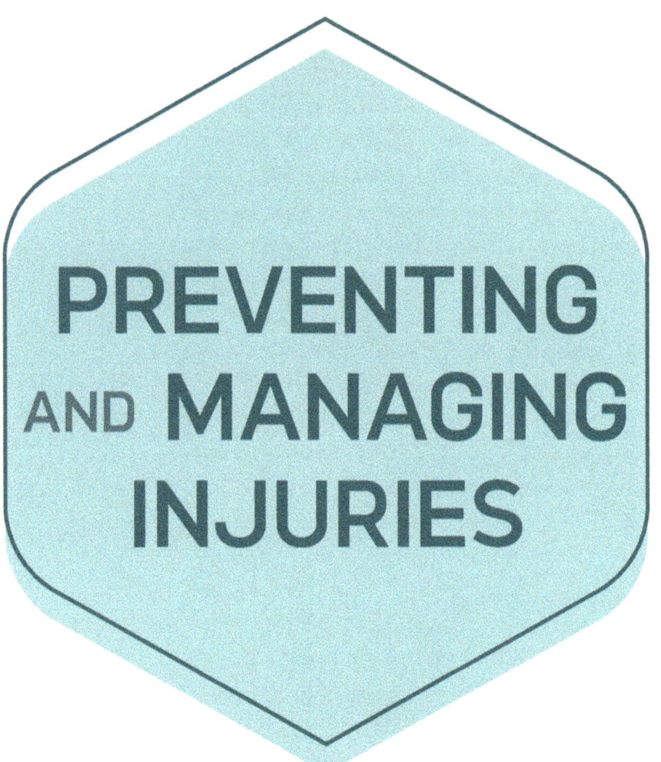

PREVENTING AND MANAGING INJURIES

One of the most dangerous myths in yoga is the belief that the harder you push your physical limits, the faster your practice will move forward. This is misguided thinking that almost always leads to injury.

That's because the key to avoiding injury in your yoga practice is to establish and maintain correct alignment and muscle recruitment in each pose. Central alignment and full muscle recruitment relieve pressure on your joints, and help prevent you from pushing them beyond their normal range of motion.

Remember, what you want is a sustainable, therapeutic yoga practice. And that can only develop gradually. Building your practice means sharpening your awareness of alignment and muscle recruitment, learning to feel when you can push a little harder and when you should ease off. Most importantly, yoga is not about accomplishing physical feats of strength and flexibility for their own sake. It's about honing your awareness of what you're doing right this second, and learning how to get the most possible benefit from that awareness.

Why Injuries Happen

The majority of injuries in yoga are to the muscles and joints; it's very rare—though not impossible—to break a bone or damage a nerve or blood vessel when practicing yoga. In any case, generally speaking, yoga injuries are primarily caused by these three behaviors:

- Putting extreme tension or pressure on a muscle or joint.
- Moving a joint beyond its normal range of motion (known as subluxation, or distracting the joint).
- Overuse; that is, repeatedly putting pressure on a joint from a particular angle that makes it become inflamed, painful, or restricted.

Avoiding Overuse

A good yoga instructor can help you avoid injuries from extreme pressure or tension and subluxation. However, ultimately you are your body's keeper. Developing your own awareness of correct alignment and muscle recruitment will go a long way toward protecting yourself from these types of injuries. Preventing overuse injuries, on the other hand, is completely up to you. Here are some principles to follow:

Be mindful of the limits of your strength and flexibility as you practice.

Take care of small aches and pains before they become injuries.

Take a temporary break from certain poses if they irritate a particular body part.

Learn several variations of poses you do often, so you can regularly vary your practice.

Pause your practice when you're tired or injured. That means: skip a class or two this week, take more breaks during class, or practice at half-power.

Learn to turn down the physicality of your practice some days, and focus more intensely on having a steady gazing point (drishti) and breathing deeply.

Don't Force It

Introducing extreme tension or pressure into a joint risks damaging the soft-tissue structures that support it, such as ligaments, tendons, and cartilage. Over-zealous use of arm binds, and forcing your way into bound variations (where your hands are clasped, or your arms and legs are folded into a restricted or "locked" position), can put your muscles and joints at risk. When you see someone else clasp their hands behind their back, or use their elbow to lever further into a pose, do not blindly copy them. If you don't have the strength and flexibility to establish and maintain proper (central) alignment, moving further into the pose by attempting the bound variation is not appropriate.

Protect your joints and tissues by avoiding these bad habits:

Overreaching. In standing and seated poses, do not sacrifice proper alignment by straining to put your hand on the floor or grab hold of your feet. Only touch what your hands can easily reach. Struggling to touch some landmark almost always involves letting go of some aspect of your alignment. Overreaching locks your body into an intense, misaligned position where you can't focus on your breathing. You're not only risking injury, you can't access the full strengthening and stretching benefits of the pose because, you're practicing it out of alignment.

Cranking. Do not use your arms or hands to crank yourself into twisted or revolved poses. You must learn to turn further by engaging your deep core muscles and the muscular locks (called *bandas*) of your low belly and pelvic floor muscles. This takes time. Be patient, and pay attention to what muscles are working or switching off as you practice. A good instructor will give you verbal cues to help you start finding these deep, muscular actions. Listen and explore what their suggestions feel like.

Hefting and heaving. In learning inversions and arm balances, many people are tempted to heave their body weight up onto their arms, shoulders, or neck before they have the strength and flexibility to do these poses with control and correct, central alignment. This action not only risks injury, it bypasses the more appropriate variations which could build your strength and flexibility. There are several steps to entering every arm balance and inversion. If you can't calmly move from one step to the next with control and a sense of calm, you don't yet have the strength and flexibility to do the pose safely. There should be no kicking, jumping, or flinging to get into or out of these poses. If you aren't sure what stage (krama) you need to work on, ask a good instructor to help you.

It's particularly important to work your way up to doing inverted poses like Shoulder Stand (Salamba Sarvangasana), Fish (Matsyasana), Head Stand (Sirsasana), Plow (Halasana), and Hand Stand (Adho Mukha Vrksasana) in a step-by-step manner. You should become comfortable in each stage of a pose before adding more weight above your head. You will gain nothing by hefting yourself into inverted poses and hoping for the best. Find a variation or krama that challenges your strength and flexibility, but allows you to still breathe steadily. Work there.

Over time, the multiple, preparatory stages for every yoga pose will build the strength and flexibility you need to do the full pose safely and correctly. These kramas give you the same benefits as the full variation, but with less intensity and less risk for injury. Start with stage one (krama one). When you can do it easily with steady, calm breathing move on to krama two.

Mental Management

Disciplining yourself to approach difficult poses slowly is a tremendous challenge, especially when you're in a class where others are doing variations that look very different (and maybe more exciting) than yours. Be intelligent about your yoga practice. Avoid mistaken paths that can put you on the road to an injury. Work on your preparatory poses. Be curious about the variations that are easy for you, as well as the ones that are difficult. Notice when something that used to be difficult has gotten easier, because your body has gradually gotten stronger and more flexible. Be amazed by that! You're amazing. Good job.

Along with the physical guidelines we've covered in this chapter, also notice your mental self-talk in class. Are you bored and easily distracted in poses you find easy? Do you fidget, and crave more physically challenging positions? Why is that? Why can't you be content and stay focused when you're at ease? Why can't you simply enjoy taking deep full breaths with a steady focused mind?

By contrast, in difficult poses, is your mind angry and argumentative? Do you give up after a few breaths? Do you grit your teeth and suffer until it's over? Why is that? Why can't you be content and focused during physical difficulty?

This exploration of your mental chit-chat is where your true yoga practice, and some of your hardest work, lies. Practicing yoga poses is really about learning to notice and manage your mental and emotional states. Frustration, boredom, irritation, annoyance, contentment, anxiety, fear, pride, and peace will all come up while you practice.

Yoga classes are designed to help you develop balance in your body *and* mind. So your yoga practice should be not only about developing symmetrical strength and flexibility in your body, but also in your psyche. That may sound like a tall order. But the path to success is simple: Keep getting on your mat. Build your practice persistently and patiently. Notice what's happening in your mind. Go slow. Practice with intelligence. Tune out that nagging ego. Breathe and move. Move and breathe.

You'll discover that practicing yoga poses is often about learning to manage your mental and emotional states.

Managing Injuries: Five Principles to Follow

Students often ask me for advice about managing an injury, or a new ache or pain that's cropped up during practice. I'll first remind them, and you, that I am not a physician. I cannot diagnose what's wrong with your back, shoulder, wrist, or knee. That said, I've been practicing yoga for over 25 years in my own body, and I have a solid working knowledge of human anatomy. So I can offer you these helpful tips for managing your bodily aches and pains.

1 **Rest is your best friend.** This is the first and most important tip. If a joint or muscle is consistently painful during your yoga practice, take two weeks of complete rest. Yes, you heard me. Two whole weeks with absolutely no asana practice, no gym workouts, no running or

MECHANIC'S NOTE

Over the years, I've notice that some people have difficulty taking responsibility for themselves during class. Please understand that this is a crucial aspect of your yoga development. Taking responsibility for your practice acknowledges that you have choices about the physical demands you put on your body, and about how to handle any mental or emotional discomfort that comes up. When you take full responsibility for your practice, you accept that managing your own discomfort, happiness, or challenges is completely up to you. A good way to start taking charge of your own practice is by asking for one-on-one help, before or after class, for a pose you are struggling with. Or take a private lesson or a special workshop to help you move forward with your goals.

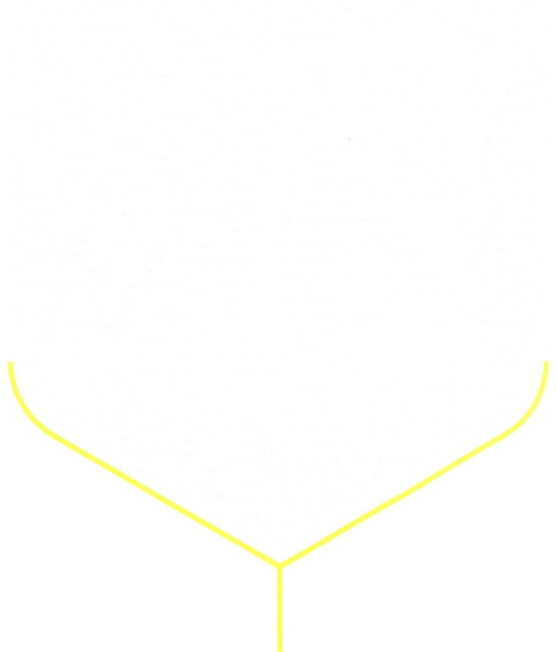

vigorous walking. ZERO. Do nothing that uses the affected area at all.

Many people—especially dedicated yoga practitioners—find the thought of complete physical rest horrifying. If that's your reaction, you might want to explore why. Stridently resisting the reasonable suggestion that you should rest an injury can tell you something about yourself. Remember, yoga is a practice of self-exploration. The refusal to physically rest your body when it's injured can give you a naked view of some of your deepest attachments and fears.

Here are some reasons students have given me for why they don't want to rest an injury:

- I'll get fat.
- I'll lose my asana practice.
- I'll be bored.
- I'll go crazy just sitting around the house.
- I'll miss my friends at class.

Does any of that sound familiar? These conversations always stir up my deepest compassion. We all have our demons. What I hear in these responses is: I have body image issues, I'm attached to my physical abilities on the mat, I need distraction to keep my mind occupied, I can't be present and peaceful, I'm lonely.

But rest is the most important thing you can do for an injury, and it gives you critical information you'll need to make your next decision. If you rest an injury for two weeks and the irritated area feels better, you've learned that it can get better and heal. If you rest for two weeks and it stays about the same or gets worse, you've learned that you need to have your injury assessed by a healthcare professional.

Resting an injury is a reasonable, helpful way to honor your body and support your health. Be sensible. Rest when you're injured. Respecting your body in sickness will support its return to full health.

2 Injuries are excellent teachers. But you have to stop arguing and learn to listen to what they're telling you. Think of your injury like a trusted advisor. Physical pain is your body's voice speaking to you in the firmest language it knows.

When you take time to listen to your body and care for an injury, you have to change your daily habits. Injuries are one of those proverbial "blessings in disguise." Changing your routine gives you space to take stock, to look around at your life and see what's really going on. What have you missed while you were rushing through the days by rote? Do you find it difficult to actually take care of yourself, have compassion for yourself, and give yourself space and time to heal? These are just some of the important lessons your new teacher has to offer.

By allowing your body to rest and heal when it's injured, you're recognizing that your body is a miraculous system with its own internal intelligence. Very often, your body will heal itself if you simply create the conditions it needs to do that. Rest and listen. Notice if you have self-denying, harmful impulses. Acknowledge them. Look at them clearly when they come up, and then wrap them in velvet and put them aside. Love yourself enough to give your body space and time to work its invisible miracles. Resting is an act of faith in yourself.

3 Try something new. While you rest and wait for an injury to heal, you have an excellent opportunity to try some of the other yoga practices. Remember, doing the physical poses (asanas) is just one small fraction of the yoga-sphere.

Maybe look into some of the other practices that may contribute to helping heal your injury. There's the practice of chanting mantras (jappa yoga), doing good deeds (bhakti yoga), regulated breathing practices (pranayama), meditation, and conscious relaxation (yoga nidra). Finding a studio that offers these types of classes can really help you if you miss the social aspects of going to a studio and practicing with others while recuperating from an injury. You can also try them at home on your own, using a book or video for guidance on how to get started.

4 Find a knowledgeable, supportive instructor. If you have a chronic condition or have recently had surgery or recovered from an injury, find an experienced instructor who has studied anatomy to help you adjust your practice accordingly. That said, don't forget that your best teacher will always be inside your own body. Ignoring the wisdom of your body is irrational and risks further injury.

When you're recovering from an injury, you must practice yoga with an additional level of mindfulness and humility. An experienced instructor with a good understanding of anatomy and alignment can teach you pose variations that provide similar strengthening and flexibility benefits without irritating your injury. That said, it's important not to expect in-depth, individual attention during a regular yoga class. Ask your instructor before or after to give you one-on-one help. Better yet, schedule a private session to get specific, personalized assistance.

5 Become skilled in using yoga tools. As we've discussed, a good instructor can guide you, but you must take responsibility for developing your own safe and effective yoga practice. That includes learning the practical ins and outs of using yoga tools like a strap, block, bolster, or blanket during class.

Place your tools beside your mat before class starts; don't wait until you need something and then run off and go get it. Have a foam block or two, a folded blanket, a strap, or a bolster within reach, so you can get them quickly as class moves along. If the studio you regularly go to doesn't have many of these tools available, invest in buying your own and bring them with you.

Like any tool, you need to practice using your yoga tools so that placing and removing them becomes second nature. In no time, you'll find you're able to slide them into place and move them aside quickly and easily—with hardly a second thought.

Finally, remember that it's unreasonable to expect every instructor to know exactly what tools you need in each pose—especially if they've rarely or never seen you practice before. You're in charge of building your own sustainable, safe, and effective yoga practice. Your practice belongs to you. Instructors can guide you and suggest variations that might work better for your body, but ultimately, you're in control of what happens on your mat. Learn to use your tools. Practice with them wisely. Your body will thank you.

Mechanic's Note: Your Yoga Toolbox

Sometimes yoga tools like blocks, straps, and bolsters are called "props." I don't like that term, because it implies that these tools are for "propping up your body," which is not the correct way to use them (with the exception of a yin-yoga class). In a general yoga asana class, these tools can actually make many poses much more demanding, by correcting your alignment to isolate the muscle groups that should be doing the work. Using blocks, straps, and bolsters helps ensure that you have correct (central) alignment, and that you're using the muscles that the pose is meant to stretch and strengthen.

MECHANIC'S NOTE: The Role of the Instructor

Although your yoga practice is deeply personal, you don't have to go it alone. There are lots of experienced, knowledgeable instructors who are generally happy to help you make progress.

The instructor's job is to guide everyone in the room through class safely and effectively by:

- Providing appropriate variations of each pose.
- Emphasizing important points of alignment.
- Encouraging you to breathe deeply.
- Cuing and explaining each step as you enter, hold, and exit each pose.

A good instructor constantly scans the room and adjusts as needed, based on the responses and abilities of the class overall. Good instructors vary their words, offer specific variations, and give verbal and physical cues based on what they see happening during class.

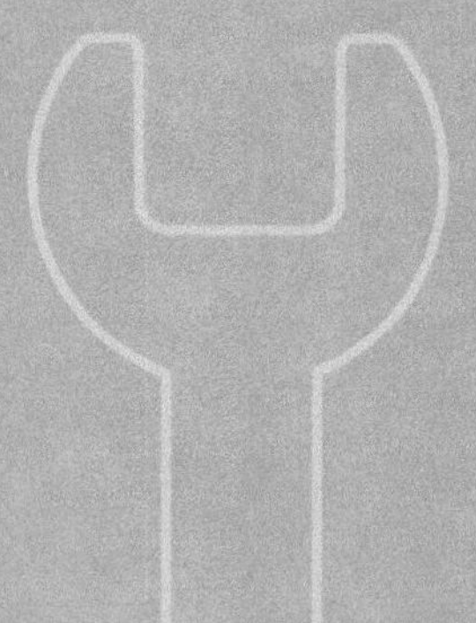

If you're confused about an instruction, or feel you need a different variation to accommodate your body, the best time to ask is before or after class. It's OK to ask for a quick pointer during class, but remember you're not the only person in the room—the instructor is trying to maintain a breath-connected flow for everyone to follow. That said, don't be shy. Most instructors are happy to give you one-on-one help before or after class. After all, their chosen vocation is to help you develop a safe and sustainable yoga practice.

If you have a lot of questions, or a specific physical challenge, it's a good idea to sign up for a private class with your instructor. A private session or two can be very helpful for figuring out which variations will be most beneficial for you to work on. Then, next time that pose comes up in a class, you'll know exactly what you should do. Special workshops on certain types of poses like inversions or back bends, or that isolate particular aspects like meditation or breathing practices, are another great place to explore and take responsibility for your practice.

Having an instructor in class doesn't mean you're absolved from making decisions. Instructors should gently but consistently communicate how important it is for students to take responsibility for their own practice. Sometimes it works. One student came to my classes regularly for about seven years. As an endurance athlete, she'd accumulated joint damage and chronic knee and hip pain. After class, she often remarked that this or that pose had hurt her. My reply was always: "I'm so sorry that the way you did that pose hurt you. Let's take a look at how you need to adjust it." The fact was, I'd instructed several variations of the pose during class with this exact student in mind, but she would only attempt the most intense version. After many years of going through this same routine, during one consultation she stopped herself mid-sentence, smiled, and said, "I know! I know! I hurt myself. Will you show me again how I should do it?" We both had a good laugh.

SOME NOTES FOR TEACHERS

It's a wonderful thing to become a yoga instructor, and make a commitment to helping other people make progress toward improving their mental, physical, and emotional health and wellness. However, you need to develop a special mindset to effectively help a roomful of people with different abilities, personalities, habits, and goals. Here are some tips I've learned over the hundreds of classes and workshops I've taken as a student or taught.

Clearly explaining the physical actions and muscles used in a pose helps students have "light-bulb" moments in their practice.

Because I'm an anatomy instructor and a science writer, my mind is geared to think about the anatomical pathways we use in yoga. And many years of teaching yoga anatomy workshops has taught me that for anyone who does yoga, understanding how your physical body works is immeasurably helpful to deepen your practice and avoid injuries. I've seen for myself that when I clearly explain the physical actions and muscles being used in a pose, the light bulb comes on for students. Seeing them make discoveries about how their bodies work in various positions is one of my greatest joys. So I highly recommend becoming familiar with where the basic muscle groups are, and which ones are stretching, stabilizing, or strengthening in a particular pose.

This is an ongoing process (like yoga!). I keep a couple of anatomy books on the kitchen counter, and flip through them while I have my morning tea. Every so often I'll take a class or workshop with a yoga teacher who specializes in anatomy. I always get lots of great ideas for my own teaching. Finally, don't forget to observe and explore your own body while you practice—be curious. How does your breathing change when you raise your arms in Chair Pose? Does using a tool like a strap or a block activate new muscle groups? These discoveries are a never-ending spring of insights, and you can share sips from it with your students.

Speaking without intelligence and critical thinking is the opposite of what practicing yoga is meant to cultivate.

As a science-minded person, I'm bothered by some instructions I've heard in yoga classes over the years—sometimes because it's anatomically incorrect, but mostly because it's not particularly useful to the students. For example: "Inhale through the soles of your feet." Since your feet are not part of your respiratory system, it's unclear what the instructor really wants you to do. Lift your arches? Imagine a breezy sensation in your feet? Spread out your toes? I believe it's always more helpful when the instructor clearly tells students what they should do. "Inhale and lift the arches of your feet" would be a more useful cue.

Don't get me wrong, I understand that instructors often use this kind of language as a figure of speech. My point is that as instructors, we should ask ourselves: What are we actually trying to say? What concept do we mean to express? Often when I ask an instructor about this, they can't clearly explain what they mean, or tell me how they know if their students are doing it or not. What does "Inhale through your soles" look like?

I get it; in the middle of teaching a class, it's really easy to repeat a catch phrase you heard somewhere. I've caught myself doing it. But speaking without applying your critical thinking skills is the opposite of what practicing yoga means to show us: How to refine our thoughts, words, and actions to make them more intentional.

The average person does not come to yoga to get religion.

Simply repeating what you've heard other yoga instructors say—even "famous" ones—without bothering to figure out what you mean to communicate is at best lazy, and at worst arrogant. Not only can ill-considered language be unhelpful for students, I've often seen overly esoteric or religious language repel people who are new to yoga. It puts them off from continuing; they write yoga off and move on. To me, that's a great shame.

I'm also troubled by classes where there's a lot of talk about "purifying" your body. The concept of purification starts from an assumption that students are somehow dirty or impure. I'm bothered by instructors who assume the authority to make this type of broad, negative judgment about an entire roomful of people. Not to mention that the idea of "purity" (spiritual or physical) springs from a deeply-rooted religiosity (think, Puritanism) that I don't think belongs in a general level yoga asana class.

Similarly, I suggest that we yoga instructors be mindful of using punishing words like "wring," "squeeze," "detoxify," "cleanse," "stoke," and "burn," which are rooted in a very subtle form of criticism and a puritanical spirit of self-flagellation. This language supports an unspoken judgment that something deep inside a student is broken, dirty, toxic, or stuck and must be wrenched, scorched, or otherwise driven out.

It all comes down to this: The average person does not come to yoga class to get religion. I think it's a much better idea to save the religious philosophy and spiritual discussions about who is "pure" and who needs "purifying" for specific cleansing (kriya) classes and workshops, where students know what they're in for. Frankly, I find that in a general level yoga asana class, exhorting students to "purify" themselves comes off as preachy and judgmental.

Yoga class is not an exorcism. It's a therapeutic place of healing. I believe that using these kinds of intense, punishing words for instruction in a yoga class is disrespectful and potentially harmful. Disrespectful, because the underlying communication is that the wonderful people who have come to take your class are unacceptable as they are. Harmful, because these critical words can reinforce that harsh inner voice that so many people already struggle with—the one that tells them, daily, how broken they are.

The most important thing we do is to create a safe, non-judgmental space.

In my opinion, the most important thing a yoga instructor can do is create a safe, accepting, non-judgmental space, where people can come and explore how practicing yoga might help make their lives a little easier–physically, mentally, and emotionally. The most effective yoga instructors I've ever met do not see themselves as their student's savior or guru, but as their friend, companion, and guide. I strongly believe that messages in class should be positive: Congratulations for getting here. You're not faulty or broken. Your body is a living breathing miracle. You're a good person. You deserve compassion. You fit in here. We are equals. You're worthy of love and respect exactly as you are.

Are you teaching what's useful?

It's fine that some instructors have a more esoteric style than others. Different strokes for different folks, right? I'm not saying that there's only one acceptable way to instruct a yoga class. But I do think instructions in class should be immediately useful and anatomically correct. What I mean by "immediately useful" is that students should be able to put the instruction to use right then and there.

A general, all-levels yoga class is not the place to pontificate about personal lifestyle choices such as eating a vegetarian or vegan diet, about religious philosophy, or about political issues. Save that content for workshops and special-interest classes. That way, people can sign up if they're interested and, if they're not, won't feel like it was forced on them while they were a "captive audience" so to speak. It makes me sad when an instructor's style puts someone off from starting or continuing their yoga practice. Because that means they've contributed to closing—instead of opening—an avenue to health and wellness for that person.

Always remember that students have a lot to keep up with in a yoga asana class. They have to follow the sequences, attend to their alignment, breathe deeply, steady their drishti, and focus their mind on the present moment. That's plenty! All of those tasks help cultivate an inner calm. An additional layer of tangential rhetoric is usually too much. Besides, students who are already working hard to keep their physical asana practice focused and flowing are likely to just tune out the sermon.

If someone wants to explore ancient texts, philosophies, mantras, energy centers (chakras), or any of the other many aspects of yoga, that's great. There are lots of excellent workshops, special classes, study groups, books, and online resources for that.

It's useful to reflect on why we instruct the way we do.

Whenever I encounter a "font of esoteric wisdom" teaching style in a regular class, I always wonder about the instructor's motive. Does he or she feel a need to appear more holy, spiritual, enlightened, or pure than others? Is it driven by a deeper insecurity? If you instruct this way, I humbly suggest giving your motive some quiet consideration. After all, yoga is a practice of self-exploration. We should always ask ourselves: Why do I teach the way I do? Could my teaching style be more beneficial to students if I made some changes?

CLOSING THOUGHTS

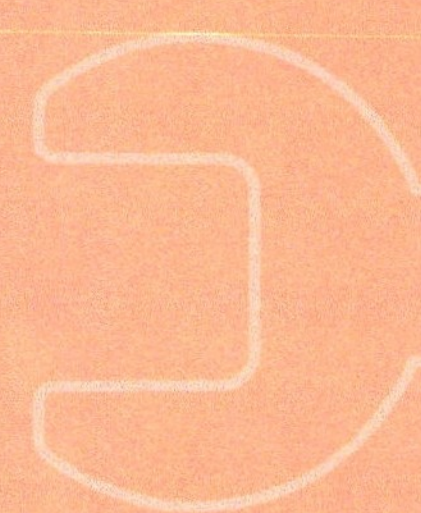

I hope this book has given you a clearer picture of the nuts and bolts of doing yoga—from how your anatomy is put together, to how you can customize your practice to fit your own body and goals. While we didn't cover every aspect of yoga by any means, I trust sticking to the practical ins and outs—identifying a good instructor and a class style that works for you, understanding how various poses stretch and strengthen different muscle groups, and focusing on your breathing and thinking patterns while you practice—has empowered you with some valuable advice that will help you on your way.

The most important take-home message I have for you is this: Yoga is a personal journey. It's like a long, slow rafting trip down your own inner river, where you can explore and discover yourself. It's not formal therapy, but many people find the time they spend on their yoga mat to be very therapeutic. And the scenery is always changing. After a while, you'll notice that aspects of your practice which used to be hard get easier . . . and that other aspects, now that you have a deeper understanding, get harder. You'll gain the confidence and strength to try poses you never thought you'd consider. As this happens, I hope you'll return to this book as an ongoing reference to draw on as your practice develops and shifts.

My wish is that you will be well, live fully, and have more peace than stress on this crazy ride we call life.

Pose Index

Acknowledgements

When I first sat down to organize my thoughts for this book, I had no idea how many people would come to my rescue over the next two years as I stumbled around trying to coax it into being. Without their generosity, support, guidance, and encouragement, I would have never finished. To my dear friend, Lea Austen, I am beyond grateful for your photographic talent and kindness. When you said, "Sure, I'll help you," I know you didn't expect to spend so many weekends wrangling lights as you lay on the floor of my guest room to capture each pose from the best angle. You're a wonder. To my editor, Rick Chillot, thank you for your infinite desire to understand convoluted yoga terminology and your spectacular editorial chops. Your patient game of whack-a-mole with my gerunds, em dashes, and repetitions made this book make sense. Namaste. To my designer, Andie Reid, thank you for putting it all together and making a useful thing of beauty from a massive beast of a manuscript. To my brother, Grady Hendrix, thank you for not blocking my number and finding a million spare minutes to steer me away from the abyss. To my friends who modelled the poses, you are the very heart of it, literally and figuratively. Thank you from the bottom of my heart to: Martha Criscuolo, Freida Sokol, Paul Sykes, Cliff Woods, Maria Kelly, Genise Dawkins, Kenny Dawkins, Cherna Bednarsh, Annie Lee, Mike Huffman, Lyn Huffman, Marty Rivers, AJ Dales, John Gaskins, Jocelyn Chateauvert, Heidi Crotts, Shoba Kousik, Erin Kosak, Paul Ferrari, Hannah Weber, and Jack Lynch. Thanks also to my fellow anatomist Dr. Eric Lacey for being an early reader. Finally, my endless gratitude to to Trace Bonner and the yoga community at Holy Cow Yoga Center in Charleston, South Carolina. Thanks for putting the 'Om' in my home. You guys are awesome.